The Ecology of Purposeful Living Across the Lifespan

Anthony L. Burrow · Patrick L. Hill
Editors

The Ecology of Purposeful Living Across the Lifespan

Developmental, Educational, and Social Perspectives

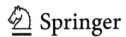 Springer

Editors
Anthony L. Burrow
Department of Human Development
College of Human Ecology
Cornell University
Ithaca, NY, USA

Patrick L. Hill
Department of Psychological
and Brain Sciences
Washington University in St. Louis
Saint Louis, MO, USA

ISBN 978-3-030-52077-9   ISBN 978-3-030-52078-6   (eBook)
https://doi.org/10.1007/978-3-030-52078-6

This Springer imprint is published by the registered company Springer Nature Switzerland AG
The registered company address is: Gewerbestrasse 11, 6330 Cham, Switzerland

Acknowledgements

The current volume represents the product of multiple workshops hosted across the USA, through the generous funding from sources including the Program for Research on Youth Development and Engagement (PRYDE) at Cornell University, made possible by a gift from Rebecca Q. Morgan.

Contents

Chapter 1
Introduction: The Purpose of Studying Purpose and the Need for an Ecological Perspective

Patrick L. Hill and Anthony L. Burrow

> Research is formalized curiosity. It is poking and prying with a purpose.
> —Zora Neale Hurston (1942).

Abstract The empirical study of purpose in life has been a booming industry over recent decades. As such, the current volume provides a reflection on this past work with an eye toward future endeavors across academic disciplines. To start, this introductory chapter provides a brief overview of central topics in the field of purpose. First, we discuss what it means to have a purpose in life, providing different academic lenses through which to consider the construct. Second, we describe the value of purpose in life, as a construct that appears to be associated with wide ranging benefits for individuals across the lifespan. Third, we conclude by setting the stage for the upcoming chapters, providing an organizational scheme that builds from ecological perspectives on human development.

The value of living a life with direction and purpose is not difficult to communicate to most audiences. Indeed, in our work on the topic, we have spoken with groups across the world, both in the academic realm and very far from it, and it is a rare occurrence that anyone contradicts the suggestion that having a purpose promotes personal well-being and development. However, while discussions on the value of purposeful living date back to Aristotelian times, the academic conversation around purpose has grown considerably in recent years. After multiple, relatively "simple" demonstrations that having a purpose (or a sense of purpose and direction in life) is a valuable commodity, academics have started to poke and pry at the construct of purpose along three primary fronts. First, definitional issues remain at the forefront, with inquiry centering on

P. L. Hill (✉)
Department of Psychological and Brain Sciences, Washington University in St. Louis, St. Louis, MO, USA
e-mail: patrick.hill@wustl.edu

A. L. Burrow
Department of Human Development, Cornell University, Ithaca, NY, USA

© Springer Nature Switzerland AG 2020
A. L. Burrow and P. Hill (eds.), *The Ecology of Purposeful Living Across the Lifespan*,
https://doi.org/10.1007/978-3-030-52078-6_1

1

how purpose is distinct from related constructs, particularly when efforts are made to extend purpose into a new research guild. Second, researchers have examined why purpose appears so vital and valuable to successful development across the lifespan. Third, and perhaps most important, what can we do to help others develop a sense of purpose, while properly taking into account their given context and background? The "we" in this case goes far beyond the authors of this and the other chapters in this volume, and instead speaks to the far-reaching implications for society and its prominent institutions.

The current volume reflects our efforts over the years to bring together prominent thinkers and scholars from multiple seemingly disparate fields, to have an open discussion across these and other important questions regarding the construct of purpose. As such, this book reflects a formalization of the multiple researchers' curiosity into the construct of purpose. We begin here with a brief overview of the extant literature on purpose in life. First, we provide the reader with multiple perspectives on the construct, several of which are echoed in the chapters that follow, with the understanding that there is no one dominant definition of what it means to have a purpose or feel purposeful. Second, we discuss why this construct has accrued greater attention in recent years, by briefly outlining some of work linking purpose to valuable life outcomes. Third, we conclude with an organizational framework for the chapters that follow, and the types of questions the authors in this volume seek to address.

1.1   What Is Purpose?

This question alone could take the entire book to answer, and indeed others have written volumes that are significantly dedicated to address this question (e.g., Bronk, 2014; Damon, 2008). Given the variety of perspectives taken by authors in the current volume, here we describe two important perspectives on defining purpose. One comes from a lifespan developmental perspective that starts with considering how children develop purposeful action and the perception that their actions have consequence on the world. The second recognizes perhaps the most well-known account of purpose in life, namely as a facet of psychological well-being and marker of adaptive development. These perspectives overlap to significant degrees, and both have roots in the seminal work of Viktor Frankl (1959), whose powerful narrative provided a first-hand account of why living a purpose-driven life can provide hope in even the most desperate of circumstances. However, in addition to their commonalities, we hope that briefly describing these perspectives provides the reader with insight into how different guilds have handled the construct, a theme relevant to the rest of the volume.

1.1.1 Purpose Through a Lifespan Developmental Lens

Erikson's (1959, 1968) classic theory of identity development across the lifespan provides a valuable context for considering the precursors of having a purpose in life. To start, Erikson suggests that the development of purposeful living starts prior to even entering kindergarten. Specifically, the ability to develop goal-directed action is the successful resolution of identity development for children as young as four-to-six years of age, reflecting the potential for personal initiative. The knowledge that one's actions have consequences is an important, but often overlooked starting point to setting goals that direct one's short- and long-term activities. As such, the roots of purposeful living start very early insofar that Erikson uses the term "purpose" to describe the positive outcome obtained via the successful resolution of this early identity crisis of initiative.

However, most people likely think about purpose more in line with how it is treated during Erikson's later discussion of how individuals develop a fuller sense of identity during adolescence and young adulthood. At this point, the discussion turns to how determining where one wants to go is an integral component of knowing who one is (see also Burrow & Hill, 2011; Hill & Burrow, 2012; Sumner, Burrow, & Hill, 2015); in other words, finding a direction in life may help individuals commit to a personal identity. In this sense, purpose in life can be described as the identification of the life direction that one deems personally meaningful, to the extent that individuals view this life path as self-defining and self-descriptive. Support for the claim that this period is formative for finding a life path comes from the developmental trends ongoing with respect to how people are setting personal goals. During adolescence and emerging adulthood, individuals appear to start winnowing down their goal pursuits to focus on those goals of greater personal relevance (Roberts, O'Donnell, & Robins, 2004), counter to earlier developmental period where individuals have a tendency for widespread, rather than focused goal endorsement. The purpose development process likely occurs as an ebb-and-flow between focused activity on certain personally-important goals, with reduced engagement regarding those goals that provide less personal definition (see also Moran, this volume).

Accordingly, this lifespan developmental perspective alerts us to three important points regarding what it means to have a purpose in life. First, the precursors to purpose manifest early in the lifespan, perhaps even starting with merely the understanding that one can initiate purposeful action with consequence to the world. Second, individuals may start to deliberate on what their personal purpose is in earnest during adolescence and emerging adulthood, given that this period is a point of profound self and identity development, as well as a time of more focused goal endorsement. Third, committing to a purpose in life involves deciding upon a critical element of what one deems personally meaningful and valuable, and disengaging from those activities and goals that are less descriptive of the self.

1.1.2 Purpose as a Component of Psychological Well-Being

Another perspective is perhaps the one most widely adopted in recent scientific inquiry around the construct of purpose, namely that having a sense of purpose has been described as one component of psychological well-being in adulthood (Ryff, 1989a; 1989b; Ryff & Keyes, 1995). In her effort to provide the field with a context for understanding individual well-being beyond only the discussion of hedonic well-being, Carol Ryff's model of psychological well-being has provided the starting point for most empirical studies of purpose in the past three decades. Indeed, Ryff's measures have been included in several of the most prominent large-scale studies of aging and development across the world.

We leave the bulk of the discussion of psychological well-being to the progenitor herself (see Ryff & Kim, this volume). However, this view of purpose brings three new definitional elements that merit attention. First, as mentioned earlier, this view of purpose (or at least the typical measurements associated with it) focuses primarily on the extent to which individuals feel they have a purpose and direction, rather than on the content of the direction itself. Though there is a clear tradeoff in the idiographic depth acquired about participants, this measurement strategy has provided the opportunity for researchers to delve into the topic of purpose with more cost- and time-effective methods that avoid the need for thematic coding of specific purpose contents. Indeed, the value of this approach comes from the assumption that regardless of the path one chooses, and the extent to which one can fully describe that path, purposeful living involves believing that one has a direction in life, and that one's activities are personally meaningful. By focusing on this measurement strategy, researchers were given the opportunity to examine the correlates of sense of purpose in large-scale samples, which has directed much of the work described below.

Second, this view of purpose couches it within the realm of "well-being." Though not orthogonal to the lifespan developmental perspective, this terminology does carry some new implications for researchers. Given that constructs like happiness and positive affect hold positive effects on health and life outcomes (Pressman & Cohen, 2005), as do other components of Ryff's psychological well-being scale (see Ryff, 2014), researchers are left with the challenge of demonstrating that benefits associated with purposeful living are not better described as simply the artifacts of positive well-being more broadly. Research using bi-factor modeling approaches (see Hill, Allemand, & Burrow, 2018 for discussion) has demonstrated that sense of purpose appears uniquely associated with early family relationships, distinct from the effects of these relationships on life satisfaction and (lack of) perceived stress (Hill, Schultz, Jackson, & Andrews, 2019). What this work suggests is that sense of purpose captures something unique from general subjective well-being, a point that merits further attention in future empirical studies on the construct. In sum, the psychological well-being perspective on purpose brings both great value for researchers, and some unique challenges for rigorous scientific inquiry.

As you will see, authors throughout the volume will borrow from these perspectives throughout their entries, with some guilds focusing more on one perspective than others. Other chapters will add to this brief review by presenting entirely different theoretical and scientific perspectives on what purpose means for individuals (e.g., Moran, this volume; Pfund, this volume; Wingfield, this volume). Although the field benefits considerably from having multiple viewpoints and perspectives on what purpose means, one overarching challenge for future research remains the issue of how to measure purpose, as the reader will see how different authors have dealt with this challenge in unique ways.

1.2 Why Study Purpose?

Though defining purpose is difficult, the task proves well worth the challenge given the multitude of benefits associated with the construct. We highlight a few of these points below, but they are sprinkled across every chapter in the volume, with the authors providing new insights into the value of a purposeful life. Moreover, we alert the reader to our recent reviews of these benefits for additional details (e.g., Hill, Burrow, & Sumner, 2013; Pfund & Hill, 2018). For now, we will focus on the value of purpose for leading individuals toward promoting health, wealth, and cognitive functioning, support for the centuries' long claims that leading a purposeful life is a sign of adaptive development (see Ryff, 2014 for a review).

First, sense of purpose predicts a reduced risk for a wide array of health issues, including cardiovascular problems and stroke (Kim, Sun, Park, Kubzansky, & Peterson, 2013; Kim, Sun, Park, & Peterson, 2013), infirmity and disability (Mota et al., 2016), and even sleep issues (Kim, Hershner, & Strecher, 2015). Moreover, it even appears associated with greater longevity across multiple samples (Boyle, Barnes, Buchman, & Bennett, 2009; Cohen, Bavishi, & Rozanski, 2016; Hill & Turiano, 2014). Having a purpose in life may lead individuals to focus on health maintenance, because regardless of the purpose one holds, being in better health will likely assist in any type of goal pursuit. One rationale for these effects comes from evidence suggesting that purposeful individuals have healthier lifestyles; sense of purpose has been associated with engagement with positive health behaviors, such as eating a healthier diet and oral health care (Hill, Edmonds, & Hampson, 2019), having regular checkups (Kim, Strecher, & Ryff, 2014), and being more active as assessed by pedometer counts (Hooker & Masters, 2016).

Second, living a purpose-driven life requires that individuals possess the ability to allocate resources, tangible and intangible, toward their goal pursuits (McKnight & Kashdan, 2009). Toward this end, researchers have investigated the role of purposeful living on financial asset accrual (Hill, Turiano, Mroczek, & Burrow, 2016). In a longitudinal study of adults, individuals who reported a higher sense of purpose tended to have higher income and net worth. Moreover, purposeful individuals tended to increase their wealth more over the nine years following the first assessment. These effects held over known predictors of wealth, such as personality dispositions and demographics. Interestingly, research also shows that positive associations between purposefulness and economic outcomes are present at the level of individual states in the U. S. (Baugh, Pfund, Hill, & Cheung, in press) and broader societies and nations (Hill, Cheung, Kube, & Burrow, 2019). Collectives with more purposeful citizens, at multiple levels of aggregation, thus appear to benefit financially. Though work is needed to better understand the directionality and mechanisms involved in these associations, one explanation follows a similar logic to the purpose-health connection. Namely, regardless of whether one's purpose is focused on financial and occupational success, building financial assets is likely to help scaffold progress toward a life direction.

Third, having a purpose requires switching between more or less goal-relevant tasks, as well as remembering next steps toward short- and long-term goals (McKnight & Kashdan, 2009). In line with these propositions, researchers have found that individuals who report a higher sense of purpose tend also to score higher on objective tests of memory and executive functioning (Lewis, Turiano, Payne, & Hill, 2017; Windsor, Curtis, & Luszcz, 2015). Moreover, research has suggested that sense of purpose may prove a resilience factor against risk for later dementia (Boyle, Buchman, Barnes, & Bennett, 2010). Greater discussion of this point will come in later chapters as well (Wynn, Dewitte, & Hill, this volume), but this research points to how purposeful living may help build cognitive resilience, as well as health and wealth resources.

1.3 Outline of the Book

These findings provide broad support for the notion that purposeful living may produce a wide array of positive life outcomes. Building from this empirical foundation, the following chapters will provide additional details on how people develop a purpose and the value of doing so across life domains. The volume has been organized in a format befitting a more ecological perspective on human development (e.g., Bronfenbrenner, 1979), which underscores the importance of contextualizing developmental trajectories as interactions between the individual and broader social, sociological, and societal structures.

To start, we present three chapters focusing primarily on how purpose impacts the "person in the center of the circles" (Darling, 2007). Pfund starts by describing how purpose in life fits within personality science, a discipline sometimes referred to as the "study of the person" (Funder, 1997). Ryff and Kim then discuss how purpose plays a role in the virtuous development of individuals, and what it means for one to hold a prosocial or noble purpose. Wynn, Dewitte, and Hill conclude this section by underscoring the importance of purpose in life for older adults, ending with a description of what social structures can do to impact the purposefulness of persons later in the lifespan. Indeed, though these chapters are primarily focused on the purposeful *person*, all allude to fact that the discussion of purpose cannot be contained solely at the person-level.

The four chapters that follow consider the role of close relationships in the purpose development process. Larson begins by describing the potential impact of one-on-one apprenticeship programs on helping youth find a purpose. Kiang, Malin, and Sandoz then describe how these purpose-building interactions play out within the school context. Yu and Deutsch continue this theme with respect to adult-child relationships more broadly. MacTavish then bridges the arenas of close relationships with broader sociological factors, in considering whether and how youth develop purposeful aims when growing up in more culturally-closed, impoverished settings. This final chapter provides an interesting counterpoint wherein the ecological context shapes whether close relationships are in fact valuable to maintain, insofar that MacTavish's work also presents occasions where youth may be better served by leaving their developed social ties.

The next section considers societal and ideological structures and their influence on purpose in life. Sumner explores the context of gender identity and how society may press individuals into circumscribed purposes based on their gender. Rogers builds from the discussion of gender, adding an intersectionality angle by presenting evidence of the challenges for Black boys to disconfirm the negative stereotypes attributed to them. Wingfield enhances this conversation by describing her research with adult samples, noting the challenges faced by Black professionals and the potential scaffolding provided by social networks. Combined, these three chapters provide perspective into how our societal demands and expectations differentially impact individual's purpose development based on their social identities.

The final two chapters provide efforts to capture purpose development at the intersection of multiple ecological levels. To start, Moran presents a theoretical foundation for how future research can incorporate dynamical systems approaches to understanding how individuals advance their purpose development through interactions across levels. Bronk and Mitchell then provide an overview of their lab's efforts to understand purpose from cultural and historical lenses, developing upon the themes presented earlier with respect to how the individual person's development is impacted by their close associates, social identities, and broader societal structures. Overall, this volume showcases the widespread curiosity into purpose in life, with a demonstration of different methods, perspectives, and directions future researchers can take for poking and prying further into the construct.

References

Baugh, G. A., Pfund, G. N., Hill, P. L., & Cheung, F. (In press). Fifty states of purpose: Examining sense of purpose across the United States. *The Journal of Positive Psychology*.

Boyle, P. A., Barnes, L. L., Buchman, A. S., & Bennett, D. A. (2009). Purpose in life is associated with mortality among community-dwelling older persons. *Psychosomatic Medicine, 71*(5), 574–579.

Boyle, P. A., Buchman, A. S., Barnes, L. L., & Bennett, D. A. (2010). Effect of a purpose in life on risk of incident Alzheimer disease and mild cognitive impairment in community-dwelling older persons. *Archives of General Psychiatry, 67*(3), 304–310.

Bronfenbrenner, U. (1979). *The ecology of human development.* Cambridge, MA: Harvard University Press.

Bronk, K. C. (2014). *Purpose in life: A critical component of optimal youth development.* Dordrecht: Springer.

Burrow, A. L., & Hill, P. L. (2011). Purpose as a form of identity capital for positive youth development. *Developmental Psychology, 47,* 1196–1206.

Cohen, R., Bavishi, C., & Rozanski, A. (2016). Purpose in life and its relationship to all-cause mortality and cardiovascular events: A meta-analysis. *Psychosomatic Medicine, 78*(2), 122–133.

Damon, W. (2008). *The path to purpose: Helping our children find their calling in life.* New York: Free Press.

Darling, N. (2007). Ecological systems theory: The person in the center of the circles. *Research in Human Development, 4*(3–4), 203–217.

Erikson, E. H. (1959). *Identity and the life cycle.* W. W. New York: International University Press.

Erikson, E. H. (1968). *Identity, youth and crisis.* New York: Norton.

Frankl, V. E. (1959). *Man's search for meaning.* New York: Pocket Books.

Funder, D. C. (1997). *The personality puzzle.* New York: Norton.

Hill, P. L., & Burrow, A. L. (2012). Viewing purpose through an Eriksonian lens. *Journal of Identity, 12*(1), 74–91.

Hill, P. L., & Turiano, N. A. (2014). Purpose in life as a predictor of mortality across adulthood. *Psychological Science, 25*(7), 1482–1486.

Hill, P. L., Allemand, M., & Burrow, A. L. (2018). Considering multiple methods for differentiating conceptually close constructs: Examples from the field of positive psychology. *Social and Personality Psychology Compass, 12,* np.

Hill, P. L., Burrow, A. L., & Sumner, R. A. (2013). Addressing important questions in the field of adolescent purpose. *Child Development Perspectives, 7,* 232–236.

Hill, P. L., Cheung, F., Kube, A., & Burrow, A. L. (2019a). Life engagement is associated with higher GDP among societies. *Journal of Research in Personality, 78,* 210–214.

Hill, P. L., Edmonds, G. W., & Hampson, S. E. (2019b). A purposeful lifestyle is a healthful lifestyle: Linking sense of purpose to self-rated health through multiple health behaviors. *Journal of Health Psychology, 24,* 1392–1400.

Hill, P. L., Schultz, L. H., Jackson, J. J., & Andrews, J. A. (2019c). Parent-child conflict during elementary school as a longitudinal predictor of sense of purpose in emerging adulthood. *Journal of Youth and Adolescence, 48,* 145–153.

Hill, P. L., Turiano, N. A., Mroczek, D. K., & Burrow, A. L. (2016). The value of a purposeful life: Sense of purpose predicts greater income and net worth. *Journal of Research in Personality, 65,* 38–42.

Hooker, S. A., & Masters, K. S. (2016). Purpose in life is associated with physical activity measured by accelerometer. *Journal of Health Psychology, 21*(6), 962–971.

Hurston, Z. N. (1942). *Dust tracks on a road: an autobiography.* London: Hutchinson & Co.

Kim, E. S., Strecher, V. J., & Ryff, C. D. (2014). Purpose in life and use of preventive health care services. *Proceedings of the National Academy of Sciences, 111*(46), 16331–16336.

Kim, E. S., Sun, J. K., Park, N., & Peterson, C. (2013a). Purpose in life and reduced incidence of stroke in older adults: 'The Health and Retirement Study'. *Journal of Psychosomatic Research, 74*(5), 427–432.

Kim, E. S., Sun, J. K., Park, N., Kubzansky, L. D., & Peterson, C. (2013b). Purpose in life and reduced risk of myocardial infarction among older US adults with coronary heart disease: a two-year follow-up. *Journal of Behavioral Medicine, 36*(2), 124–133.

Lewis, N. A., Turiano, N. A., Payne, B. R., & Hill, P. L. (2017). Purpose in life and cognitive functioning in adulthood. *Aging, Neuropsychology, and Cognition, 24*(6), 662–671.

McKnight, P. E., & Kashdan, T. B. (2009). Purpose in life as a system that creates and sustains health and well-being: An integrative, testable theory. *Review of General Psychology, 13*(3), 242–251.

Pfund, G. N., & Hill, P. L. (2018). The multifaceted benefits of purpose in life. *The International Forum for Logotherapy, 41,* 27–37.

Pressman, S. D., & Cohen, S. (2005). Does positive affect influence health? *Psychological Bulletin, 131*(6), 925–971.

Roberts, B. W., O'Donnell, M., & Robins, R. W. (2004). Goal and personality trait development in emerging adulthood. *Journal of Personality and Social Psychology, 87*(4), 541–550.

Ryff, C. D. (1989a). Beyond Ponce de Leon and life satisfaction: New directions in quest of successful ageing. *International Journal of Behavioral Development, 12*(1), 35–55.

Ryff, C. D. (1989b). Happiness is everything, or is it? Explorations on the meaning of psychological well-being. *Journal of Personality and Social Psychology, 57,* 1069–1081.

Ryff, C. D. (2014). Psychological well-being revisited: Advances in the science and practice of eudaimonia. *Psychotherapy and Psychosomatics, 83*(1), 10–28.

Ryff, C. D., & Keyes, C. L. M. (1995). The structure of psychological well-being revisited. *Journal of Personality and Social Psychology, 69*(4), 719–727.

Sumner, R., Burrow, A. L., & Hill, P. L. (2015). Identity and purpose as predictors of subjective well-being in emerging adulthood. *Emerging Adulthood, 3*(1), 46–54.

Windsor, T. D., Curtis, R. G., & Luszcz, M. A. (2015). Sense of purpose as a psychological resource for aging well. *Developmental Psychology, 51*(7), 975–986.

Chapter 2
We Meet Again: The Reintroduction and Reintegration of Purpose into Personality Psychology

Gabrielle N. Pfund

Abstract The current chapter posits that sense of purpose and purpose in life are individual differences that find a natural home in personality science. Situating these constructs within personality psychology allows for an abundance of future research opportunities to illuminate clearer answers to questions such as what the daily life of a purposeful person looks like, what behaviors purposeful people enact, and the unique lifespan trajectories of purpose. Before discussing the research questions personality psychology methodology will support answering, I begin by defining the two main purpose constructs of interest: sense of purpose and purpose in life. From there, I integrate these constructs into three main personality frameworks to provide initial evidence for purpose being an important factor in personality theory. I then discuss the history of purpose within personality science, and why it is distinct from the work that has previously been done in the field. I close the chapter by describing essential questions that exist in purpose research, and offering recommendations for addressing them using personality methodology.

Keywords Sense of purpose · Purpose in life · Personality psychology · Personality science · Traits

The current chapter posits two simple, but potentially transformative, ideas. The first idea is that what you want for your life—the goals that move you and the extent to which you feel that they propel for you forward—is not simply a desire you have, but is actually part of who you are. Articulating that you have a purpose in life, or that you are a purposeful person, are actually inherent to what makes you "you." The second idea is that by taking this perspective—by embracing purpose as a part of oneself, i.e. one's personality—the current trajectory of purpose research can be elevated. By turning to personality science, some of the inconsistent definitions, unclear mechanisms, and unanswered questions prevalent in purpose research can be addressed. We can gain construct clarity, methodological advancement, and an

G. N. Pfund (✉)
Washington University in St. Louis, St. Louis, MO, USA
e-mail: gabrielle.pfund@wustl.edu

© Springer Nature Switzerland AG 2020
A. L. Burrow and P. Hill (eds.), *The Ecology of Purposeful Living Across the Lifespan*,
https://doi.org/10.1007/978-3-030-52078-6_2

abundance of empirical opportunities when viewing purpose through a personality psychology lens.

Personality psychologists work to define what makes up an individual, and what these differences within and between individuals mean for our life outcomes. With purpose being something that differs between people, both in the extent to which they feel purposeful as well as the specific purposes one pursues, personality psychology becomes a natural mold for these constructs. The chapter begins by discussing two main components of purpose research: sense of purpose and purpose in life. From there, I posit why these components can fit into personality science by integrating them into well-known personality psychology models. By doing this, a foundation is created to investigate purpose using a personality psychology framework. I also discuss the history of purpose in personality psychology. I mention previous misconceptions of where purpose fits into common personality theory, as well as provide evidence to show that purpose is distinct. Finally, this chapter concludes by considering specific personality psychology methodologies that could be utilized to answer possible research questions, such as how purpose functions and fluctuates in day-to-day life, the kind of behaviors a purposeful person enacts, and the consequences of atypical purpose lifespan trajectories. However, before delving into these questions, I first define what I mean by purpose.

2.1   Conceptualizing Purpose

Purpose is a multifaceted construct that has previously displayed its aptitude to promote desirable outcomes, as well as to mitigate negative effects (see Pfund & Hill, 2018 for review). In order to appreciate its predictive abilities, it is first important to understand the nature of it as a construct. Purpose is composed of two main components: purpose in life and sense of purpose. *Purpose in life* is often more challenging for both individuals to articulate and researchers to empirically evaluate. Someone's purpose in life can be understood as the large-scale goal or goals that generate an individual's sense of purpose. Put more concretely by McKnight and Kashdan (2009), "Purpose is a central, self-organizing life aim that organizes and stimulates goals, manages behaviors, and provides a sense of meaning" (p. 242). Researchers can assess purpose in life by 1) simply asking participants for its presence or absence, or by 2) taking a more qualitative approach and focusing on the content of one's purpose in life (Hill, Burrow, Brandenberger, Lapsley, & Quaranto, 2010). In this regard, some have suggested that purpose in life should not be accomplishable, but rather more of a general intention that directs smaller goals as one pursues it (Damon et al., 2003; McKnight & Kashdan, 2009). For example, becoming a medical doctor may not qualify as a purpose in life, whereas aspiring to help heal sick people would. In this way, purpose in life is the overarching goal that guides us as we journey through the pursuits of our lives.

Relatedly, *sense of purpose* can be understood as the extent to which an individual feels that they have personally meaningful goals and directions guiding them through life (Ryff, 1989). It is often assessed via self-report, wherein individuals respond the extent of their agreement to items such as "I have a sense of direction and purpose in my life" (Ryff, 1989), or "To me, the things I do are worthwhile" (Scheier et al., 2006). Because of the quantitative assessment approach for this construct, sense of purpose is often the focal point of research evaluating the implications of purpose and different outcomes it may promote. While the measurement and nature of these constructs differ, both components of purpose are consistently associated with desirable well-being, health, and social outcomes throughout the lifespan (Pfund & Hill, 2018; Pfund & Lewis, 2020). Both components of purpose also fit into prominent theories of personality psychology.

Before diving into the ways in which purpose fits into a personality paradigm, it is important to discuss how this construct has been categorized up until this point. Currently, there is no consensus. While Ryff's work is a cornerstone for the broader field, sense of purpose is but one of several indicators of psychological well-being (Ryff, 1989; Ryff & Keyes, 1995). Although purpose is consistently predictive of well-being components like positive affect and life satisfaction (Hill et al., 2018; Sumner, Burrow, & Hill, 2015), more recent sense of purpose measures have specifically tried to measure purpose without conflating it with well-being (Scheier et al., 2006). A personality psychology framework will allow for this construct to both be understood as a promoter of well-being, while also giving it opportunities to flourish in a variety of other life domains. Some scholars have characterized purpose a virtue or a character strength (e.g., Damon, Menon, & Bronk, 2003; Han, 2015), which often invites construing the contents of one's aspirations as either good and nobel or bad and ignoble. Personality psychology, by contrast, allows for the existence of these individual differences without moral implications regarding where one falls on the purposefulness spectrum. Others still have suggested purpose is a component of one's identity (Bronk, 2011; Burrow & Hill, 2011). This perspective may not be entirely discrepent from the view discussed below, given identity is often part of personality frameworks (Roberts & Nickel, 2017). However, taking a broader view of purpose will likely allow for a wider range of research opportunities. Besides the new empirical endeavors a personality science framework will provide, this framework will also create a united and less constrained narrative around the purpose construct itself.

2.2 Purpose and Personality

Personality science focuses on the study of individual differences, that make up a person, ranging from tendencies toward certain thoughts, feelings, and behaviors to values, motives, and abilities (Roberts, 2009; Roberts, Kuncel, Shiner, Caspi, & Goldberg, 2007). Understanding the ways in which purpose fits into personality science theory allows for utilization of personality science's unique approaches, methods, and techniques to broaden future research endeavors. To illustrate that purpose can function from a personality psychology perspective, I will discuss three related but distinct models of personality: the Neo-Socioanalytic Model of Personality (Roberts & Nickel, 2017), the Five Principles of Personality Psychology (McAdams & Pals, 2006), and the Systems Framework of Personality (Mayer, 2005).

2.2.1 Neo-Socioanalytic Model of Personality

When considering the Neo-Socioanalytic Model of Personality, the way in which purpose fits into personality psychology is quite complex. This model posits that there are four unique domains that capture the main aspects of our individual differences: traits, motives, abilities, and narratives. Though these four domains of personality are generally argued to be separate entities (Roberts & Nickel, 2017), purpose finds a place in each of them. When discussing each of these components, I will mention how purpose conceptually fits into it, how purpose connects to constructs typically assessed in that domain, and how it predicts related outcomes.

Traits. The first domain in this theory is *traits*, which are dispositional characteristics that maintain relative consistency of thoughts, feelings, and behaviors throughout similar situations across time (Roberts & Nickel, 2017; Roberts, 2009). Sense of purpose finds its niche in the personality science literature due to its dispositional nature, with differential levels of purposefulness promoting distinct thoughts, feelings, and behaviors. Regarding thoughts, people with a higher sense of purpose generally feel greater hope (Bronk, Hill, Lapsley, Talib & Finch, 2009), which is comprised of individuals feeling that they can think of clearer pathways to overcome obstacles as well as believing that they have the agency to take those pathways (Snyder, Rand & Sigmon, 2005). Furthermore, the affective nature of purpose is captured by work that has found individuals who report a higher sense of purpose feel more positive affect, less negative affect, and also are less reactive to stress (Bronk et al., 2009; Hill, Sin, Turiano, Burrow, & Almeida, 2018). Fewer studies have evaluated the behavioral nature of sense of purpose, though theory has suggested that purposeful individuals may be more effective in organizing their daily and long-term activities than their less purposeful counterparts (McKnight & Kashdan, 2009).

Motives. Purpose also finds a natural categorization in the domain of *motives*, or the things we want to do, pursue, and have (Roberts & Nickel, 2017). Purpose in life is not simply a goal; it also "provides a broader motivational component that stimulates goals and influences behavior" (McKnight & Kashdan, 2009, p. 243). If individual differences in motives are captured by the things we desire to do and have, purpose in life is a direct influencer of an individual's motives, guiding their short-term goals as they follow their long-term desires. The role of purpose on motives can also be understood through purpose orientations, which reflect the general nature of one's purpose in life. Purpose orientations are defined as the broader content of one's purpose in life. Examples include having a *prosocial orientation*, which focuses on helping others, or a *personal recognition orientation*, which emphasizes the desire to be recognized and respected by others (Hill et al., 2010). Referring back to the example of the medical doctor's purpose in life, their overarching goal was to heal sick individuals, which would fit into the prosocial purpose orientation. However, if they decided to become a medical doctor due to the desire to become a world-renowned brain surgeon, their purpose in life would better fit under the personal recognition orientation. While the presence of a purpose in life exists in both cases, the motivations and smaller actions that the pursuit of that purpose guides will shift depending on the purpose orientation itself. Purpose influences motives both narrowly, in the daily goals an individual sets as they pursue their purpose, as well as broadly, in the large purpose orientations they have.

Abilities. The third domain of the Neo-Socioanalytic Model is *abilities*, or our cognitive, physical, and emotional aptitudes (Roberts & Nickel, 2017). While purpose itself is not necessarily an ability, previous research has found associations between purpose and different kinds of abilities. For example, a higher sense of purpose is positively associated with better memory, executive functioning, and general cognitive ability in adults (Lewis, Turiano, Payne & Hill, 2017). Furthermore, some work has shown higher cognitive ability in adolescence to be associated with a higher sense of purpose (Minehan, Newcomb, & Galaif, 2000). Other work, meanwhile, has found that differences in ability are rooted in an adolescent's purpose orientation, not the presence of a purpose in life. In particular, while ability did not predict the presence of a purpose, specific purpose orientations differed in a study of high ability youth, which was defined as adolescents attending schools that required students to score two standard deviations about the mean on a common youth-oriented intelligence test. Those who were high ability youth were more likely to subscribe to a more other-focused purpose than adolescents tending non-selective schools (Bronk, Finch, & Talib, 2010). Research has indicated that sense of purpose is associated with abilities such as better cognitive functioning, and one's purpose orientation may differ based on one's abilities.

Narratives. Purpose can also fit into the fourth domain of the Neo-Socioanalytic Model. *Narratives* are rooted in how someone authors and understands their own life story (Roberts & Nickel, 2017), a part of which is determining the events that someone defines as significant and important (McAdams, 2013). There is a foundation of literature showing that sense of purpose is related to individuals' narratives (Bauer, McAdams, & Sakaeda, 2005; McAdams & Guo, 2015), with the kinds of memories people express relating differently to sense of purpose. For example, memories that reflect experiences that are more personally meaningful to an individual are more strongly associated with a higher sense of purpose than memories focusing on integrating one's life experiences (Bauer et al., 2005). The kind of narrative someone creates may influence how purposeful they are, or how purposeful they are may shape the way they develop and understand their own narrative.

Bringing the domains together. Each of these domains influence, and are also influenced by, our *identity* (how we see ourselves) and our *reputation* (how others see us). To have an identity, individuals often explore different aspects of themselves before committing to the personal and social identities that they feel best describes them (Brewer & Gardner, 1996; Kroger & Marcia, 2011; Sim, Goyle, McKedy, Eidelman, & Correll, 2014). Alongside this process occurs purpose development, wherein individuals explore goals and causes that are important to them before narrowing in on and committing to their specific purpose in life (Sumner, Burrow, & Hill, 2015). Research has illustrated that these processes co-occur, and that individuals who are high on purpose commitment also report being more committed to their identity (Hill & Burrow, 2012). In fact, some preliminary findings have shown that purpose may be higher on days in which individuals participate in activities related to their identities (Kiang, 2012). The structure of the Neo-Socioanalytic Model provides a valuable reference to understand how and why purpose predicts life outcomes.

The way in which purpose is easily and systematically interwoven into this model extends beyond its simple categorization and into the way in which these domains, perceptions of self and others, and even social roles influence each other. The fluidity of this model allows for the same flexibility that individuals might encounter in their own experience of purpose. For example, if someone greatly values family and is motivated to prioritize their familial relations, they could identify themselves as family-oriented, which may lead them to taking on roles in which they support and take care of their relatives. Then, if a parent were to get sick, this scenario could lend an individual to embracing the role of caretaker, which would further solidify their identity as family-oriented and now the caretaker of their parent. This new development could then influence some of the main personality domains: their narrative may be impacted as the diagnosis of their parent's sickness becomes a significant memory for them, their motives and values may further shift toward this family-oriented caretaking role, and possibly even become their purpose in life, which would further heighten their trait-level sense of purpose. While this situation is hypothetical, it encapsulates the thoroughness with which purpose as a multifaceted construct can be integrated into the Neo-Socioanalytic Model.

2.2.2   Five Principles of Personality Psychology

Another theory of personality to consider is the Five Principles of Personality Psychology (McAdams & Pals, 2006). This model contains two components that are similar to the model just reviewed: *dispositional traits* and *life narratives*. In addition, the model mentions characteristic adaptations, human nature, and differential role of culture. *Characteristic adaptions* envelope individual differences like goals and motives, as well as an individual's plans. This extends beyond the motives piece captured in the previous model and considers how an individual characteristically interacts with their environment. This principle integrates well with McKnight and Kashdan's (2009) description of a purpose in life as something that directs behaviors and may influence the organization of one's day-to-day life.

Another principle proposed by McAdams and Pals (2006) focuses on *human nature*, which posits that we share a basic human design that has experienced slight variations throughout evolution. When discussing evolutionary needs that individuals share, McAdams and Pals (2006) mention innate desires to *get along* with others as well as a basic need to *get ahead*. Previous theory has connected the purpose literature to evolutionary work by suggesting that purpose may promote more effective resource allocation (McKnight & Kashdan, 2009). With sense of purpose being positively associated with better personal relations with others and better romantic relationship outcomes (Pfund et al., 2020; Ryff & Keyes, 1995), there is support for the purposeful resource allocation that promotes getting along. Furthermore, earlier sense of purpose is positively associated with income and net worth later on (Hill, Turiano, Mroczek, & Burrow, 2016), which may lend support to the way purpose helps in the evolutionary desire to get ahead. Finally, the fifth principle is the *differential role of culture*, which elaborates on the impact culture can have on the rest of this personality model (McAdams & Pals, 2006). With a growing literature on the cross-cultural context of purpose, there is accruing evidence that both the development and manifestation of purpose can differ across countries, but having a purpose is not bound to the culture from which an individual is (Damon & Malin, 2020). Purpose can be more thoroughly understood through the lens of the Five Principles of Personality.

2.2.3   Systems Framework of Personality

Purpose also fits within Mayer's (2005) Systems Framework of Personality. This framework incorporates the larger ecology surrounding individuals, such as their social groups and overarching cultures. As previously mentioned, past work has found that purpose is a valued construct in a variety of cultures, though its definition and the specific purposes in life individuals articulate may vary cross-culturally (Damon & Malin, 2020). After taking this bigger picture context into account, Mayer (2005) posits we can then begin to understand an individual's personality. Mayer believes one's personality is comprised of *major psychological subsystems.* Recognizing the challenge of summarizing and separating these subsystems, Mayer took a more fluid route in crafting this theory. This fluidity, in turn, allows for other models of personality as described above to be incorporated into it rather than be superseded by it.

The major psychological subsystems are broken into four broad areas within which they are organized working on two spectrums, one of which reflects smaller, simpler subsystems versus complex, learned systems, while the other reflects internal processing subsystems versus external aspects of personality. However, due to the expansive and exhaustive nature of this model, I will highlight factors of the model that are most relevant to purpose research. For example, the *models of the self* subsystem from the *knowledge works* area is broken into components such as self-concept and life-story memory. These aspects relate back to the *identity* and *narratives* components of the Neo-Socioanalytic model, as well as the *life narratives* component of the Five Principles of Personality Psychology. As previously mentioned, purpose and identity development co-occur (Hill & Burrow, 2012), and purpose is related to the narratives we create (Bauer et al., 2005). Purpose plays a clear role in the different facets of the model of the self subsystem.

Another relevant aspect of this model focuses on the more people-oriented parts of personality. Specifically, the *social actor* area is described as "the expression of personality in a socially adaptive fashion," (Mayer, 2005, p. 10), as is comprised of elements such as *social role knowledge* and *attachment systems*. Social role knowledge refers to one's own understanding of their roles, such as being a parent, their job at work, etc. These roles could be used to derive a greater sense of purpose. For example, collegiate volunteerism predicts a higher sense of purpose later on (Bowman, Brandenberger, Lapsley, Hill, & Quaranto, 2010), and greater support from friends, children, and spouses predicts greater sense of purpose in older adulthood (Weston, Lewis, & Hill, 2020). In general, there is a consistent association between social connections and purpose. People with a higher sense of purpose report better relations with other and better romantic relationship quality (Ryff & Keyes, 1995; Pfund et al., 2020), and, in fact, those who are married report a higher sense of purpose than those who are not (Hill & Weston, 2019). Unsurprisingly then, purpose fits into the attachment system of the social actor, given sense of purpose is associated with less conflictual parental relationships as well as more secure attachment to parental figures (Hill, Burrow, & Sumner, 2016; Hill, Schultz, Jackson, & Andrews, 2019). Purpose both shapes and is shaped by who we are as social actors.

These examples are a few of the more basic ways purpose can be embraced by this exhaustive personality framework. These three personality models have commonalities off of which purpose can be built. Whether it be how purposeful an individual feels or the way their purpose in life motivates and shapes how they understand and author their own life story, purpose fits into a variety of components both within and across these models. With all three theories, purpose is a construct that has a far reach in the way in which it can be smoothly integrated into personality research, pointing to personality science as a reliable foundation from which research on purpose can be further built.

2.2.4 Narrowing in on Trait Purpose

The current chapter will focus most of its review and suggestions on the more trait-like nature of sense of purpose. It is important to note two limitations before further discussing the history of purpose in personality literature. First, though conceptually sense of purpose appears to be fairly trait-like (Ko, Hooker, Geldhof, & McAdams, 2016; Pinquart, 2002), future research endeavors are necessary to investigate the extent to which sense of purpose is, in fact, a trait. Second, purpose is an intricate construct that can fit into a variety of components of personality theories as discussed above. Therefore, handling it solely as a trait has its limitations when working to exhaustively understand the role it plays in individuals' lives. Within personality psychology, though, traits are the most studied construct of the various personality models and predict a variety of outcomes. Thus, personality traits give us the clearest direction for next steps in purpose research. However, we must first discuss the history of traits and how sense of purpose fits into it before diving into how trait theory can inform future research endeavors.

2.3   The Misunderstood History of Personality Traits and Purpose

While these models have worked to capture individual differences in people, personality science has generally focused on understanding what traits exist and what those traits mean. Nearly a century ago, researchers began to evaluate what adjectives could effectively describe a person (Allport & Odbert, 1936; Cattell, 1943). Through this process, research began to narrow in on five general traits that are now deemed the Big Five personality traits (McCrae & Costa, 1987; Peabody & Goldberg, 1989): extraversion, neuroticism, conscientiousness, agreeableness, and openness. Though these traits have slightly varied definitions across research groups, John, Naumann, and Soto (2008) identified common aspects amongst them. For example, those who are high in extraversion are considered to be more sociable, gregarious, and assertive. High agreeableness is comprised of modesty, empathy, and trust. High conscientiousness is consistently shown with high orderliness, industriousness, and self-discipline. High neuroticism, which is often understood as low emotional stability, is represented by greater anxiety, depression, and irritability (John et al., 2008). Finally, openness, sometimes called intellect (Goldberg, 1990), is represented by intellectualism, imagination, and, sometimes, adventurousness (John et al., 2008). There are other components of these traits that are less agreed upon, and, the lack of unanimity regarding these definitions, is one of the main reasons there is a need to consider other traits beyond the Big Five.

While some have stated that these five traits fully capture a person (Digman & Inouye, 1986), others have argued these traits are not exhaustive, and work should consider narrower traits in order to understand a person (Condon, 2018; Paunonen & Ashton, 2001). With this in mind, personality scientists have turned to considering the facets that comprise these traits in order to most effectively capture individual differences and have more precise predictions of experiencing certain life outcomes (Costa & McCrae, 1995; DeYoung, Quilty, & Peterson, 2007; Soto & John, 2017). Other work has taken it a step further to consider traits that are separate from the Big Five, rather than smaller aspects of which a Big Five trait is comprised (Condon, 2018). For example, going outside the context of the Big Five, researchers have begun to consider other non-facet Big Five traits, like narcissism (Foster, 2009; Wurst et al., 2017), optimism (Assad, Donnellan, & Conger, 2007; Lemola, Räikkönen, Gomez, & Allemand, 2013), and gratitude (Hill, Allemand, & Roberts, 2013), in order to understand how our dispositions predict different life outcomes. While this evaluation of narrower traits is an improvement in understanding both what makes up a person and greater specificity in trait-related predictions, some of these narrower traits have been misunderstood or overlooked, such as sense of purpose.

Given the prominence of the Big Five, it is worth discussing how purpose does and does not fit in, which has been debated over the years. Some have suggested that sense of purpose is a facet of conscientiousness (Goldberg, 1999). Conscientiousness has been defined as "a spectrum of constructs that describe individual differences in the propensity to be self-controlled, responsible to others, hardworking, orderly, and rule-abiding," (Roberts, Lejuez, Krueger, Richards, & Hill, 2014). While someone who is high on conscientiousness would be hardworking and industrious (Peabody & Goldberg, 1989; Goldberg, 1990), an individual who is high on sense of purpose does not necessarily just work hard, but would also report that they feel greater direction in life and that the activities with which they engage are important to them (Ryff, 1989; Scheier et al., 2006). With some theory suggesting that someone who is high on conscientiousness might be more likely to be passionless (Goldberg, 1990), these traits, though they may appear to lead to similar behaviors regarding the pursuit of goals, likely stem from different motivations regarding those pursuits. Purpose itself is not simply passion, but people with a higher sense of purpose find their activities meaningful (Scheier et al., 2006), something that would likely not be the case for someone without passion. Other work that has evaluated the association between sense of purpose and the aspects of the Big Five found that people who were more purposeful were also more industrious, an aspect of conscientiousness, as well as enthusiastic, an aspect of extraversion (Sun, Kaufman, & Smillie, 2018). However, organization (the other aspect of conscientiousness) and assertiveness (the other aspect of extraversion), were not associated with purpose, indicating that purposeful people may appear to be higher on extraversion and conscientiousness due to their hardworking and enthusiastic natures even when they do not report higher scores on the other aspects of those traits.

Beyond the semantic distinctions between conscientiousness and sense of purpose, research also suggests they are empirically distinguishable. In a recent meta-analysis (Anglim, Horwood, Smillie, Marrerro, & Wood, 2020), researchers evaluated the associations between various aspects of Ryff's (1989) psychological well-being subscales and the Big Five personality traits. One of these subscales is Ryff's measure of Purpose in Life (1989), which conceptually maps onto the current chapter's definition of sense of purpose. In this meta-analysis, when looking at two prominent models of personality trait theory, the Big Five and HEXACO (which includes Honesty/Humility alongside the other Big Five traits), sense of purpose *was* positively associated with conscientiousness. However, with associations of 0.50 (number of people = 5699, number of studies = 15) and 0.47 (number of people = 2003, number of studies = 5) between sense of purpose and the two conscientiousness models (Anglim, Horwood, Smillie, Marrerro, & Wood, 2020), there is clear evidence that sense of purpose is not simply conscientiousness as previously suggested. This quantitative distinction maps on well to other work that has evaluated the predictive ability of sense of purpose predicting desirable outcomes above and beyond conscientiousness as well as the other Big Five traits. To highlight a few examples, work has illustrated that sense of purpose is positively associated with romantic relationship satisfaction and commitment when controlling for the Big Five (Pfund, Brazeau, Allemand, & Hill, 2020). Furthermore, emerging adults with a higher sense of purpose experienced greater well-being, had better self-image, and less delinquent acts when accounting for the Big Five (Hill, Edmonds, Peterson, Luyckx, & Andrews, 2016). Regarding financial matters, when controlling for the Big Five, purposeful people cross-sectionally had greater household wealth and net worth initially, and they also incurred greater wealth longitudinally after approximately a decade (Hill, Turiano, et al., 2016). From love to happiness to wealth, sense of purpose has proven itself to be a trait that need not be swept under the rug to be ignored or thrown under the umbrella of a more commonly known personality trait. Sense of purpose has proven that it can stand on its own, and that it necessitates research as its own discrete entity. While there is evidence that sense of purpose is a predictive construct distinct from the Big Five, previous theory and methodology used to understand the Big Five can inform and enhance future research questions involving purpose.

2.4 Future Opportunities for Purpose Researchers Through Personality Science

Understanding that purpose can be integrated into personality psychology models while still remaining a distinct construct that functions above and beyond the well-known Big Five personality traits is important for two reasons. First, it provides evidence that purpose is a construct that is unique from past personality trait work and warrants further research consideration by both purpose researchers and personality psychologists alike. Second, it creates a bridge between these two disparate areas of research, which, in turn, creates novel opportunities for purpose researchers to adapt novel personality science theory and methodology. The final section of this chapter notes just a few of many potential research avenues that could open up through change in perspective.

2.4.1 Purpose in Daily Life

A fruitful opportunity in the purpose literature would be to understand short-term variability within an individual's sense of purpose. Work in personality psychology has considered states, which are considered temporary thoughts, feelings, and behaviors (Fleeson, 2001), that may deviate from one's normal trait tendencies. While a large proportion of variance in personality traits can often be explained as between-person differences, there is evidence of within-person variability in the daily or even momentary experiences of a trait (Fleeson, 2001, 2004). The frequency with which an individual fluctuates from their general trait-level, as well as the magnitude of the deviation from the trait itself, may have implications for related outcomes.

With the possibility of state-level changes in purpose, a valuable next step is understanding what could lead to these short-term deviations. Some work has shown that the kinds of tasks and activities in which an individual participates from day-to-day are related to one's experience of daily positive emotions, with some activities being more highly associated with positive emotions than others (Cantor et al., 1991).

With a core part of some sense of purpose measures including items such as "I value my activities a lot" (high purpose) and "Most of what I do seems trivial and unimportant to me" (low purpose; Scheier et al., 2006), it is possible that there will be daily purpose variability just like there is positive emotion variability based on activity engagement. In fact, some preliminary findings indicate that daily purpose could change based on one's daily activities (Kiang, 2012). Future work should consider if one's sense of purpose varies from day-to-day based on the activities with which they engage, or if more purposeful individuals are selecting activities that better align with their specific purpose orientation.

More broadly, research is needed to understand how much purpose can vary between and within days for an individual, as well as what greater variability in this state-level purpose means for both short- and long-term outcomes. Daily diary methodology and ecological momentary assessments with questions regarding purposefulness and outcomes of interest at each measurement occasion can be utilized to assess the presence and possible reasoning behind these short-term deviations. By more clearly grasping the potentially dynamic nature of purpose, future work can then consider how to intervene on these temporary purposeful states so individuals can feel greater trait-level sense of purpose in the future. Past trait intervention work has recommended a bottom-up approach, suggesting that if we want to change something at the trait-level, it is best to intervene at the state-level (Magidson, Roberts, Collado-Rodriguez, & Lejuez, 2014). If we know purpose is variable and potentially plastic, there is foundational research in the personality literature that recommends continuous state intervention could someday actually change someone's trait-level purpose, giving hope that just because an individual currently does not feel purposeful does not mean they always will not.

2.4.2   The Behaviors of Purpose

The breadth of benefits that purpose promotes is vast, though the mechanisms through which it works remain unclear. With traits being comprised of thoughts, feelings, and behaviors (Roberts, 2009), considering these three components in purpose research gives a foundation for further exploring why purpose leads to desirable outcomes. Some of these components have been examined more than others. With respect to feelings, sense of purpose consistently is linked to greater positive affect and less negative affect (Scheier et al., 2006; Sumner et al., 2015). Regarding thoughts, purposeful people report a greater sense of pathways they can take to overcome an obstacle, as well as more agency that they can take those pathways (Bronk et al., 2009). Furthermore, purposeful people experience less stress reactivity to stressors compared to their less purposeful peers (Hill et al., 2018), implicating a potential cognitive component in the way purposeful people perceive and understand daily challenges. Perhaps the reason people with a higher sense of purpose experience less stress when they experience an obstacle is because they think they are able to overcome it, or they do not think of the stressor in the same way as someone with a lower sense of purpose. While there is a growing literature on the thoughts and feelings of purpose, the behaviors that purpose promotes still require research.

One method to begin this process would be the Act Frequency Approach to Personality (Buss & Craik, 1983), wherein individuals would be asked to imagine the most purposeful person they know, then to describe the behaviors of that person. These descriptions could be utilized to determine behaviors commonly mentioned across individuals. This method previously supported other commonly studied traits in personality psychology (Botwin & Buss, 1989), indicating that this process would likely lead to a first step in understanding the more action-oriented component of purpose. This method, in turn, would lay the groundwork necessary for understanding why purpose does what it does. When considering the previous associations found with purpose, such as better romantic relationship outcomes (Pfund et al. 2020), better financial outcomes (Hill, Turiano, et al., 2016), and even greater longevity (Hill & Turiano, 2014), it is possible that understanding the behavioral nature of purpose could lead to a better grasp on the actions that lead to these desirable outcomes.

2.4.3   Purpose Across the Lifespan

Personality psychology seeks to understanding the developmental trajectories of traits throughout the lifespan, as well as the implications of intraindividual differences in those trajectories. Past work has shown that, while there are degrees of rank order stability in the Big Five personality traits (with stability increasing with age), these traits experience unique mean-level change from adolescence to older adulthood (Caspi, Roberts, & Shiner, 2005; Roberts & DeVecchio, 2000). Some of these traits, such as neuroticism, show the biggest change in young adulthood, with individuals becoming more emotionally stable during this time. Other traits, like openness and the sociability component of extraversion, experience large mean-level changes in older adulthood, while agreeableness and conscientiousness increase in young adulthood and through middle adulthood (Caspi, Roberts, & Shiner, 2005). Based on this work, it is likely that sense of purpose would have similar trajectories throughout the lifespan.

There is a basic understanding of lifespan developmental purpose trajectories. Past work has shown that purpose development occurs throughout adolescence and emerging adulthood as people explore and later commit to a purpose in life (Bronk et al., 2009; Burrow, O'Dell, & Hill, 2010; Sumner et al., 2015). Work also has shown that middle adults experience fairly high, stable levels of sense of purpose (Ko et al., 2016; Pinquart, 2002), and that those who are still exploring their purpose in life in middle adulthood experience poorer outcomes relative to their same-age peers, such as lower life satisfaction (Bronk et al., 2009). Furthermore, older adulthood is associated with a decrease in sense of purpose (Pinquart, 2002; Ryff, 1989), as individuals face decline in cognitive and physical functioning, retirement, and loss of life partners. Though there is some understanding about the mean-level lifespan trajectories, work has also found significant heterogeneity between subjects in their longitudinal purpose trajectories in middle to older adulthood (Hill & Weston, 2019), with the reasons for these atypical purpose patterns remaining unclear. With higher sense of purpose predicting desirable outcomes across the lifespan (Pfund & Lewis, 2020), it is important to understand at what points developmentally purpose is likely to be lower, as well as why certain individuals are able to maintain higher purpose while others in their age group are experiencing a lull.

Personality frameworks can set the stage for understanding why individuals' sense of purpose may further develop or decline. The Neo-Socioanalytic Model in particular gives an effective context to evaluate what may lead to trait change (Roberts & Nickel, 2017). This model suggests that traits are influenced by our identities and reputations, which both impact and are impacted by our social roles. When considering the general decline in sense of purpose among older adults (Pinquart, 2002; Ryff, 1989), as well as the heterogeneity in purpose trajectories among older adults (Hill & Weston, 2019), this personality framework may help understand why decline does—or does not—occur. Perhaps the reason some older adults decline in purpose while others do not is due to shifts in roles, whether relational or work-related, which may lead to a change in their own conceptualization of their identity and, in turn, affect their sense of purpose. Personality frameworks such as the Neo-Socioanalytic Model creates a theoretical pathway for future work to investigate deviations from typical lifespan developmental purpose trajectories.

2.5   Conclusion

Research on purpose has shown the construct as a consistent promoter of desirable outcomes across the lifespan (Pfund & Hill, 2018; Pfund & Lewis, 2020). By integrating purpose throughout prominent personality frameworks, its intricate nature becomes apparent. Also what becomes clear is that purpose is, in fact, a multifaceted individual difference that is not simply about having a goal, or pursuing a goal. For future personality researchers to continue exploring the nature and life of a person without considering this construct will mean for them to miss a fantastic opportunity as well as to encounter a blind spot regarding who that person may be. Purpose is a complex construct that warrants future research, both from personality researchers and purpose researchers alike.

Purpose is a powerful construct. However, to effectively capitalize on its power, we must fully fathom what it is and how it works. Personality psychology, a field focused on understanding the nature of an individual, and the implications of their nature, gives a foundation that can elevate the way we comprehend, evaluate, and utilize purpose. This chapter is a call to reframe purpose, not in a way that disregards all of the incredible research on this construct to this point, but to expand on that vital work with new scientific approaches that may be impossible without the reintroduction and reintegration of purpose into personality psychology.

References

Allport, G. W. & Odbert, H. S. (1936). Trait-names: A psycho-lexical study. *Psychological Monographs, 47*(1).

Anglim, J., Horwood, S., Smillie, L. D., Marrero, R. J., & Wood, J. K. (2020). Predicting psychological and subjective well-being from personality: A meta-analysis. *Psychological Bulletin.*

Assad, K. K., Donnellan, M. B., & Conger, R. D. (2007). Optimism: An enduring resource for romantic relationships. *Journal of Personality and Social Psychology, 93*(2), 285.

Bauer, J. J., McAdams, D. P., & Sakeda, A. R. (2005). Interpreting the good life: Growth memories in the lives of mature, happy people. *Journal of Personality and Social Psychology, 8*(1), 203–217.

Brewer, M. B., & Gardner, W. (1996). Who is this "We"? Levels of collective identity and self representations. *Journal of Personality and Social Psychology, 71*(1), 83.

Bronk, K. C. (2011). The role of purpose in life in healthy identity formation: A grounded model. *New Directions for Youth Development, 2011*(132), 31–44.

Bronk, K. C., Finch, W. H., & Talib, T. L. (2010). Purpose in life among high ability adolescents. *High Ability Studies, 21*(2), 133–145.

Bronk, K. C., Hill, P. L., Lapsley, D. K., Talib, T. L., & Finch, H. (2009). Purpose, hope, and life satisfaction in three age groups. *The Journal of Positive Psychology, 4*(6), 500–510.

Botwin, M. D., & Buss, D. M. (1989). Structure of act-report data: Is the five-factor model of personality recaptured? *Journal of Personality and Social Psychology, 56*(6), 988–1001.

Bowman, N., Brandenberger, J., Lapsley, D., Hill, P. L., & Quaranto, J. (2010). Serving in college, flourishing in adulthood: Does community engagement during the college years predict adult well-being? *Applied Psychology: Health and Well-being, 2*(1), 14–34.

Burrow, A. L., & Hill, P. L. (2011). Purpose as a form of identity capital for positive youth adjustment. *Developmental Psychology, 47*(4), 1196–1206.

Burrow, A. L., O'Dell, A. C., & Hill, P. L. (2010). Profiles of a developmental asset: Youth purpose as a context for hope and well-being. *Journal of Youth and Adolescence, 39*, 1265–1273.

Buss, D. M., & Craik, K. H. (1983). The act frequency approach to personality. *Psychological Review, 90*(2), 105–126.

Cantor, N., Norem, J., Langston, C., Zirkel, S., Fleeson, W., & Cook-Flannagan, C. (1991). Life tasks and daily life experience. *Journal of Personality, 59*(3), 425–451.

Caspi, A., Roberts, B. W., & Shiner, R. L. (2005). Personality development: Stability and change. *Annual Review of Psychology, 56*, 453–484.

Cattell, R. B. (1943). The description of personality: Basic traits resolved into clusters. *Journal of Abnormal and Social Psychology, 38*, 69–90.

Condon, D. M. (2018). The SAPA personality inventory: An empirically-derived, hierarchically-organized self-report personality assessment model. Preprint at https://psyarxiv.com/sc4p9/.

Costa, P. T., Jr., & McCrae, R. R. (1995). Domains and facets: Hierarchical personality assessment using the revised NEO personality inventory. *Journal of Personality Assessment, 64*(1), 21–50.

Damon, W., & Malin, H. (2020). The development of purpose: An international perspective. In *The oxford handbook of moral development: An interdisciplinary perspective* (pp. 110–127). New York, NY: Oxford University Press.

Damon, W., Menon, J., & Bronk, K. C. (2003). The development of purpose during adolescence. *Applied Developmental Science, 7*(3), 119–128.

DeYoung, C. G., Quilty, L. C., & Peterson, J. B. (2007). Between facets and domains: 10 aspects of the Big Five. *Journal of Personality and Social Psychology, 93*(5), 880–896.

Digman, J. M., & Inouye, J. (1986). Further specification of the five robust factors of personality. *Journal of Personality and Social Psychology, 50*, 116–123.

Fleeson, W. (2001). Toward a structure- and process-integrated view of personality: Traits as density distributions of states. *Journal of Personality and Social Psychology, 80*(6), 1011–1027.

Fleeson, W. (2004). Moving personality beyond the person-situation debate: The challenge and opportunity of within-person variability. *Current Directions in Psychological Science, 13*(2), 83–87.

Foster, J. D. (2009). Incorporating personality into the investment model: Probing commitment processes across individual differences in narcissism. *Journal of Social and Personal Relationships, 25*(2), 211–223.

Goldberg, L. R. (1999). A broad-bandwidth, public-domain, personality inventory measuring the lower-level facets of several Five-Factor models. *Personality Psychology in Europe, 7*, 7–28.

Goldberg, L. R. (1990). An alternative "description of personality": The big-five factor structure. *Journal of Personality and Social Psychology, 59*(6), 1216–1229.

Han, H. (2015). Purpose as a moral virtue for flourishing. *Journal of Moral Education, 44*(3), 291–309.

Hill, P. L., Allemand, M., & Roberts, B. W. (2013). Examining the pathways between gratitude and self-rated physical health across adulthood. *Personality and Individual Differences, 54*(1), 92–96.

Hill, P. L., & Burrow, A. L. (2012). Viewing purpose through an Eriksonian lens. *Identity, 12*(1), 74–91.

Hill, P. L., Burrow, A. L., Brandenberger, J. W., Lapsley, D. K., & Quaranto, J. C. (2010). Collegiate purpose orientations and well-being in early and middle adulthood. *Journal of Applied Developmental Psychology, 31*(2), 173–179.

Hill, P. L., Burrow, A. L., & Sumner, R. (2016). Sense of purpose and parent–child relationships in emerging adulthood. *Emerging Adulthood, 4*(6), 436–439.

Hill, P. L., Edmonds, G. W., Peterson, M., Luyckx, K., & Andrews, J. A. (2016). Purpose in life in emerging adulthood: Development and validation of a new brief measure. *The Journal of Positive Psychology, 11*(3), 237–245.

Hill, P. L., Schultz, L. H., Jackson, J. J., & Andrews, J. A. (2019). Parent-child conflict during elementary school as a longitudinal predictor of sense of purpose in emerging adulthood. *Journal of Youth and Adolescence, 48*(1), 145–153.

Hill, P. L., Sin, N. L., Turiano, N. A., Burrow, A. L., & Almeida, D. M. (2018). Sense of purpose moderates the associations between daily stressors and daily well-being. *Annals of Behavioral Medicine, 52*(8), 724–729.

Hill, P. L., & Turiano, N. A. (2014). Purpose in life as a predictor of mortality across adulthood. *Psychological Science, 25*(7), 1482–1486.

Hill, P. L., Turiano, N. A., Mroczek, D. K., & Burrow, A. L. (2016). The value of a purposeful life: Sense of purpose predicts greater income and net worth. *Journal of Research in Personality, 65*, 38–42.

Hill, P. L., & Weston, S. J. (2019). Evaluating eight-year trajectories for sense of purpose in the Health and Retirement Study. *Aging & Mental Health, 23*(2), 233–237.

John, O. P., Naumann, L. P., & Soto, C. J. (2008). Paradigm shift to the integrative big five trait taxonomy. In *Handbook of personality: Theory and research* (pp. 114–158).

Kiang, L. (2012). Deriving daily purpose through daily event and role fulfillment among Asian American youth. *Journal of Research on Adolescence, 22*(1), 185–198.

Ko, H. J., Hooker, K., Geldhof, G. J., & McAdams, D. P. (2016). Longitudinal purpose in life trajectories: Examining predictors in late midlife. *Psychology and Aging, 31*(7), 693.

Kroger, J., & Marcia, J. E. (2011). The identity statuses: Origins, meanings, and interpretations. In *Handbook of Identity Theory and Research* (pp. 31–53). New York, NY: Springer.

Lemola, S., Räikkönen, Katri, Gomez, V., & Allemand, M. (2013). Optimism and self-esteem are related to sleep. Results from a large community-based sample. *International Journal of Behavioral Medicine, 20*(4), 567–571.

Lewis, N. A., Turiano, N. A., Payne, B. R., & Hill, P. L. (2017). Purpose in life and cognitive functioning in adulthood. *Aging, Neuropsychology, and Cognition, 24*(6), 662–671.

Mayer, J. D. (2005). A tale of two visions: Can a new view of personality help integrate psychology? *American Psychologist, 60*(4), 294.

Magidson, J. F., Roberts, B., Collado-Rodriguez, A., & Lejuez, C. W. (2014). Theory-driven intervention for changing personality: Expectancy value theory, behavioral activation, and conscientiousness. *Developmental Psychology, 50*(5), 1442–1450.

McAdams, D. P. (2013). The psychological self as actor, agent, and author. *Perspectives on Psychological Science, 8*(3), 272–295.

McAdams, D. P., & Guo, J. (2015). Narrating the generative life. *Psychological Science, 26*(4), 475–483.

McAdams, D. P., & Pals, J. L. (2006). A new big five: Fundamental principles for an integrative science of personality. *American Psychologist, 61*(3), 204.

McCrae, R. R., & Costa, P. T. (1987). Validation of the five-factor model of personality across instruments and observers. *Journal of Personality and Social Psychology, 52*(1), 81–90.

McKnight, P. E., & Kashdan, T. B. (2009). Purpose in life as a system that creates and sustains health and well-being: An integrative, testable theory. *Review of General Psychology, 13*(3), 242–251.

Minehan, J. A., Newcomb, M. D., & Galaif, E. R. (2000). Predictors of adolescent drug use: Cognitive abilities, coping strategies, and purpose in life. *Journal of Child & Adolescent Substance Abuse, 10*(2), 33–52.

Paunonen, S. V., & Ashton, M. C. (2001). Big five factors and facets and the prediction of behavior. *Journal of Personality and Social Psychology, 81*(3), 524–539.

Peabody, D., & Goldberg, L. R. (1989). Some determinants of factor structures from personality-trait descriptors. *Journal of Personality and Social Psychology, 57*(3), 552–567.

Pfund, G. N., Brazeau, H., Allemand, M., & Hill. P. L. (2020). Associations between sense of purpose and romantic relationship quality in adulthood. *Journal of Social and Personal Relationships*.

Pfund, G. N., & Hill, P. L. (2018). The multifaceted benefits of purpose in life. *The International Forum for Logotherapy, 41*, 27–37.

Pfund, G. N., & Lewis, N. L. (2020). Aging with purpose: Developmental changes and benefits of purpose in life throughout the lifespan. In P. L. Hill & M. Allemand (Eds.), *Personality and healthy aging in adulthood: New directions and techniques*. Cham: Springer.

Pinquart, M. (2002). Creating and maintaining purpose in life in old age: A meta-analysis. *Ageing International, 27*(2), 90–114.

Roberts, B. W. (2009). Back to the future: Personality and assessment and personality development. *Journal of Research in Personality, 43*(2), 137–145.

Roberts, B. W., & DelVecchio, W. F. (2000). The rank-order consistency of personality traits from childhood to old age: A quantitative review of longitudinal studies. *Psychological Bulletin, 126*(1), 3–25.

Roberts, B. W., Kuncel, N. R., Shiner, R., Caspi, A., & Goldberg, L. R. (2007). The power of personality: The comparative validity of personality traits, socioeconomic status, and cognitive ability for predicting important life outcomes. *Perspectives on Psychological Science, 2*(4), 313–345.

Roberts, B. W., Lejuez, C., Krueger, R. F., Richards, J. M., & Hill, P. L. (2014). What is conscientiousness and how can it be assessed? *Developmental Psychology, 50*(5), 1315–1330.

Roberts, B. W., & Nickel, L. B. (2017). A critical evaluation of the Neo-Socioanalytic Model of personality. In *Personality development across the lifespan* (pp. 157–177). London: Academic Press.

Ryff, C. D. (1989). Happiness is everything, or is it? Explorations on the meaning of psychological well-being. *Journal of Personality and Social Psychology, 57*(6), 1069.

Ryff, C. D., & Keyes, C. L. M. (1995). The structure of psychological well-being revisited. *Journal of Personality and Social Psychology, 69*(4), 719.

Scheier, M. F., Wrosch, C., Baum, A., Cohen, S., Martire, L. M., Matthews, K. A., … Zdaniuk, B. (2006). The life engagement test: Assessing purpose in life. *Journal of Behavioral Medicine, 29*(3), 291.

Sim, J. J., Goyle, A., McKedy, W., Eidelman, S., & Correll, J. (2014). How social identity shapes the working self-concept. *Journal of Experimental Social Psychology, 55*, 271–277.

Snyder, C. R., Rand, L. K., & Sigmon, D. R. (2005). Hope theory: A member of the positive psychology family, In C. R. Snyder & S. J. Lopes (Eds.), *Handbook of positive psychology* (pp. 257–276). Oxford: Oxford University Press.

Soto, C. J., & John, O. P. (2017). The next big five inventory (BFI-2): Developing and assessing a hierarchical model with 15 facets to enhance bandwidth, fidelity, and predictive power. *Journal of Personality and Social Psychology, 113*(1), 117–143.

Sumner, R., Burrow, A. L., & Hill, P. L. (2015). Identity and purpose as predictors of subjective well-being in emerging adulthood. *Emerging Adulthood, 3*(1), 46–54.

Sun, J., Kaufman, S. B., & Smillie, L. D. (2018). Unique associations between big five personality aspects and multiple dimensions of well-being. *Journal of Personality, 86*(2), 158–172.

Weston, S. J., Lewis, N. A., & Hill, P. L. (2020). Building sense of purpose in older adulthood: Examining the role of supportive relationships. *The Journal of Positive Psychology.*

Wurst, S. N., Gerlach, T. M., Dufner, M., Rauthmann, J. F., Grosz, M. P., Küfner, A. C. P., et al. (2017). Narcissism and romantic relationships: The differential impact of narcissistic admiration and rivalry. *Journal of Personality and Social Psychology, 112*(2), 280–306.

Chapter 3
Extending Research Linking Purpose in Life to Health: The Challenges of Inequality, the Potential of the Arts, and the Imperative of Virtue

Carol D. Ryff and Eric S. Kim

Abstract Empirical studies of purpose in life are flourishing. However, in light of a rapidly changing social milieu, there are pressing but understudied issues to address if purpose research is to realize its potential in impacting people's lives. We first distill what has been learned from prior research on age variation in purpose in life and briefly review accumulating evidence linking higher levels of purpose to better physical health. Possible biobehavioral mechanisms underlying the purpose-health connection are noted. We then build upon this evidence to examine an array of factors that might undermine or nurture purposeful life engagement. Growing societal inequality may be critical in limiting people's capacities to pursue meaningful lives, but more research is needed. Alternatively, growing research now links the arts and humanities to health. We focus on possible influences these realms might have in cultivating purpose. The role of education in nurturing exposure to the arts is examined, along with problems of elitism in higher education (thereby re-invoking themes of inequality). Our final section calls for research that more explicitly links purpose in life to human virtues and values. Theoretical approaches and tractable empirical topics are delineated. Our overall objective is to offer innovative future paths to deepen understanding of how health and well-being at individual and societal levels are tied to purpose in life.

Keyword Purpose in Life · Meaning in Life · Inequality · Arts · Virtue

3.1 Introduction

Empirical studies of purpose in life have flourished in recent years. We focus this chapter on what has been learned in targeted areas of inquiry, and then build upon that knowledge to expand the depth and diversity of questions contemporary science

C. D. Ryff (✉)
Institute on Aging/Department of Psychology, University of Wisconsin-Madison, Madison, USA
e-mail: cryff@wisc.edu

E. S. Kim
University of British Columbia, Vancouver, Canada

© Springer Nature Switzerland AG 2020
A. L. Burrow and P. Hill (eds.), *The Ecology of Purposeful Living Across the Lifespan*,
https://doi.org/10.1007/978-3-030-52078-6_3

can bring to the existential challenges of leading purposeful lives. We begin by considering age variation in purpose, which on average shows decline from midlife to old age—although there is notable variability within age groups. Accumulating evidence suggests that adults who maintain high levels of purposeful engagement show better physical health and greater longevity. We consider possible biobehavioral mechanisms that might explain such observations. Building on these findings, the remainder of the chapter articulates several new scientific directions.

A first focus is on obstacles to purposeful living ensuing from the problems of inequality, which represent societal chasms that have deepened in recent decades. One's position in the social structural hierarchy, typically indexed by socioeconomic status (education, income, occupational standing) brings into high relief issues that have received limited attention in prior studies of purpose in life. Because inequality is growing, key questions going forward are whether purposeful engagement will increasingly become an experience of more privileged segments of society, while those lacking educational and economic opportunity will be left behind, increasingly unable to lead purposeful and meaningful lives.

The next section is less dystopian in tone. We highlight ways in which two rapidly growing but relatively separate strands of research—arts/humanities-health research and purpose in life-health research—might converge in synergistic ways. Of particular interest is how people's encounters with the arts and humanities may be important sources of nourishment for human development, vitality, and particularly, the ability to cultivate purposeful engagements in life. Along the way, we examine core questions about the crucial role higher education in nurturing the sensibilities needed to partake in the arts, broadly defined. Also considered are problems of elitism in higher education, which signal a return to the growing problems of inequality considered in the prior section.

We then move toward a cornerstone, but as yet under-evaluated question in scientific studies of purpose in life among adults: namely, whether the content of people's purposeful engagements reflect human virtues. As envisioned by Aristotle, the realization of one's true capacities, what he called eudaimonia, involves "activities of the soul in accord with virtue." Drawing on historical exemplars, we distinguish between benevolent and malevolent life purpose. So doing requires consideration of how purposeful actions impact others in proximal contexts, but also possibly at community and societal levels. We advocate for attending more closely to ideal and desirable ends in human virtues and values in hopes of illuminating the broader impacts, for self and others, of purposeful life engagement. Aiming for tractable empirical questions, multiple examples of virtuous purpose are considered through diverse forms of "doing" such as volunteering, caring for others (social responsibility), and work pursuits (entrepreneurial activities). A concluding section briefly recapitulates key messages from each main section of the chapter.

3.2 Aging Trajectories of Purpose and Linkages to Physical Health

Adult age variation in purpose in life was first studied in small community samples, but over time research shifted to longitudinal population-based samples. Both types of studies have shown that, on average, levels of purpose decline as people age—although some are nonetheless able to maintain a high sense of purpose into later life. Growing research has shown that those who maintain purpose typically display better health behaviors and better physiological regulation as well as reduced stress reactivity, which may, in turn, help explain why a higher sense of purpose is associated with reduced risk of several chronic conditions and pre-mature mortality. We briefly summarize this work below.

3.2.1 Age Trajectories of Purpose in Life

Initial cross-sectional comparisons of purpose in life among young-, middle-, and older-aged adults generally revealed declining trajectories of purpose as people aged (Clarke, Marshall, Ryff, & Rosenthal, 2000; Ryff, 1989; Ryff & Keyes, 1995). Subsequent studies that leveraged large longitudinal samples, some of which were representative of the U.S. population, offered converging evidence that purpose in life declines as individuals grow older (Hill & Weston, 2019; Springer, Pudrovska, & Hauser, 2011). An important question is why such later life decline in purpose occurs. Multiple forces likely shape this trajectory; we emphasize two intertwined macro-trends.

The first is that in the last 100 years, average life expectancies have increased by nearly thirty years (Martin et al., 2013). The second is that core societal institutions (family, work, education, healthcare, housing) may not be keeping up with the increasingly older distribution of the population. Riley, Kahn, Foner, and Mack (1994) described this as the problem of "structural lag." The idea is that societal norms, values, and laws have not yet adapted to the realities of growing numbers of older adults, many of whom are physically and cognitively healthier than those in prior generations. Thus, they may experience diminished opportunities for meaningful life engagement and continued self-realization because societal institutions lag behind the reality of their abilities.

In light of average trajectories of purpose as people age, empirical studies also reveal notable *variability within aging adults*. Although average levels of purpose decline with age, some are able to maintain a high sense of purpose into later life. More importantly, a growing literature documents notable health benefits among such individuals. We highlight these findings in the next sections, focusing first on the evidence linking purpose in life to longevity, followed by studies linking purpose to other health outcomes, then we end with consideration of possible biobehavioral mechanisms that might explain these associations.

3.2.2 Purpose and Mortality

Longitudinal evidence that purpose in life matters for longevity was first evident in the Rush Memory and Aging Project (MAP), which showed that those who displayed higher levels of purpose in life at baseline displayed substantially reduced levels of mortality over a six-year period (after adjusting for key covariates; Boyle et al., 2009). Subsequent findings from the Midlife in the U.S. (MIDUS) study (Hill & Turiano, 2014) showed that purposeful individuals lived longer than their lower purpose counterparts over a 14-year period (again, after adjusting for key covariates). Then, in 2016, a meta-analysis of ten prospective studies (pooled n = 136,265; mean follow-up duration: 7.3 years, mean age 67 years) observed that people with a higher sense of purpose had reduced risk of mortality (RR:0.83, 95% CI: 0.75, 0.91) (Cohen, Bavishi, & Rozanski, 2016). According to the Newcastle-Ottawa Scale (developed to assess the quality of observational studies), the quality of these 10 purpose studies was excellent (mean score was 8 out of 9)—all studies were longitudinal with reasonably long follow-up times, all controlled for key confounders (demographics, physical health, psychological distress), and most used validated multi-item purpose in life assessments. The meta-analysis also evaluated 5 studies that specifically considered cardiovascular events (pooled n = 124,948; age range: 57–72 years), and results showed that the relative risk for cardiovascular events among people with a higher sense of purpose was 0.83 (95% CI: 0.75, 0.92) in models adjusting for demographics, conventional cardiovascular risk factors, and psychological distress. Additional evidence linking purpose in life to health outcomes follows below.

3.2.3 Purpose and Other Health Outcomes

Since the meta-analysis appeared, other studies evaluating the purpose-health connection have been published with highly consistent findings. For example, one study of 6985 older adults from the Health and Retirement Study, expanded on past work by evaluating specific causes of mortality over a 4-year follow-up period (Alimujiang et al., 2019). Compared to those with the highest levels of purpose in life, those with the lowest levels of purpose (compared to those with the highest purpose) had reduced risk of all-cause mortality (HR:2.43, 95% CI: 1.57–3.75) and reduced risk of mortality from heart, circulatory, and blood conditions (HR:2.66, 95% CI: 1.62–4.38), after adjusting for sociodemographics, and a wide array of health behaviors as well as several other dimensions of psychosocial well-being and psychological distress.

However, a higher sense of purpose was not associated with mortality from the other causes of death including: cancer and tumors (HR:1.16, 95% CI: 0.60–2.25), respiratory tract system conditions (HR:1.83, 95% CI: 0.80–4.20), or digestive tract system conditions (HR:2.05, 95% CI: 0.52–8.13). These null findings may be attributable to other factors. For example, if the true effect of purpose in life on other causes of death is somewhat small, it may be difficult to detect associations without substantially more cases for each specific cause. Alternatively, sense of purpose might confer protective benefits on only some systems of the body (e.g., cardiovascular system), and not others. Further work that widens the aperture beyond cardiovascular outcomes is an important future direction.

Research evaluating other health outcomes, such as Alzheimer's disease, decline in physical function, and other chronic diseases, has begun, but more studies are needed (Alimujiang et al., 2019; Boyle et al., 2012; Kim, Kawachi, Chen, & Kubzansky, 2017). As an illustration, one study of 246 people with Alzheimer's Disease (AD) in the Rush Memory and Aging Project, autopsied participants upon death and found higher amounts of global AD pathologic changes, amyloid, and tangles were associated with lower cognitive function measured approximately one year prior to death (Boyle et al., 2012). However, among individuals with a higher sense of purpose, these factors were weakly linked with cognitive function, suggesting that a sense of purpose may potentially "dampen" the effects of pernicious biological forces, perhaps by recruiting other compensatory neural mechanisms. Below we expand on mechanisms that might underlie the health-protective influence of purpose in life.

3.2.4 Potential Underlying Mechanisms

Purpose in life may influence physical health outcomes through at least three different biobehavioral pathways. First, purpose might indirectly effect health through health behaviors. For example, a higher sense of purpose has been associated with healthier amounts/use of: preventive healthcare services, physical activity, and diet (Chen, Kim, Koh, Frazier, & VanderWeele, 2019; Hill, Edmonds, & Hampson, 2019; Hooker & Masters, 2016; Kim, Delaney, & Kubzansky, 2019; Kim, Strecher, & Ryff, 2014; Steptoe & Fancourt, 2019). Alternatively, evidence for sleep is mixed: higher purpose has been linked with higher sleep quality (Kim, Hershner, & Strecher, 2015; Turner, Smith, & Ong, 2017), but not healthier sleep quantity (Chen et al., 2019; Ryff, Singer, & Love, 2004).

Evidence for smoking is also mixed, with larger prospective studies generally observing no association, but cross-sectional studies show an inverse association (Chen et al., 2019; Konkolÿ Thege, Stauder, & Kopp, 2010; Lappan, Thorne, Long, & Hendricks, 2018; Morimoto et al., 2018; Steptoe & Fancourt, 2019). However, most existing studies have evaluated purpose after individuals already initiated smoking, and cessation might entail a different psychological process than smoking initiation, underscoring the need for more prospective research around smoking initiation. Interestingly, a growing body of research has observed that people with a higher sense of purpose have a lower likelihood of misusing both prescription drugs and illegal substances (Abramoski, Pierce, Hauck, & Stoddard, 2018; Harlow, Newcomb, & Bentler, 1986; Kinnier, Metha, Keim, Okey, & et al, 1994; Newcomb & Harlow, 1986; Nicholson et al., 1994).

Although the evidence around purpose and health behaviors is mixed, people with a higher sense of purpose generally tend to behave in healthier ways and this might attributable to a variety of reasons. For example, adhering to healthy behaviors requires the ability to make healthy choices consistently in the midst of competing options. One recent study suggests that people with higher purpose experience less neural conflict when confronted with competing decisions. Participants that were overweight/obese and sedentary viewed health messages promoting physical activity while blood flow to various brain regions (including those activated when feeling conflict) was measured via a MRI scanner. Participants with a higher sense of purpose were less likely to show neural conflict processing and also reported increased receptivity to health advice (Kang et al., 2019). Thus, people with higher purpose might make healthier behavioral decisions with more cognitive ease.

A second possible pathway linking purpose to health may be enhancement of other psychological and social resources that buffer against the toxic effects of excessive stress. For example, several studies suggest that people with higher purpose are less vulnerable to life stressors via dampened stress reactivity. These effects might result in less frequent activation of the sympathetic-adrenal medullary system and hypothalamic-pituitary-adrenocortical axis as well less frequent dampening of the parasympathetic nervous system, both systems of which contribute to development of chronic conditions. To illustrate, a daily diary study tracked 1949 middle-aged adults up to 8 days and obtained daily assessments of stressors and affect. On days when higher amounts of daily stressors were experienced, those with higher purpose showed less pronounced spikes in negative affect (Hill, Sin, Turiano, Burrow, & Almeida, 2018). Further, van Reekum et al., (2007) used functional MRI techniques to show that those with higher psychological well-being, including purpose in life, had less amygdala activation in response to negative stimuli as well as more activation of regions (ventral anterior cingulate cortex) that help regulate emotions. Schaefer et al., (2013) also showed that higher purpose in life predicted less reactivity (eye-blink startle response) to negative stimuli, while Heller et al., (2013), observed more sustained activation of reward circuitry (striatal activity) in response to positive stimuli among those with higher eudaimonic well-being, including sense of purpose.

Finally, purpose might influence physical health by directly impacting biological pathways. A higher sense of purpose has been associated with better glucose regulation and lower metabolic syndrome, as well as lower allostatic load (Boylan & Ryff, 2015; Hafez et al., 2018; Zilioli, Slatcher, Ong, & Gruenewald, 2015). Evidence around inflammation (IL-6, CRP, triglycerides) and lipids (HDL, LDL, cholesterol) is mixed (Boylan & Ryff, 2015; Friedman, Hayney, Love, Singer, & Ryff, 2007; Friedman & Ryff, 2012; Morozink, Friedman, Coe, & Ryff, 2010; Steptoe & Fancourt, 2019) and more prospective research is needed. A related study evaluated the relation between purpose in life with a gene expression pattern identified as a conserved transcriptional response to adversity (CTRA). Researchers hypothesized that CTRA gene expression pattern results from experiencing stress, and then the accompanying activation of stress hormones trigger increased transcription of genes involved in inflammation. One study found a strong link between a higher sense of purpose in life and down-regulation of CTRA gene expression after adjusting for health conditions and other potential confounders (Cole et al., 2015). Importantly, there have been null associations with other biological markers and processes such as heart rate variability and markers of atherosclerosis, carotid intima thickness, and coronary artery calcification (Low, Matthews, Kuller, & Edmundowicz, 2011; Shahabi et al., 2016).

Taken together, studies in this section suggest that a higher sense of purpose in life is associated with reduced risk of several chronic diseases and mortality. Accumulating observational and experimental evidence also implicates potential biobehavioral pathways underlying the purpose-health association. Thus, purpose in life is provisionally a target for interventions and policies aimed at enhancing biobehavioral pathways to maintain health in adulthood and later life. That said, other lines of inquiry that consider the impact of rapidly changing social structural realities are needed, such as the growing plight of disadvantaged segments of society. These concerns are addressed in the next section.

3.3 Purposeful Lives and Widening Inequalities: Understanding Obstacles to Fulfillment of Human Potential

The preceding evidence that purpose in life likely benefits health, including: reduced risk of disease, good health behaviors, better physiological regulation, and extended longevity, calls for critical next questions—namely, what factors nurture or undermine purposeful life engagement? There is much to consider on this front. We first acknowledge prior literatures that have examined sources (antecedents) of people's meaning and purpose, such as social connections and family ties (Lambert, et al., 2010; Martela, Ryan & Steger, 2018; Stavrova & Luhmann, 2016) as well as the role of prosocial behaviors (Klein, 2017). In the spirit of Victor Frankl (1959), we also note work examining the impact of difficult life challenges on purpose, growth, and meaning, such as studies conducted in the post-traumatic growth (Aldwin & Sutton, 1998; Tedeschi, Park, & Calhoun, 1998) and resilience literatures (Masten, Best, & Garmezy, 1990; Ryff, et al., 2012) where dealing with targeted life challenges, such as cancer survival (Jim, Richardson, Golden-Kreutz & Andersen, 2006; Kernan & Lepore, 2009; Pinquart, Silbereisen, & Fröhlich, 2009), have advanced our knowledge base tremendously.

Mindful of these important topics, we shift the focus to less considered influences on purposeful life engagement that emanate from one's position in the social structural hierarchy. So doing brings a sociodemographic perspective to factors that facilitate or impede purposeful life pursuits. In survey research, it has long been known that educational status and income matter for well-being, distress, and health (Lynch, Kaplan, & Shema, 1997; Marmot, 2015; Ross & Wu, 1995). We note that many scientific findings summarized in the preceding section include indicators of socioeconomic status (SES) as covariates in reported findings, but few give central interest to questions of inequality. Alternatively, psychological variables have been formulated as essential for understanding how health inequalities emerge (Adler, 2009; Kirsch, et al., 2019; Matthews & Gallo, 2011).

The changing historical context heightens the importance of such queries. Contemporary life in many countries, especially in the U.S., reveals dramatic deepening of economic inequality. The Great Recession of 2007–2009 radically changed the U.S. economy with poverty rates rising from 33 million in 2005 to more than 48 million in 2012 (Bishaw, 2013), with further evidence documenting the consequences of job loss, unemployment, financial strain and Recession hardships on health outcomes (Burgard & Kalousova, 2015). A prominent theme in such work is that low SES individuals and minorities experienced the largest declines in wealth following the Great Recession (Pfeffer, Danziger, & Schoeni, 2013), and less educated adults experienced more economic hardships and also experienced greater difficulty recovering (Carnevale, Jayasundera, & Gulish, 2016; Hoynes, Miller, & Schaller, 2012). Further, *annual* income growth has been unequally distributed in recent years, estimated to be as high as 6% for the richest Americans, a mere 1% for those in the middle class, and nearly 0% among those at the bottom of the income distribution (Piketty, Saez, & Zucman, 2018).

When comparing the U.S. and Europe, Reeves (2017) described heightened income inequality as the "hoarding" of the American dream wherein the top 20% of income earners have privileged access to better: educations, jobs, income, and wealth as well as greater likelihood of benefiting from: stable marriages to successful partners, thriving neighborhoods, and healthier lifestyles. Graham (2017) has linked discrepancies in economic and life opportunities to ever-more-compromised levels of optimism, life satisfaction, and happiness among disadvantaged segments of society. Recent findings implicate these factors in the opioid epidemic and related increases in "deaths of despair" (i.e., increasing numbers of death due to drug and alcohol poisoning, suicide, and chronic liver disease) (Case & Deaton, 2015) among middle-aged whites. Related work documents declining mental health among disadvantaged Americans (Goldman, Glei, & Weinstein, 2018), many of whom report heightened perceptions of economic distress (Glei, Goldman, & Weinstein, 2018).

A variety of factors likely contribute to growing deaths of despair, including loss of, or impaired access to economic opportunities and financial supports (savings, pensions), meaningful work, environmental supports (shelter, transport, sanitation), and social support (networks, affiliation, reciprocity, trust). We submit that a diminished sense of purpose in life may be an important part of this malaise increasingly experienced by disadvantaged Americans. Prior research, in fact, shows that a higher sense of purpose is associated with lower rates of the 3 main causes of deaths of despair including: suicide (e.g., reduced ideations and attempts), drug and alcohol poisoning, and excessive alcohol consumption (Abramoski et al., 2018; Harlow et al., 1986; Heisel, Neufeld, & Flett, 2016; Kinnier et al., 1994; Kleiman & Beaver, 2013; Newcomb & Harlow, 1986; Nicholson et al., 1994). Such findings underscore the future importance of tracking who in American society is experiencing a diminished sense of purpose in their day-to-day lives as well as identifying what forms of socioeconomic hardship and distress predict such existential despair, and of course of fundamental importance is what health sequelae follow from these profiles of disadvantage.

Put succinctly, a critical issue going forward is whether purpose in life will be ever more compromised among less educated and economically vulnerable segments of society. Such vulnerability may emerge in early adult life when individuals are striving to formulate and implement their life plans, but also in middle adulthood as the challenges of managing work and family life are paramount, and in later life, when the losses of aging and the effects of structural lag come to the fore. Focusing on hardships from the Great Recession, Kirsch and Ryff (2016) showed that educationally disadvantaged adults who experienced greater hardship (job loss, home foreclosure, bankruptcy) showed poorer self-rated health and had higher levels of chronic conditions. Psychological factors (e.g., purpose in life, sense of control, conscientiousness) were examined as moderators (i.e., buffers against) such outcomes. However, the pattern of effects showed that rather than serving as aa protective resource, these psychological factors became sources of vulnerability that heightened people's risk for adverse health outcomes. Such findings converge with prior perspectives arguing that protective resources can, in fact, become "disabled" (Shanahan et al., 2014) when the forces of economic hardship are sufficiently extreme. In such contexts, the magnitude of inequality experienced effectively overpowers what would otherwise be valuable human strengths. Given growing evidence toward ever widening disparities in wealth and life opportunities, new research is needed on the import of these societal changes on people's capacities to live purposeful lives that benefit their health.

Such inquiries demand integrative health science (Ryff & Krueger, 2018). That is, although health inequalities research emerged decades ago largely within population-based fields (demography, epidemiology, sociology), it is increasingly recognized that psychological (e.g., purpose in life, optimism, sense of control) and social factors (e.g., social ties and social support) play critical roles in understanding how inequality perniciously compromises health. Kirsch et al., (2019) offered a recent synthesis of such research from the MIDUS (Midlife in the U.S.) national study data. Purpose in life and other aspects of well-being were shown to buffer against the adverse effects of low educational status on biological factors, such as interleukin-6 (IL-6), an inflammatory marker implicated in multiple disease outcomes (Morozink, Friedman, Coe, & Ryff, 2010). Alternatively, anger was shown to exacerbate links between low educational standing and inflammatory markers (Boylan & Ryff, 2013). Key future questions are whether heightened economic disparities will increasingly undermine the health benefits of psychological resources, while also possibly amplify the health costs of psychological vulnerabilities. Related questions are whether these disablement processes are accentuated by perceptions of stigma tied to lower class identities. These questions demand attention to the historical stage on which health inequalities are unfolding and whether evidence from past cohorts will generalize to future cohorts. As a counterpart to this grim scenario, the next section considers factors that might nurture purposeful lives, even in contexts of adversity.

3.4   Connecting Purpose in Life to the Arts and Humanities

Recent advances underscore the positive impact of the arts and humanities, broadly defined, on well-being and health. In 2013 the Royal Society for Public Health in the United Kingdom published a report titled "The Arts, Health, and Well-Being" that summarized the benefits of philosophy, theology, literature, music, poetry, and film for human health, while also considering implications for public policies designed to promote healthier societies. The report also distilled the considerable accruing evidence which points to the useful role that the arts play in therapy, healthcare, community life, and professional education (medical training). Around the same time, a new field called "health humanities" (Crawford et al., 2015) began examining how the application of the arts, literature, languages, history, philosophy, and religion can promote health and well-being. Relatedly, a new journal titled *Arts and Health* was launched in 2009. A review at the time (Stuckey & Nobel, 2010) examined relationships between engagement with the creative arts (music, visual arts therapy, movement-based creative expression, expressive writing) and various health outcomes.

Within research universities, the Alliance for the Arts in Research Universities (www.a2ru.org), was founded in 2012 with the goal of promoting arts-integrative research, curricula, and programs in higher education. Another initiative emphasized the creation of healthy communities via collaboration between fields of public health, the arts and culture, and community development (Sonke, et al., 2019). Embracing a global perspective, the World Health Organization initiative recently issued a synthesis report (Fancourt & Finn, 2019) summarizing evidence on the role of the arts in improving health and well-being in many countries.

Most of these endeavors fill an important void in extant health research and practice by acknowledging major societal ills (e.g., inequality, racism, xenophobia, varieties of trauma) and demanding fresh responses and novel solutions. Below we offer multiple venues for future research intended to stimulate work linking the arts to purposeful life engagement.

3.4.1   Finding Purpose Through the Arts and Humanities

Psychologists are increasingly interested in how the visual arts, music, literature, and drama can: enrich experience, entertain, build aesthetic appreciation, facilitate sense-making (Lomas, 2016) and promote positive emotions, growth, vitality, and life satisfaction (Shim, Tay, Ward, Pawelski, 2019; Tay, Pawelski, & Keith, 2017). To consider such ideas, we draw insights from university professors who teach great literature and poetry to undergraduates. How do such educators conceptualize the arts and humanities as key sources of influence that nurture aspects of self-making, including finding one's way in life? Harold Bloom, in *How to Read and Why* (2000), says great literature and poetry strengthen the self and help one learn authentic interests. Such results squarely align with helping people find goals and directions for how to live, a key element of building a sense of purpose in life. In Bloom's view, great literature and poetry also help people cultivate a sense of purpose by clearing the mind of cant (dogma), helping one recover a sense of the ironic (vis-à-vis the contradictions and paradoxes of life), and prepare people for change.

Similarly, Mark Edmondson, in *Why Read?* (2004) believes that vitality can be nurtured through great literature and poetry, even though many humanities educators shy away from teaching literature for this purpose. Instead, critical thinking skills are often the prized outcome of reading (e.g., knowing how to deconstruct or take apart great works). Edmondson sees such efforts as teaching a disassociation of intellect from feeling, arguing that Derrida's deconstructions (which take apart the meaning of texts by showing they are irreducibly complex, unstable, impossible) clear away but offer nothing in return. In contrast, in a world where young people are inundated with ceaseless stimuli from the internet and advertising, Edmonson asserts that there is no better medium to help young people learn how to pursue meaningful lives, than immersion in great literature and poetry. He draws on the philosopher Richard Rorty who calls for narratives about personal lives to help justify actions and beliefs as well as to articulate one's highest hopes and deepest doubts.

Teaching literature to serve such ends, Edmondson regularly asks his students who are in the throes of reading great novels and poems: *can you live it?* So doing pushes them to consider whether the works offer new or better ways of understanding themselves and others, and whether they reveal paths to a better life. Values and ideals, often implicit in creative works, are thus put into action via such reflective activities. For example, Wordsworth's poetry is described as ministering to the dull ache in the poet's heart. His poems are known to have helped John Stuart Mill recover from an emotional crisis in his early adulthood (1893/1989). Literature thus becomes a preeminent means for shaping lives, thereby extending Aristotle's view of eudaimonia as becoming the best one can be. So doing requires engaging deeply with many forms of the arts and humanities, not only literature and poetry, but also painting, music, sculpture, and nature. The point, Edmondson reminds, is not to cheer oneself up but to pursue truths: "It's not about being born again, but about growing up a second time, this time around as your own educator and guide, Virgil to yourself." (p. 122).

Another educator, Deresiewicz (2015) frames the job of college as starting one on the path of soul-making via books, ideas, art, and thought. These mediums provide incitements and disruptions that raise questions about everything, thereby building capacities for introspection needed to formulate a defensible self that is guided by more than the bromides exchanged on Facebook or Twitter. The ability to grasp abstract concepts, engage in deep philosophical questions, perceive and probe hidden layers of meaning and emotion are critically needed to interpret and shape reality, and to make defensible life choices. These observations elevate questions about higher education.

3.4.2   What Is Higher Education for?

Advocacy for the arts and humanities raises fundamental questions why we need higher education and what it does for us. Although education is a ubiquitous variable in health research—almost always included as a covariate in analytic models, or as a substantive predictor in studies of inequality - remarkably little is known about how the content and substance of higher education facilitates meaningful, well-lived—i.e., purposeful—lives. A recent essay (Ryff, 2019a) written for the Mellon Foundation's initiative on the Value and Effectiveness of a Liberal Arts Education probed such issues. The guiding hypothesis was that a liberal education, rich in exposure to the arts and humanities, including philosophy and history, offers key nutrients for psychological well-being, and thereby, for health.

Extensive prior research on social stratification (e.g., Chetty, et al., 2017; Sewell et al., 1976, 2004) documents the role of higher education in achieving desirable positions (high status and income) in the economic hierarchy. Knowledge of how to achieve social mobility alone does not, however, illuminate how a liberal education might foster meaningful, purposeful lives, including those rich in civic and social responsibility (topics considered in Sect. 3.4). Distant arguments for a liberal education in America (see Roth, 2014) have been echoed by prominent thinkers throughout modern history. Thomas Jefferson, founder of the University of Virginia in 1819, envisioned a curriculum that would provide useful knowledge, which is capacious, open-ended, and serves as a means to improve private and public lives. Ralph Waldo Emerson thought the point of education was not just accumulation of knowledge, or even the building of character, but rather the transformation of the self (as elucidated by other educators above). Regarding what kind of education should be made available to the freed slaves, W. E. B. Dubois wrote eloquently about the capacity-building dimensions of liberal learning, which he saw as nurturing human development and human freedom, in contrast to the molding of an individual into one capable of performing a particular task.

In our era, Nussbaum (1997, 2010), has underscored the critical role of the liberal arts in producing capable and competent citizens. Also notable is a recent National Academies of Sciences report, *Branches From the Same Tree* (2018), that decries problems in higher education characterized by disciplinary silos preoccupied with learning as a conduit to well-paying jobs. Those trained in STEMM (science, technology, engineering, mathematics, medicine) fields are described as lacking adequate exposure to the humanities and the arts which are crucial for nurturing people's capacity to think critically, problem-solve creatively, and communicate effectively. Other new initiatives supported by the Mellon Foundation are investigating whether the actual content of what is studied in undergraduate training might shape the lives of students in terms of their later well-being, civic responsibility, and community engagement. These inquiries implicate another issue—namely, elitism in higher education—which signals a return to growing problems of inequality.

3.4.3 Elitism in Higher Education

A grave consequence of higher education in its current form is that it routinely social-izes young generations to give outsized importance to prestigious job placements and high income. In this regard, *where* the education was obtained has become ever more critical. This trend is of concern given what happens at elite private institutions (defined by prestige ratings, acceptance rates, and the socioeconomic backgrounds of students) relative to public universities and "lower-tier colleges." These dynamics play a key role in the forces that fuel today's growing socioeconomic inequalities. Interestingly, Benjamin Franklin (see Roth, 2014) was an outspoken critic of inherited privilege that cemented unearned advantages. He satirized idle students at Harvard, stating that their education taught them mostly how to carry themselves handsomely and enter a room genteelly. Deresiewicz (2015) also lamented the miseducation of the American elite, describing how such privileged environments nurture a false sense of self-worth, including narrow views of intelligence (defined by grades needed for success in business, science, and medicine), while also undermining people's capacity to effectively relate to non-elites. These ideas align with the work of Pierre Bourdieu (Bourdieu & Passeron, 1997, 1990), who decades earlier, framed higher education in France as the systematic process whereby elite institutions serve as mechanisms through which status hierarchies are maintained.

These arguments are carried to new heights in Markovits' (2019) *The Meritoc-racy Trap: How America's Foundational Feeds Inequality, Dismantles the Middle Class, and Devours the Elite.* A Law Professor from Yale, he asserts that the deeply embedded ideology of the American dream—i.e., social and economic rewards follow effort and talent, not breeding and inherited privilege—is a sham. With detailed support, much coming from the field of economics, he argues that instead of meritoc-racy emerging from internal attributes, we have elite institutions that are effectively ensuring dynastic transmission of wealth and privilege. The educational tournaments that define this system begin early in kindergarten and continue throughout higher education.

Meanwhile, the embattled middle class is sinking, such that upward mobility has become an increasingly distant fantasy, with life worse still for working class Americans. Notably, Markovits conveys that those at the top are suffering, too. Not only have they sacrificed and endured much to gain admission into the most elite schools in order to increase their likelihood of obtaining prestigious positions with salaries to support privileged lifestyles (e.g., gold handcuffs), they then find them-selves burdened with crushing workloads and incessant job demands, which possibly contribute to deteriorating psychological, social, and physical health. Contrary to prior conceptions of aristocrats whose "conspicuous consumption" happened amidst gracious, easy living (Veblen, 1889), the lives of present-day elites are the antithesis of leisure.

New research brings into high relief socialization processes at elite institutions, which illuminate what lies behind the growing acceptance of inequality. Analyses from a large panel study of ~65,000 students from over 350 schools (Mendelberg,

McCabe, & Thal, 2016) examine responses to a single question, namely, the strength of agreement with the following statement: "Wealthy people should pay a larger share of taxes than they do now." Findings showed that during the current era of growing income inequality, students at affluent colleges (defined by the SES background of the students) showed the highest levels of opposition to this statement when compared students at non-affluent colleges. Further, those embedded in certain aspects of campus social life (membership in fraternities and sororities), showed even higher opposition to the statement. The authors note this pattern contrasts with prior eras in which affluent colleges tended to have a liberalizing influence on students from conservative backgrounds. The research findings also converge with Markovits' (2019) emphasis on how immersion into the social environments of elite school are engines of socialization processes that normalize pursuits of affluence, often at the expense of values needed to foster just and equitable societies. If anything, students from privileged backgrounds at elite institutions are increasingly likely to emerge with economic outlooks that distinctly favor the wealthy.

In sum, higher educational attainment, including its role in creating sensibilities to partake of the arts and humanities, does not inevitably translate to beneficent life purposes. Sometimes the opposite occurs. We bring these complex issues into high relief in the final section, which calls for greater focus on the content of people's purposeful engagements and what they mean for the lives of others—which unavoidably takes us to doorstep of virtue, a topic we explore in the next section.

3.5   Purpose and Virtue

Examples from human history reveal that deeply-held life purposes are sometimes profoundly malignant in their impact on others. This observation underscores the need to connect purpose in life to the weighty matter of virtue. Given widespread societal ills unfolding around the world, the idea of *"virtuous purpose"* underscores the importance of nurturing varieties of purposeful engagement that benefit not just individuals and their own health, but their families, communities, and the larger society within which they exist. In addressing these issues, we first juxtapose benevolent versus malevolent life purpose to bring attention to the content of people's life purposes, which are largely neglected in the extant literature linking purpose with health and well-being outcomes. We also seek to illuminate the values that sit behind such intentional actions and objectives, including possible tensions among them, such as between promoting social cohesion versus fostering social change.

These issues take us back to theoretical and philosophical underpinnings of purpose in life, arguably the central strengths of this realm of inquiry. That said, it is equally important to advance these ideas in ways that are empirically tractable. Thus, the latter part of this section delineates multiple concrete examples of behavioral "doing" that exemplify blends of both purpose and virtue. Overall, the intent is to infuse research with new questions designed to augment self-reports purpose in adulthood with behaviors and actions that embody how their values and intentions are lived.

3.5.1 Distinguishing Benevolent from Malevolent Life Purposes

We posit that the *content of an individual's life purpose* is key to understanding how this construct influences personal health and possibly the well-being and health of others. Aristotle saw eudaimonia as the highest of all human goods and defined it as "activities of the soul in accord with virtue" (Aristotle, 349 B.C., 1925). Of central concern was achieving one's true potential, seen as a kind of personal excellence to be accomplished, by: (1) identifying virtues, (2) cultivating them, and (3) living in accord with them. He thus emphasized that virtue is not an isolated action but a habit of acting well. Multiple virtues were explicated in his *Nichomachean Ethics*, including bravery, temperance, generosity, munificence, magnanimity, honor, good temper, friendliness, truthfulness, amusement, and justice. Each represented a "golden mean" between other qualities representing excess or deficiency in specific domains of life.

A modern-day articulation of several of Aristotle's ideas is evident in Peterson and Seligman's (2004) *Character Strengths and Virtue* that has been operationalized with self-report measures that assess numerous strengths. Relatedly, in the field of aging, Laceulle (2017) offers a thoughtful formulation of virtue drawn from multiple philosophical sources (Aristotle, MacIntyre, Swanton). Of central interest is existential vulnerability that emerges from the tragic and inescapable realities of the human condition. Most contemporary science, however, is focused on what she labels contingent vulnerability that involves problematic life circumstances (financial concerns, care arrangements, health risks). Laceulle makes the case that throughout the life course, it is the challenges of existential vulnerability that lead to deeper meanings and practices of virtue.

Both virtues and values can explicate morally praiseworthy behavior, though virtues tend to be regarded as internal qualities, while values are viewed as external standards (Holmes 2014; Rachels, 1999). We posit that purpose in life research is enriched by considering links to both domains. At its best, purpose is a self-created, higher-order framework, that helps people achieve and maintain personal excellence (eudaimonia) by generating and managing life objectives congruent with their virtues and values. Scientifically, we conjecture that virtue may amplify the salubrious effects of purpose on health.

For example, one who pursues a virtuous self-transcending purpose consistent with established social values may pursue goals that are generally facilitated and rewarded by society. However, one who pursues overarching goals that reflect self-oriented values with little regard for impact on others (thus contradicting social values) may face more socially constructed barriers (McKnight & Kashdan, 2009), possibly resulting in more frequent experiences of overwhelming stress that stimulates the cardiotoxic stress axis; over time this could heighten a person's risk of several chronic conditions. We acknowledge thorny caveats to these ideas, such as when considering those who champion social justice concerns that run against established social norms of a given era (e.g., racism). In such cases, those who pursue such virtuous aims aligned with self-transcendent values may experience both health benefits (linked with living in accord with one's daimon) while also suffering the health burdens associated with pursuing social causes that are disparaged and even despised by others. Stated otherwise, bringing guiding virtues and values into the scientific enterprise adds to the complexity of the investigative task, but leaving out issues underscores the costs of failing to differentiate between benevolent and malevolent life purposes.

Social scientists have proposed several classification systems of values that show substantial agreement with one another, differing chiefly in levels of abstraction (e.g., Allport, Vernon & Lindzey, 1960; Bok, 1995; Hofstede, 2001; Inglehart, 1990; Rokeach, 1973; Schwartz & Bilsky, 1987, 1990; Scott, 1959). Nearly all values are endorsed as ideals by all people, but what differs is how they are prioritized. Among the many value classifications, the model put forth by Shalom Schwartz (2012) has been among the most prominent. Surveying individuals from 70 different nations, he articulated values that were universally endorsed and functioned to help both individuals and groups survive. From their rankings of values in relation to one another, a circumplex model was generated that included four primary groups of values: (1) self-transcending values, such as benevolence (preservation and enhancement of the welfare of those in close networks) and universalism (understanding, appreciating, tolerating, protecting all people and nature); (2) self-enhancement values, such as achievement (personal success through demonstrating competence in domains valued by society), power (social status, prestige, dominance, and control over others and resources); (3) openness to change, such as self-direction (autonomous thought and action), stimulation (excitement, novelty, and challenge in life); and (4) conservation, including tradition (respect and acceptance of one's cultural and/or religious customs), conformity (restraint of actions and impulses that violate social norms or expectations), security (safety, harmony, stability of society).

We see self-transcending versus self-enhancing values as particularly helpful in distinguishing between life purposes that are benevolent versus malevolent. We first acknowledge prior work by Damon and colleagues who operationalized purpose itself as a, "a stable and generalized intention to accomplish something that is at once meaningful to the self and of consequence to the world beyond the self" (Damon et al., 2003, p. 121). They also differentiated noble purposes (e.g., purposes that promote good) from ignoble purposes (e.g., purposes that promote antisocial, inhumane, and destructive acts) (Colby, Bundick, Remington, & Morton, 2020). We invoke notable exemplars from human history whose guiding life purposes were transformative in promoting better lives for many include Abraham Lincoln, Gandhi, Mother Teresa, Eleanor Roosevelt, Martin Luther King, Mikhail Gorbachev, and Nelson Mandela. Although imperfect, as all humans are, their overarching commitments were about preservation and enhancement of the welfare of others, along with tolerance and appreciation of all people. Alternatively, history also includes those whose core purposes were responsible for massive suffering and death: Stalin, Hitler, or more recently, Saddam Hussein and Muammar Gaddafi. Their core purposes were the pursuit of power, dominance, and control over others, enacted with dramatic cruelty and heartlessness.

Those not so famous are also worth noting. Colby and Damon (1992) conducted in-depth interviews with 23 contemporary Americans in *Some Do Care* to illustrate varieties of virtue, such as those who worked for the poor, fought for civil rights, or promoted peace and protection of the environment. All impacted their communities and society by their moral leadership. Additionally, acclaiming virtuous purpose in later life, the Purpose Prize is now awarded annually to numerous older adults who devote their time and talents to helping their communities by mentoring children, including those with incarcerated parents, working for affordable housing for seniors, and creating fitness programs for those with health problems (see https://purposepr ize.encore.org/).

Alternatively, on the side of self-enhancing values and the antithesis of generosity (greed), it is important to consider malevolent pursuits in contemporary life. Here we note *Winners Take All* (Giridharadas, 2019), which showcased "predatory philanthropy." Among the global elite are some who use their wealth and power to preserve economic and social systems engineered to concentrate and sustain their wealth, usually at the expense of broader societal progress. Numerous examples are provided in the volume. What we underscore is that these contemporary manifestations of malevolent purpose may well be related to growing problems of inequality and deaths of despair emphasized in the section above.

To summarize, we invoke ideas of virtue and human values to bring emphasis to the content of people's purposeful life engagements. Some deeply held life commitments do not exemplify moral goodness and may even do great harm to others. Thankfully many behavioral enactments of purpose embody at least some of Aristotle's virtues as well as self-transcendent values. Such qualities are likely needed to foster just and fair societies. In the section below we consider how these ideals can be made empirically tractable.

3.5.2 Empirical Translations: Assessing Virtuous Purpose Through Doing

When we contemplate gaps in existing research and scan the scientific horizon, we see promising new directions for empirical studies of virtuous life purpose. However, at the outset, we observe that self-report methodologies may be inherently limited in capturing ideas of virtue and self-transcendent values in people's life engagements. The reason is that these honorific qualities may be particularly prone to bias when assessed from the respondents' point of view. Some individuals may be vulnerable to lauding their own generosity, magnanimity, and honor, even while others who know them might disagree. As an alternative, we favor assessing virtuous purpose through what people *do—i.e., the behaviors and actions in which they engage.* These ideas are illustrated with several substantive domains, each of which constitute extant realms of empirical inquiry: volunteering, generativity, social responsibility, and work pursuits (illustrated with entrepreneurship). The objective with all of them, which are somewhat overlapping in content, is to infuse scientific research on purpose in life with new assessments of virtuous doing. Several studies described below draw on data from MIDUS, a national longitudinal study that includes not only cross-time assessments of purpose in life (self-reported), sociodemographic variables, and diverse indicators of health, but also measures of virtuous doing.

3.5.2.1 Volunteering

Contributing one's time and energy to assist others (volunteering) has been associated with a wide array of psychological, social, and physical health benefits (selective evidence provided below). However, we begin by noting values-based moderators of the volunteering-health/well-being association. Compared to non-volunteers, those who volunteered had reduced risk of mortality, but these effects varied depending on motives for volunteering. Those who volunteered for self-transcendent reasons (values of social connection, altruism, learning/understanding) had reduced mortality compared to those who volunteered for self-protection reasons. Their mortality was also higher than that of non-volunteers (see Fig. 3) (Konrath et al., 2012). Another study found that only those who viewed others positively (not cynically) benefited from the stress-buffering effects of volunteering (Poulin, 2014). These values-based windows on volunteering may also be accompanied by high levels of purpose in life, queries that are ripe for future analysis.

Using data from MIDUS, multiple investigators have examined links between volunteering and well-being. Son and Wilson (2012) found that volunteering (measured as a binary or continuous variable) prospectively predicted greater eudai-monic and social well-being, but not hedonic well-being, though number of hours contributed made no difference. They also found that those with higher well-being were more likely to volunteer. Choi and Kim (2011) used a eudaimonic composite and found after controlling for baseline well-being and other resources that time volunteering (up to 10 hours monthly) and charitable giving had direct positive asso-ciations with subsequent well-being. Greenfield and Marks (2004) examined formal volunteering as moderator of links between later life role loss and psychological well-being, with findings most strongly evident for purpose in life. Another study also examined volunteering as a moderating influence (Russell et al., 2019) and found that among adults with low self-esteem, those who volunteered had higher levels of life satisfaction. Son and Wilson (2015) brought economic factors into the query, finding no direct association between household income and volunteering once chronic financial strain and social and eudaimonic well-being were taken into account. Other MIDUS findings have linked volunteering to physical health: Han, Kim, and Burr (2018) found that volunteering buffered against the adverse effects of daily stress on diurnal cortisol output, while Whillans et al. (2016) found that spending money on others was subsequently linked with lower levels of systolic and diastolic blood pressure.

The above studies point to promising lines of future inquiry in which various indices (giving time or money to others) could be investigated as examples of virtuous doing that may moderate (or mediate) how the challenges of aging (or inequality or other stresses) are linked with reports of purpose in life. Such works thus pave the way for inquiries to examine virtuous doing as a direct influence on purpose in life and various aspects of physical health as well as a possible indirect influence (virtuous doing as mediator) linking the difficulties of aging or the challenges of inequality to health.

3.5.2.2 Generativity

As formulated by Erikson (1959), generativity involves having a concern for guiding and directing the next generation, which can be expressed behaviorally in contexts of family, work, or community. Keyes and Ryff (1998) first used baseline data from MIDUS to show social structural influences on expressions of generativity—namely, those with more education displayed higher levels of multiple aspects of generativity (self-conceptions, norms, behaviors). These aspects of caring and doing for others were also predictive of multiple aspects of psychological and social well-being. Generativity was also found to partially explain socioeconomic disparities in well-being, thus underscoring our previous emphasis on how heightened inequality may undermine purposeful life engagements of future generations of U.S. adults who lack the wherewithal to help guide and direct the lives of others. Another study (Son & Wilson (2011) found that generativity (a desire to leave a legacy and provide for the welfare of others) mediated the influence of both religion beliefs and educational status on volunteering. Bringing physical health into the query, Gruenewald, Liao, and Seeman (2012) reported that greater levels of generative concern and generative contributions predicted lower odds of declining physical function or death 10 years later. Finally, Homan, Greenberg, and Mailick (2020) focused on the challenges of parenting a child with developmental problems or mental disorder and found that the associations between parenting such a child and psychological (e.g., positive and negative affect) and as well as physical health outcomes was moderated by parents' gender and levels of generativity. Mothers experienced greater adverse effects of parenting a child with developmental or mental problems, but these adverse effects were buffered by high levels of generativity.

Building on these illustrative examples of virtuous doing concerned with guiding and directing others (generativity), we posit that these activities (expressed as attitudes and behaviors) are key factors that may moderate impacts of aging or inequality or non-normative parenting on reported levels of purpose in life. In addition, generativity profiles may also amplify or mediate how purpose in life matters for diverse health outcomes.

3.5.2.3 Social Responsibility

Seeking to illuminate profiles of social responsibility in midlife and older adults, Alice Rossi (2001) brought multiple measures to the MIDUS baseline survey to assess social responsibility in domains of family and community life as well as to probe social responsibility in terms of normative obligations, time commitments, and financial contributions. She also examined the developmental roots (e.g., early socialization experiences) of adult social responsibility as well as how it is impacted by family problems or by the interplay between work and family life. Two additional chapters in the volume brought in-depth, qualitative interviews to the topic of social responsibility. In one, Colby, Sippola, and Phelps (2001) considered whether the social fabric of modern society, as suggested by mass media at the time, is fraying, possibly due to heightened concerns with self-interest, individualism, and moral relativism. A subsample of MIDUS participants were interviewed about how they understood the personal meaning of their paid work and its relation to their other values and goals. Most reported that their work was meaningful and that it contributed to the well-being of others and society. Those who described their work in terms of social responsibility also displayed higher scores on measures of civic obligation and altruism.

In a second chapter, Markus et al., (2001) conducted qualitative interviews aimed at probing how Americans of different educational backgrounds conceptualize and talk about adult responsibility (e.g., protecting individual rights). Findings were discussed to underscore that core perceptions of what it means to be socially responsible vary by one's position in the educational hierarchy. For example, among high-school educated adults, many emphasized that being responsible involved meeting obligations to others and being dependable. Additionally, high school educated adults gave greater emphasis to the importance of adjusting to circumstances in thinking about social responsibility. College-educated adults, in contrast, gave greater emphasis to juggling and balancing many different tasks, taking initiative or control of situations, and taking care of oneself.

Returning to guiding themes of this chapter, important queries going forward are whether various indicators of social responsibility described above serve as modifiers of links between aging and inequality on reported levels of purpose in life and possibly various health outcomes. For example, those who more strongly endorse normative obligations in doing for others, or give greater time or money to others may also report higher levels of purpose in life and thereby, show better physical health via their engagement in activities that reflect doing for others. We reiterate there is some overlap, conceptually and empirically, between our categories of virtuous doing (volunteering, generativity, social responsibility) considered above. Future research will help to determine the unique and joint effects of these various indicators of virtuous doing on purpose in life and health. Below we consider virtuous doing in the context of work.

3.5.2.4 Doing Work that Benefits Others: The Case of Entrepreneurship

The last topic considered under the heading of virtuous doing involves activities related to adult work pursuits. We focus specifically on the topic of entrepreneurship, often operationalized as self-employment. Some of the largest companies today such as the FAANG companies (Facebook, Apple, Amazon, Netflix, Google) make up ~15% of the S&P 500, but did not exist a mere 20 years ago. They have an outsized influence on society, with young startups having the ability to grow at unprecedented speed. Further, many startups consciously formulate value systems and ways of operating, and are often more open to new ways of operating compared to large corporations that have existed for several decades. Thus, entrepreneurship constitutes an interesting societal leverage point that can and should be scientifically targeted.

We note that entrepreneurship has been linked to the health of entrepreneurs, including studies conducted in MIDUS (Patel, Wolfe, & Williams, 2019). We showcase it because of growing evidence that entrepreneurship impacts well-being (Stephan, 2018). This literature is also relevant because it allows connections to previous contrasts between benevolent and malevolent life purposes. In the world of entrepreneurship there are notable examples of both virtuous and vicious entrepreneurs (Ryff, 2019b). Blackburn and McGhee (2007), in fact, distilled three key virtues that guide some entrepreneurs: creativity, beneficence, and integrity. These laudatory qualities are increasingly evident in positive organizational research (Cameron et al., 2008), which emphasizes how optimal organizations foster human strengths (virtue, gratitude, courage, positive emotions, empowerment, meaning) among their employees. In the entrepreneurial field, there is also concern with "doing well by doing good" (Williams & Shepherd, 2016) which focuses on actions intended to help relieve human suffering via an array of methods such as creating ventures that help people deal with the aftermath of environmental disasters.

The tensions between prosocial motivation and for-profit entrepreneurship constitute key directions in ongoing inquiries (Davidsson & Wiklund, 2001). That is, there is a dark side to self-initiated business ventures, including a version driven primarily by greed and self-interest. Baumol (1990) provides a broad look across multiple centuries to distinguished between productive, unproductive, and destructive entrepreneurial activities. For example, during the Middle Ages wealth and power were pursued by entrepreneurs focused on military pursuits, such as the creation of the stirrup for effective cavalry tactics. Unproductive entrepreneurship was described as prominent for centuries via rent-seeking. In contemporary science, there is need to shine a spotlight on the *consequences* that beneficent versus self-serving entrepreneurs have on the well-being and health of employees, and the surrounding community.

Entrepreneurship, as a realm of scientific inquiry, is thus ripe for new investigations that focus, for example, on distribution of profits, viewed as behavioral acts reflecting beneficence or greed at the top, and what they mean for the lives of others, measured in terms of well-being and health of those employed by the new start-up endeavors. We hypothesize that entrepreneurial pursuits driven by virtuous intentions will likely nurture the purposeful engagement of both entrepreneurs and their employees, while also likely contributing to better profiles of health of both, to say nothing of facilitating flourishing within the communities in which they are embedded.

3.6 Concluding Summary

This chapter covered expansive territories, all with the goal of generating new directions for science built on growing evidence that purpose in life, known to decline for many as they age, importantly predicts reduced risk for mortality and multiple disease outcomes as well as better regulation of multiple physiological systems. We considered possible mechanisms, including biobehavioral and brain-based processes that may help explicate the pathways through which believing one's life has purpose is salubrious for health.

We then shifted to consider growing problems of economic inequality, asking whether heightened financial strain and diminished life opportunities experienced by many are and will continue translating into ever more compromised profiles of purposeful life engagement among disadvantaged segments of society. Such questions are important to consider across the decades of adult life, including early adulthood when individuals are formulating their life plans, in middle adulthood as challenges of managing work and family life are paramount, and in old age when losses of aging and possibly structural lag may come to the fore. We emphasized the need to investigate such topics with integrative biopsychosocial research.

Our attention then shifted to consider the role of the arts and humanities in helping nurture purposeful and meaningful lives. We drew on growing evidence that the arts, broadly defined, are linked with better health and well-being. Although psychologists are increasingly interested in how the arts promote positive emotions, we focused on insights from those who teach great literature and poetry to undergraduates so as to distill how encounters with these realms might contribute to greater self-knowledge, including one's sense of direction in and vitality in life. We emphasized the need for goals in higher education that go beyond concerns for remunerative employment following graduation. Related to the theme of inequality, we noted problems of elitism in higher education and socialization for norms of affluence, perhaps at the expense of just societies.

Such issues provided a transition to our last section calling for greater linkage of purposeful life engagement to topics of virtue and related values concerned with more than self-enhancement. We reviewed differing conceptions of virtue and self-transcendent values, illustrated with examples of benevolent versus malevolent life purpose, drawing on historical figures as well as present-day individuals from multiple walks of life. Underscoring the need to translate these ideas to empirically tractable questions, we considered multiple types of "virtuous doing" via studies of volunteering, generativity, social responsibility, and entrepreneurship. Taken together, the ideas and research directions generated in this chapter aim to contribute to novel varieties of science wherein purposeful life engagements are carried to new heights in illuminating how good lives are lived and better societies promoted.

Acknowledgements The MIDUS baseline study was supported by the John D. and Catherine T. MacArthur Foundation Research Network on Successful Midlife Development. Longitudinal extensions of MIDUS have been supported by Grants from the National Institute on Aging (P01-AGO20166; U19-AGO51426). The biological research has been supported by the following grants: M01RR023942 (Georgetown), M01-RR0865 (UCLA), from the General Clinical Research Centers Program, and UL1TR000427 (University of Wisconsin) from the National Center for Advancing Translational Sciences (NCATS National Institutes of Health). Eric Kim was supported by a grant from the NIH (K99AG055696).

References

Abramoski, K., Pierce, J., Hauck, C., & Stoddard, S. (2018). Variations in adolescent purpose in life and their association with lifetime substance use. *The Journal of School Nursing, 34*(2), 114–120. https://doi.org/10.1177/1059840517696964.

Adler, N. E. (2009). Health disparities through a psychological lens. *American Psychologist, 64*(8), 663. https://doi.org/10.1037/0003-066X.64.8.663.

Aldwin, C. M., & Sutton, K. J. (1998). A developmental perspective on posttraumatic growth.

Alimujiang, A., Wiensch, A., Boss, J., Fleischer, N. L., Mondul, A. M., McLean, K., et al. (2019). Association between life purpose and mortality among US adults older than 50 years. *JAMA Network Open, 2*(5), e194270. https://doi.org/10.1001/jamanetworkopen.2019.4270.

Allport, G. W., Vernon, P., Lindzey, G. (1960). A study of values (Rev. ed.). Boston: Houghton Mifflin.

Aristotle (349 B.C./1925). *The Nicomachean Ethics* (W. D. Ross, Trans.). New York: Oxford University Press.

Baumol, W. J. (1990). Entrepreneurship: Productive, unproductive, and destructive. *Journal of Business Venturing, 11*, 3–22.

Bishaw, A. (2013). Poverty: 2000 to 2012. *American Community Survey Briefs*, 1–16.

Blackburn, M., & McGhee, P. (2007). The virtuous entrepreneur: New ventures and human flourishing. *International Journal of Entrepreneurial Innovation*, 1–25, (Paper 31–2007).

Bok, S. (1995). *Common values* (Vol. 1). University of Missouri Press.

Bourdieu, P., & Passeron, J. (1977). *Reproduction in education, society, and culture*. Beverly Hills, CA: Sage.

Bourdieu, P., & Passeron, J. (1990). *Reproduction in education, society, and culture* (2nd ed.). London: Sage.

Boylan, J. M., & Ryff, C. D. (2013). Varieties of anger and the inverse link between education and inflammation: Toward an integrated framework. *Psychosomatic Medicine, 75*, 566–574. https://doi.org/10.1097/PSY.0b013e31829683bd.

Boylan, J. M., & Ryff, C. D. (2015). Psychological well-being and metabolic syndrome: Findings from the midlife in the United States national sample. *Psychosomatic Medicine, 77*(5), 548–558. https://doi.org/10.1097/PSY.0000000000000192.

Boyle, P. A., Barnes, L. L., Buchman, A. S., & Bennett, D. A. (2009). Purpose in life is associated with mortality among community-dwelling older persons. *Psychosomatic Medicine, 71*, 574–579. https://doi.org/10.1097/PSY.0b013e3181a5a7c0.

Boyle, P. A., Buchman, A. S., Wilson, R. S., Yu, L., Schneider, J. A., & Bennett, D. A. (2012). Effect of purpose in life on the relation between alzheimer disease pathologic changes on cognitive function in advanced age. *Archives of General Psychiatry, 69*(5), 499–505. https://doi.org/10.1001/archgenpsychiatry.2011.1487.

Burgard, S. A., & Kalousova, L. (2015). Effects of the great recession: Health and well-being. *Annual Review of Sociology, 41,* 181–201.

Cameron, K. S., Dutton, J. E., & Quinn, R. E. (Eds.). (2008). *Positive organizational scholarship: Foundations of a new discipline.* San Francisco, CA: Berrett-Koehler.

Carnevale, A. P., Jayasundera, T., & Gulish, A. (2016). *America's Divided Recovery: College Haves and Have-Nots.* Center on Education and the Workforce, Georgetown Public Policy Institute, Georgetown University.

Case, A., & Deaton, A. (2015). Rising morbidity and mortality in midlife among white non-Hispanic Americans in the 21st century. *Proceedings of the National Academy of Sciences, 112*(49), 15078–15083. https://doi.org/10.1073/pnas.1518393112.

Chen, Y., Kim, E. S., Koh, H. K., Frazier, A. L., & VanderWeele, T. J. (2019). Sense of mission and subsequent health and well-being among young adults: An outcome-wide analysis. *American Journal of Epidemiology, 188*(4), 664–673. https://doi.org/10.1093/aje/kwz009.

Chetty, R., Friedman, J. N., Saez, E., Turner, N., & Yagan, D. (2017). Mobility report cards: The role of colleges in intergenerational mobility. NBER Working Paper No. 23618, Issued July, 2017.

Choi, N. G., & Kim, J. (2011). The effect of time volunteering and charitable donations in later life on psychological wellbeing. *Ageing & Society, 31*(4), 590–610.

Clarke, P. J., Marshall, V. W., Ryff, C. D., & Rosenthal, C. J. (2000). Well-being in Canadian seniors: Findings from the Canadian study of health and aging. *Canadian Journal on Aging, 19,* 139–159. https://doi.org/10.1017/S0714980800013982.

Cohen, R., Bavishi, C., & Rozanski, A. (2016). Purpose in life and its relationship to all-cause mortality and cardiovascular events: A meta-analysis. *Psychosomatic Medicine, 78,* 122–133. https://doi.org/10.1097/PSY.0000000000000274.

Colby, A., & Damon, W. (1992). *Some do care.* New York: Free Press.

Colby, A., Sippola, L., & Phelps, E. (2001). Social responsibility and paid work in contemporary American life. In A. S. Rossi (Ed.), *Caring and doing for others: Social responsibility in domains of family, work, and community* (pp. 463–501). Chicago, IL: University Chicago Press.

Colby, A., Bundick, M., Remington, K., & Morton, E. (2020). Moral flourishing in later life through purpose beyond the self. In L. A. Jensen (Ed.), *The Oxford handbook of moral development: An interdisciplinary perspective* (pp. 440–460). New York, NY: Oxford University Press.

Cole, S. W., Levine, M. E., Arevalo, J. M. G., Ma, J., Weir, D. R., & Crimmins, E. M. (2015). Loneliness, eudaimonia, and the human conserved transcriptional response to adversity. *Psychoneuroendocrinology, 62,* 11–17. https://doi.org/10.1016/j.psyneuen.2015.07.001.

Crawford, P., Brown, B., Baker, C., Tischler, V., & Abrams, B. (2015). *Health humanities.* New York: Palgrave Macmillan.

Damon, W., Menon, J., & Cotton Bronk, K. (2003). The development of purpose during adolescence. *Applied Developmental Science, 7*(3), 119–128. https://doi.org/10.1207/S1532480XADS0703_2.

Davidsson, P., & Wiklund, J. (2001). Levels of analysis in entrepreneurship research: Current research practice and suggestions for the future. *Enterp. Theory Pract., 25,* 81–100.

Deresiewicz, W. (2015). *Excellent sheep: The miseducation of the American elite.* New York: Simon & Schuster Inc.

Erikson, E. (1959). Identity and the life cycle. *Psychological Issues, 1,* 18–164.

Fancourt, D., & Finn, S. (2019). *What is the evidence on the role of the arts in improving health and well-being? A scoping review.* Copenhagen: WHO Regional Office for Europe, Health Evidence Network (HEN) synthesis report. 67.

Friedman, E. M., Hayney, M., Love, G. D., Singer, B. H., & Ryff, C. D. (2007). Plasma interleukin-6 and soluble IL-6 receptors are associated with psychological well-being in aging women. *Health Psychology, 26,* 305–313. https://doi.org/10.1037/0278-6133.26.3.305.

Friedman, E. M., & Ryff, C. D. (2012). Living well with medical comorbidities: A biopsychosocial perspective. *The Journals of Gerontology. Series B, Psychological Sciences and Social Sciences, 67*(5), 535–544. https://doi.org/10.1093/geronb/gbr152.

Edmondson, M. (2004). *Why read?*. New York, NY: Bloomsbury.

Frankl, V. E. (1959). *Man's search for meaning: An introduction to logotherapy*. Boston, MA: Beacon Press.

Giridharadas, A. (2019). *Winners take all: The elite charade of changing the world*. New York: Alfred A. Knopf.

Glei, D. A., Goldman, N., & Weinstein, M. (2018). Perception has its own reality: Subjective versus objective measures of economic distress. *Population and Development Review, 44,* 695–722. https://doi.org/10.1111/padr.12183.

Goldman, N., Glei, D., & Weinstein, M. (2018). Declining mental health among disadvantaged Americans. *Proceedings of the National Academy of Sciences of the United States of America, 115,* 7290–7295. https://doi.org/10.1073/pnas.1722023115.

Graham, C. (2017). *Happiness for All?: Unequal Hopes and Lives in Pursuit of the American Dream*. Princeton University Press.

Greenfield, E. A., & Marks, N. F. (2004). Formal volunteering as a protective factor for older adults' psychological well-being. *The Journals of Gerontology. Series B, Psychological Sciences and Social Sciences, 59*(5), S258–264.

Gruenewald, T. L., Liao, D. H., & Seeman, T. E. (2012). Contributing to others, contributing to oneself: Perceptions of generativity and health in later life. *Journals of Gerontology. Series B, Psychological Sciences and Social Sciences, 67*(6), 660–665.

Hafez, D., Heisler, M., Choi, H., Ankuda, C. K., Winkelman, T., & Kullgren, J. T. (2018). Association between purpose in life and glucose control among older adults. *Annals of Behavioral Medicine, 52*(4), 309–318. https://doi.org/10.1093/abm/kax012.

Han, S. H., Kim, K., & Burr, J. A. (2018). Stress-buffering effects of volunteering on salivary cortisol: Results from a daily diary study. *Social Science and Medicine, 1982*(201), 120–126. https://doi.org/10.1016/j.socscimed.2018.02.011.

Harlow, L. L., Newcomb, M. D., & Bentler, P. M. (1986). Depression, self-derogation, substance use, and suicide ideation: Lack of purpose in life as a mediational factor. *Journal of Clinical Psychology, 42*(1), 5–21.

Heisel, M. J., Neufeld, E., & Flett, G. L. (2016). Reasons for living, meaning in life, and suicide ideation: Investigating the roles of key positive psychological factors in reducing suicide risk in community-residing older adults. *Aging and Mental Health, 20*(2), 195–207. https://doi.org/10.1080/13607863.2015.1078279.

Heller, A. S., van Reekum, C. M., Schaefer, S. M., Lapate, R. C., Radler, B. T., Ryff, C. D., et al. (2013). Sustained striatal activity predicts eudaimonic well-being and cortisol output. *Psychological Science, 24*(11), 2191–2200. https://doi.org/10.1177/0956797613490744.

Hill, P. L., Edmonds, G. W., & Hampson, S. E. (2019). A purposeful lifestyle is a healthful lifestyle: Linking sense of purpose to self-rated health through multiple health behaviors. *Journal of Health Psychology, 24*(10), 1392–1400. https://doi.org/10.1177/1359105317708251.

Hill, P. L., & Turiano, N. A. (2014). Purpose in life as a predictor of mortality across adulthood. *Psychological Science, 25*(7), 1482–1486. https://doi.org/10.1177/0956797614531799.

Hill, P. L., Sin, N. L., Turiano, N. A., Burrow, A. L., & Almeida, D. M. (2018). Sense of purpose moderates the associations between daily stressors and daily well-being. *Annals of Behavioral Medicine, 52*(8), 724–729. https://doi.org/10.1093/abm/kax039.

Hill, P. L., & Weston, S. J. (2019). Evaluating eight-year trajectories for sense of purpose in the health and retirement study. *Aging & Mental Health, 23*(2), 233–237. https://doi.org/10.1080/13607863.2017.1399344.

Hofstede, G. (2001). *Culture's consequences: Comparing values, behaviors, institutions and organizations across nations*. Sage publications.

Holmes, R. L. (2014). *Basic moral philosophy*. Nelson Education.

Homan, K. J., Greenberg, J. S., Mailick, M. R. (2020). Generativity and well-being of midlife and aging parents with children with developmental or mentalhealth problems. *Research on Aging, 42*(3–4), 95–104. https://doi.org/10.1177/0164027519884759.

Hooker, S. A., & Masters, K. S. (2016). Purpose in life is associated with physical activity measured by accelerometer. *Journal of Health Psychology, 21*(6), 962–971. https://doi.org/10.1177/135910 5314542822.

Hoynes, Hl, Miller, D. L., & Schaller, J. (2012). Who suffers during recessions? *The Journal of Economic Perspectives, 26*, 27–47. https://doi.org/10.1257/jep.26.3.27.

Inglehart, R. (1990). Culture shift in advanced industrial society. Princeton, NJ: Princeton University Press.

Inglehart, R. F., Basanez, M., Basanez, M., & Moreno, A. (1998). *Human values and beliefs: A cross-cultural sourcebook*. University of Michigan Press.

Jim, H. S., Richardson, S. A., Golden-Kreutz, D. M., & Andersen, B. L. (2006). Strategies used in coping with a cancer diagnosis predict meaning in life for survivors. *Health Psychology, 25*(6), 753.

Kang, Y., Strecher, V. J., Kim, E. S., & Falk, E. B. (2019). Purpose in life and conflict-related neural responses during health decision making. *Health Psychology, 38*(6), 545–552.

Keyes, C. L. M., & Ryff, C. D. (1998). Generativity in adult lives: Social structural contours and quality of life consequences. In D. P. McAdams & E. de St. Aubin (Eds.), *Generativity and adult development: How and why we care for the next generation* (pp. 227–263). Washington, D.C.: American Psychological Association.

Kernan, W. D., & Lepore, S. J. (2009). Searching for and making meaning after breast cancer: Prevalence, patterns, and negative affect. *Social Science and Medicine, 68*(6), 1176–1182.

Kim, E. S., Delaney, S. W., & Kubzansky, L. D. (2019). Sense of purpose in life and cardiovascular disease: Underlying mechanisms and future directions. *Current Cardiology Reports, 21*, 135. https://doi.org/10.1007/s11886-019-1222-9.

Kim, E. S., Hershner, S. D., & Strecher, V. J. (2015). Purpose in life and incidence of sleep disturbances. *Journal of Behavioral Medicine, 38*(3), 590–597.

Kim, E. S., Kawachi, I., Chen, Y., & Kubzansky, L. D. (2017). Association between purpose in life and objective measures of physical function in older adults. *JAMA Psychiatry, 74*(10), 1039–1045. https://doi.org/10.1001/jamapsychiatry.2017.2145.

Kim, E. S., Strecher, V. J., & Ryff, C. D. (2014). Purpose in life and use of preventive health care services. *Proceedings of the National Academy of Sciences, 111*(46), 16331–16336. https://doi. org/10.1073/pnas.1414826111.

Kinnier, R. T., Metha, A. T., Keim, J. S., Okey, J. L., et al. (1994). Depression, meaninglessness, and substance abuse in "normal" and hospitalized adolescents. *Journal of Alcohol and Drug Education, 39*(2), 101–111.

Kirsch, J. A., Love, G. D., Radler, B. T., & Ryff, C. D. (2019). Scientific imperatives vis-à-vis growing inequality in America. *American Psychologist, 74*, 764–777.

Kirsch, J., & Ryff, C.D. (2016). Hardships of the Great Recession and health: Understanding varieties of vulnerability. *Health Psychology Open*, 1–15. https://doi.org/10.1177/205510291665 2390.

Kleiman, E. M., & Beaver, J. K. (2013). A meaningful life is worth living: Meaning in life as a suicide resiliency factor. *Psychiatry Research, 210*(3), 934–939. https://doi.org/10.1016/j.psy chres.2013.08.002.

Klein, N. (2017). Prosocial behavior increases perceptions of meaning in life. *The Journal of Positive Psychology, 12*(4), 354–361. https://doi.org/10.1080/17439760.2016.1209541.

Konkolÿ Thege, B., Stauder, A., & Kopp, M. S. (2010). Relationship between meaning in life and intensity of smoking: Do gender differences exist? *Psychology & Health, 25*(5), 589–599. https:// doi.org/10.1080/08870440802460442.

Konrath, S., Fuhrel-Forbis, A., Lou, A., & Brown, S. (2012). Motives for volunteering are associated with mortality risk in older adults. *Health Psychology: Official Journal of the Division of*

Health Psychology, American Psychological Association, 31(1), 87–96. https://doi.org/10.1037/a0025226.

Laceulle, H. (2017). Virtuous aging and existential vulnerability. *Journal of Aging Studies, 43,* 1–8.

Lambert, N. M., Stillman, T. F., Hicks, J. A., Kamble, S., Baumeister, R. F., & Fincham, F. D. (2013). To belong is to matter: Sense of belonging enhances meaning in life. *Personality and Social Psychology Bulletin, 39*(11), 1418–1427. https://doi.org/10.1177/0146167213499186.

Lappan, S., Thorne, C. B., Long, D., & Hendricks, P. S. (2018). Longitudinal and reciprocal relationships between psychological well-being and smoking. *Nicotine & Tobacco Research, 9815751.* https://doi.org/10.1093/ntr/nty185.

Lomas, T. (2016). Positive art: Artistic expression and appreciation as an exemplary vehicle for flourishing. *Review of General Psychology, 20,* 171–182.

Low, C. A., Matthews, K. A., Kuller, L. H., & Edmundowicz, D. (2011). Psychosocial predictors of coronary artery calcification progression in postmenopausal women. *Psychosomatic Medicine, 73*(9), 789–794. https://doi.org/10.1097/PSY.0b013e318236b68a.

Lynch, J. W., Kaplan, G. A., & Shema, S. J. (1997). Cumulative impact of sustained economic hardship on physical, cognitive, psychological, and social functioning. *New England Journal of Medicine, 26,* 1889–1895.

Markovits, D. (2019). *The meritocracy trap: How America's foundational myth feeds inequality, dismantles the middle class, and devours the elite.* New York: Penguin.

Markus, H. R., Ryff, C. D., Conner, A. L., Pudberry, E. K., & Barnett, K. L. (2001). Themes and variations in American understandings of responsibility. In A. S. Rossi (Ed.), *Caring and doing for others: Social responsibility in the domains of family, work, and community* (pp. 349–399). Chicago, IL: University of Chicago Press.

Marmot, M. (2015). The health gap: The challenge of an unequal world. *The Lancet, 386,* 2442–2444. https://doi.org/10.1016/S0140-6736(15)00150-6.

Martin, J. A., Hamilton, B. E., Ventura, S. J., Osterman, M. J., Wilson, E. C., & Mathews, T. J. (2013). National vital statistics reports. *National Vital Statistics Reports, 62*(1).

Martela, F., Ryan, R. M., & Steger, M. F. (2018). Meaningfulness as satisfaction of autonomy, competence, relatedness, and beneficence: Comparing the four satisfactions and positive affect as predictors of meaning in life. *Journal of Happiness Studies, 19*(5), 1261–1282.

Matthews, K. A., & Gallo, L. C. (2011). Psychological perspectives on pathways linking socioeconomic status and physical health. *Annual Review of Psychology, 62,* 501–530. https://doi.org/10.1146/annurev.psych.0310711.

Masten, A. S., Best, K. M., & Garmezy, N. (1990). Resilience and development: Contributions from the study of children who overcome adversity. *Development and Psychopathology, 2,* 425–444. https://doi.org/10.1017/s054580400005912.

McKnight & Kashdan. (2009). Purpose in life as a system that creates and sustains health and well-being: An integrative testable theory. *Review of General psychology, 31,* 242–251.

Mendelberg, T., McCabe, K. T., & Thal, A. (2016). College socialization and the economic views of affluent Americans. *American Journal of Political Science, 61,* 606–623.

Mill, J.S. (1989). *Autobiography.* London: Penguin. Original work published in 1893.

Morimoto, Y., Yamasaki, S., Ando, S., Koike, S., Fujikawa, S., Kanata, S., et al. (2018). Purpose in life and tobacco use among community-dwelling mothers of early adolescents. *British Medical Journal Open, 8*(4), e020586. https://doi.org/10.1136/bmjopen-2017-020586.

Morozink, J. A., Friedman, E. M., Coe, C. L., & Ryff, C. D. (2010). Socioeconomic and psychosocial predictors of interleukin-6 in the MIDUS national sample. *Health Psychology, 29*(6), 626–635. https://doi.org/10.1037/a0021360.

National Academies of Sciences, Engineering, and Medicine (2018). *The integration of the humanities and arts with sciences, engineering, and medicine in higher education: Branches from the same tree.* Washington, DC: The National Academies Press. http://doi.org/10.17226/24988.

Newcomb, M. D., & Harlow, L. L. (1986). Life events and substance use among adolescents: Mediating effects of perceived loss of control and meaninglessness in life. *Journal of Personality and Social Psychology, 51,* 564–577. https://doi.org/10.1037/0022-3514.51.3.564.

Nicholson, T., Higgins, W., Turner, P., James, S., Stickle, F., & Pruitt, T. (1994). The relation between meaning in life and the occurrence of drug abuse: A retrospective study. *Psychology of Addictive Behaviors, 8*(1), 24–28. https://doi.org/10.1037/0893-164X.8.1.24.

Nussbaum, M. D. (1997). *Cultivating humanity: A classical defense of reform in liberal education.* Cambridge, MA: Cambridge University Press.

Nussbaum, M. C. (2010). *Not for profit: Why democracy needs the humanities.* Princeton, NJ: Princeton University Press.

Patel, P. C., Wolfe, M. T., & Williams, T. A. (2019). Self-employment and allostatic load. *Journal of Business Venturing, 34,* 731–751.

Pfeffer, F. T., Danziger, S., & Schoeni, R. F. (2013). Wealth disparities before and after the Great Recession. *Annals of the American Academy of Political and Social Science, 650,* 98–123. https://doi.org/10.1177/0002716213497452.

Peterson, C., & Seligman, M. E. P. (2004). *Character strengths and virtues: A handbook and classification.* Oxford University Press. http://search.ebscohost.com/login.aspx?direct=true&db=psyh&AN=2004-13277-000&site=ehost-live.

Piketty, T., Saez, E., & Zucman, G. (2018). Distributional national accounts: Methods and estimates for the United States. *The Quarterly Journal of Economics, 133,* 553–609.

Pinquart, M., Silbereisen, R. K., & Fröhlich, C. (2009). Life goals and purpose in life in cancer patients. *Supportive Care in Cancer, 17*(3), 253–259.

Poulin, M. J. (2014). Volunteering predicts health among those who value others: Two national studies. *Health Psychology: Official Journal of the Division of Health Psychology, American Psychological Association, 33*(2), 120–129. https://doi.org/10.1037/a0031620.

Rachels, J. (1999). The elements of moral philosophy (3rd ed.). New York: McGraw-Hill.

Reeves, R. V. (2017). *Dream hoarders: How the American upper middle class is leaving everyone else in the dust, why that is a problem, and what to do about it.* Washington, D.C.: The Brookings Institution.

Riley, M. W., Kahn, R. L., Foner, A., & Mack, K. A. (1994). *Age and structural lag: Society's failure to provide meaningful opportunities in work, family, and leisure.* John Wiley & Sons.

Roth, M. S. (2014). *Beyond the university: Why liberal education matters.* New Haven: Yale University Press.

Ross, C. E., & Wu, C. (1995). The links between education and health. *American Sociological Review, 60,* 719–745.

Rossi, A. S. (Ed.). (2001). *Caring and doing for others: Social responsibility in do the domains of family, work, and community.* Chicago, IL: University of Chicago Press.

Royal Society and Public Health Working Group. (2013). *Arts, health, and wellbeing beyond the millennium: How far have we come and where do we want to go?* London, England: Royal Society for Public Health.

Rokeach, M. (1973). *The nature of human values.* Free press.

Russell, A. R., Nyame-Mensah, A., de Wit, A., & Handy, F. (2019). Volunteering and Wellbeing Among Ageing Adults: A Longitudinal Analysis. *VOLUNTAS: International Journal of Voluntary and Nonprofit Organizations, 30*(1), 115–128.

Ryff, C. D. (1989). Happiness is everything, or is it? Explorations on the meaning of psychological well-being. *Journal of Personality and Social Psychology, 57,* 1069–1081. https://doi.org/10.1037/0022-3514.57.6.1069.

Ryff, C. D. (2019a). Linking education in the arts and humanities to life-long well-being and health: New York: Andrew W. Mellon Foundation. Retrieved from https://mellon.org/resources/articles/linking-education-arts-and-humanities-life-long-well-being-and-health/.

Ryff, C. D. (2019b). Entrepreneurship and eudaimonic well-being. Five venues for new science. *Journal of Business Venturing, 34,* 646–663.

Ryff, C. D., Friedman, E., Fuller-Rowell, T., Love, G., Morozink, J., Radler, B., et al. (2012). Varieties of resilience in MIDUS. *Social and Personality Psychology Compass, 6,* 792–806. https://doi.org/10.1111/j.1751-9004.2012.00462.x.

Ryff, C. D., & Keyes, C. L. M. (1995). The structure of psychological well-being revisited. *Journal of Personality and Social Psychology, 69*, 719–727. https://doi.org/10.1037/0022-3514.69.4.719.

Ryff, C. D., & Krueger, R. F. (2018). Approaching human health as an integrative challenge: Introduction and overview. In C. D. Ryff & R. F. Krueger (Eds.), *Oxford handbook of integrative health science* (pp. 3–22). New York: Oxford University Press.

Ryff, C. D., Singer, B., & Love, G. D. (2004). Positive health: Connecting well–being with biology. *Philosophical Transactions of the Royal Society of London. Series B: Biological Sciences, 359*, 1383–1394. https://doi.org/10.1098/rstb.2004.1521.

Schaefer, S. M., Morozink Boylan, J., van Reekum, C. M., Lapate, R. C., Norris, C. J., Ryff, C. D., et al. (2013). Purpose in life predicts better emotional recovery from negative stimuli. *PLoS ONE, 8*(11), e80329. https://doi.org/10.1371/journal.pone.0080329.

Schwartz, S. H. (2012). An overview of the Schwartz theory of basic values. *Online Readings in Psychology and Culture, 2*(1), 11.

Schwartz, S. H., & Bilsky, W. (1987). Toward a universal structure of human values. *Journal of Personality and Social Psychology, 53*, 550–562.

Schwartz, S. H., & Bilsky, W. (1990). Toward a theory of the universal content and structure of values: Extensions and cross-cultural replications. *Journal of Personality and Social Psychology, 58*(5), 878.

Scott, W. A. (1959). Empirical assessment of values and ideologies. *American Sociological Review*, 299–310.

Sewell, William H., Hauser, Robert M., & Featherman, David L. (Eds.). (1976). *Schooling and Achievement in American Society*. New York: Academic Press.

Sewell, W. H., Hauser, R. M., Springer, K. W., & Hauser, T. S. (2004). As we age: A review of the Wisconsin Longitudinal Study. *Research in Social Stratification, 20*, 3–111.

Shahabi, L., Karavolos, K., Everson-Rose, S. A., Lewis, T. T., Matthews, K. A., Sutton-Tyrrell, K., et al. (2016). Associations of psychological well-being with carotid intima media thickness in African American and White middle-aged women. *Psychosomatic Medicine, 78*(4), 511–519. https://doi.org/10.1097/PSY.0000000000000293.

Shanahan, M. J., Hill, P. L., Roberts, B. W., et al. (2014). Conscientiousness, health, and aging: The life course personality model. *Developmental Psychology, 50*, 1407–1425.

Shim, Y., Tay, L., Ward, M., & Pawelski, J. O. (2019). Arts and humanities engagement: An integrative. conceptual framework for psychological research. *Review of General Psychology, 23*, 159–176.

Son, J., & Wilson, J. (2011). Generativity and volunteering. *Sociological Forum, 26*, 644–667. https://doi.org/10.1111/j.15737861.2011.01266.x.

Son, J., & Wilson, J. (2015). The psycho-social processes linking income and volunteering: Chronic financial strain and well-being. *Sociological Forum, 30*, 1059–1081.

Son, J., & Wilson, J. (2012). Volunteer work and hedonic, eudemonic, and social well-being. *Sociological Forum, 27*, 658–681.

Sonke, J., Golden, T., Francois, S., et al. (2019). *Creating healthy communities through cross-sector collaboration* [White paper]. University of Florida Center for Arts in Medicine/ArtPlace America.

Springer, K. W., Pudrovska, T., & Hauser, R. M. (2011). Does psychological well-being change with age? Longitudinal tests of age variations and further exploration of the multidimensionality of Ryff's model of psychological well-being. *Social Science Research, 40*(1), 392–398. https://doi.org/10.1016/j.ssresearch.2010.05.008.

Stavrova, O., & Luhmann, M. (2016). Social connectedness as a source and consequence of meaning in life. *The Journal of Positive Psychology, 11*(5), 470–479.

Stephan, U. (2018). Entrepreneurs' mental health and well-being: A review and research agenda. *Academy of Management Perspectives, 32*, 290–322.

Steptoe, A., & Fancourt, D. (2019). Leading a meaningful life at older ages and its relationship with social engagement, prosperity, health, biology, and time use. *Proceedings of the National Academy of Sciences, 116*(4), 1207–1212. https://doi.org/10.1073/pnas.1814723116.

Stuckey, H. L., & Nobel, J. (2010). The connection between art, healing, and public health: A review of current literature. *American Journal of Public Health, 100,* 254–263.

Tay, L., Pawelski, J. O., & Keith, M. G. (2017). The role of the arts and humanities in human flourishing: A conceptual model. *The Journal of Positive Psychology.* https://doi.org/10.1080/17439760.2017.1279207.

Tedeschi, R. G., Park, C. L., & Calhoun, L. G. (Eds.). (1998). *Posttraumatic growth: Positive changes in the aftermath of crisis.* Mahwah, NJ: Erlbaum.

Turner, A. D., Smith, C. E., & Ong, J. C. (2017). Is purpose in life associated with less sleep disturbance in older adults? *Sleep Science and Practice, 1,* 14. https://doi.org/10.1186/s41606-017-0015-6.

van Reekum, C. M., Urry, H. L., Johnstone, T., Thurow, M. E., Frye, C. J., Jackson, C. A., et al. (2007). Individual differences in amygdala and ventromedial prefrontal cortex activity are associated with evaluation speed and psychological well-being. *Journal of Cognitive Neuroscience, 19*(2), 237–248. https://doi.org/10.1162/jocn.2007.19.2.237.

Veblen, T. (1889). The theory of the leisure class: *An economic study of institutions.* Aakar Books.

Vernon, P. E., & Allport, G. W. (1931). A test for personal values. *The Journal of Abnormal and Social Psychology, 26*(3), 231.

Whillans, A. V., Dunn, E. W., Sandstrom, G. M., Dickerson, S. S., & Madden, K. M. (2016). Is spending money on others good for your heart? *Health Psychology, 35*(6), 574. https://doi.org/10.1037/hea0000332.

Williams, T. A., & Shepherd, D. A. (2016). Victim entrepreneurs doing well by doing good: Venture creation and well-being in the aftermath of a resource shock. *Journal of Business Venturing, 31,* 142–187.

Zilioli, S., Slatcher, R. B., Ong, A. D., & Gruenewald, T. L. (2015). Purpose in life predicts allostatic load ten years later. *Journal of Psychosomatic Research, 79*(5), 451–457. https://doi.org/10.1016/j.jpsychores.2015.09.013.

Chapter 4
Transitions and Opportunities: Considering Purpose in the Context of Healthy Aging

Matthew J. Wynn, Laura Dewitte, and Patrick L. Hill

Abstract The current chapter provides a foundation for considering purpose as it pertains to older adults and, in so doing, explores the implications of promoting sense of purpose for healthy aging. First, we describe what it means to have a purpose, or feel a sense of purpose, as well as the normative developmental trends for the construct during adulthood. Second, we describe the benefits associated with having a sense of purpose during older adulthood, in order to speak to the value of purpose in the context of older adults. And finally, we consider how promoting sense of purpose may be worked into the areas of role-transitions that older adults often experience such as changes in employment, living situation, health, and cognition. We conclude with future directions for exploring these considerations more fully in order to inform directives for promoting purposefulness among older adults.

Keywords Caregiving · Cognitive functioning · Older adults · Retirement

The world's population is increasingly comprised of "older" adults, namely individuals at least 60 years or older (United Nations, 2017). Though scholars have described the benefits of this change in demographics, particularly with respect to the valuable reserve of "human capital" that older adults can provide in terms of accrued knowledge and life experience (Rowe & Kahn, 2015), these trends also present a challenge for societal structures that were not designed with this population in mind. Building from structural lag theory (Riley & Riley, 2000), the age benchmarks associated with most of our societally prescribed roles were set in place during a period with a much shorter life expectancy. To demonstrate, one can compare the mandatory retirement age laws sent in some countries to the current life expectancy for those countries. For instance, Switzerland requires individuals to retire at age 65 (for men) or 64 (for women), which can leave individuals with around 16 years or 21 years (respectively)

M. J. Wynn (✉) · P. L. Hill
Department of Psychological and Brain Sciences, Washington University in St. Louis, St. Louis, MO, USA
e-mail: mjwynn@wustl.edu

L. Dewitte
School Psychology and Development in Context, KU Leuven, Leuven, Belgium

© Springer Nature Switzerland AG 2020
A. L. Burrow and P. Hill (eds.), *The Ecology of Purposeful Living Across the Lifespan*,
https://doi.org/10.1007/978-3-030-52078-6_4

of their lives in retirement, if they live to the current life expectancies (WHO, 2018). Accordingly, researchers have called for the need to revisit the societal roles and opportunities available for older adults (e.g., Rowe & Kahn, 2015).

A primary focus of this discussion has been on how we can and should change societal structures to better suit the contemporary needs of older adults. However, another component is to change the societal expectations and perceptions of older adulthood. For instance, a commonly held perception was that retirement provided a period of rest and relaxation, with the notion that the retired adult should be rewarded for the time spent serving in societally-prescribed roles. Support for this point comes from research on expectations for losses and gains during adult development. One study presented adult participants with positive, neutral, and negative characteristics, and they were asked to report when they expected those personal characteristics to be common or increase during adulthood (Heckhausen, Dixon, & Baltes, 1989). For instance, findings suggested that participants generally expected that adults continue increasing on being "leisurely" and "slow" well into their 80s; in other words, participants thought that it would common for adults to possess these traits well into older adulthood. Of interest, participants rated the traits of "purposeful" and "persevering" as becoming less common around typical retirement age (middle 60s). These conceptions, are supported in part by evidence from meta-analytic work suggesting individuals report lower levels of sense of purpose in older adulthood, with retirement itself being a predictor of declines (Pinquart, 2001). Moreover, qualitative work shows that when retirement community members are asked about their purpose in life, a common theme is the suggestion that older adults have outgrown the need for a purpose (Lewis, Reesor, & Hill, under review). In sum, across different approaches to asking the question, the answer appears to be that having a purpose, or being purposeful is not something expected of older adults. Though perhaps this point resonated in earlier cohorts with shorter time lags between retirement and typical life expectancy, these ideas seem markedly inappropriate for an era where people are now living, on average, more than a decade following the typical cessation of work roles.

The current chapter provides a foundation for reconsidering this perception, and in so doing, sets the stage for research programs focused on promoting purposeful aging. The first section will describe what it means to have a purpose, or feel a sense of purpose, as well as the normative developmental trends for the construct during adulthood. The second section describes the benefits associated with having a sense of purpose during older adulthood, to motivate the clear value of promoting purposeful living following retirement. Next, the third section considers how to carry out the purposeful aging agenda, providing specific recommendations with respect to retirement communities and caregiving experiences. We conclude with future directions for testing these recommendations and informing directives for promoting purposefulness among older adults.

4.1   Sense of Purpose Across the Lifespan

Lifespan developmental research has begun to consider trajectories in individuals' sense of purpose over time. Sense of purpose can be defined as the perception that an individual has broader life goals that provides that person with a direction, and in turn promotes engagement in life activities (Ryff, 1989; Scheier et al., 2006). This perception is distinct from one's stated purpose in life, or the goals they have stated for themselves. Though future research is sorely needed that considers intraindividual changes in one's stated purpose over time, investigations have begun to consider the extent to which normative age-graded trends are present for sense of purpose across the lifespan. For instance, several researchers have pointed to adolescence as a "starting point" for research on purpose, because it is during this period that individuals start to thoughtfully consider who they are and which goals they find most personally meaningful (Bronk, 2013; Hill, Burrow, & Sumner, 2014). As such, most longitudinal work has sought to describe changes in sense of purpose following adolescence, throughout the adult years.

Though this work comes with the caveats that (a) it often is cross-sectional in nature, and (b) there is the potential that individuals respond to purpose inventories differently depending on their current life stage (Hill & Weston, 2019), two important findings are worth underscoring with respect to the remaining discussion for this chapter. First, it appears that older adults tend to report lower levels of purpose relative to earlier points in adulthood (Ryff, 1989; Ryff & Keyes, 1995). One potential explanation is that during young and middle adulthood, individuals are committing to the occupational path, social relationships, and community roles that best suit them, in turn promoting greater purposeful engagement. Following similar logic, studies also find that older adults on average report lower levels of purposefulness compared to midlife adults. Indeed, the life tasks associated with older adulthood (see Havighurst, 1972; Hutteman, Hennecke, Orth, Reitz, & Specht, 2014) often involve dealing with losses to work, romantic, and social life, or compensating for less capacity for engagement relative to previous years.

Second, however, it is not all bad news for older adults. Even if there is a slight decline in sense of purpose due to advancing age or retirement (Pinquart, 2002), multiple studies have found evidence for inter-individual variability in intraindividual change during older adulthood. In other words, even if the mean-level trend suggests declines, not all older adults follow this trajectory and in fact some show the ability to maintain or even increase their sense of purpose in older adulthood (Hill, Turiano, Spiro, & Mroczek, 2015; Hill & Weston, 2019). This variability in trajectories holds important implications, insofar that it suggests there is opportunity to identify those older adults at risk for declines and that positive change can occur. The importance of helping older adults maintain a sense of purpose is clearly shown by the multiple studies demonstrating the health, well-being, and even economic benefits of purpose for adults.

4.2   Benefits of Sense of Purpose for Older Adults

Over recent decades, evidence for the positive role of having a sense of purpose on a wide range of health and well-being outcomes is accumulating. Two recent reviews sum up an impressive and promising list of benefits that have been demonstrated specifically for older adults (Irving, Davis, & Collier, 2017; Steptoe, 2019). Sense of purpose has been associated with lower depression, anxiety, negative affect, fear of death, and loneliness and with higher subjective well-being, positive affect, hope, and self-transcendence, among others. With regard to physical outcomes, sense of purpose has been linked to both self-reported health and objective measures of health (e.g., lower risk for stroke, myocardial and cerebral infarcts, functional disability, fewer nights spend in hospital). There is even evidence that higher levels of purpose are associated with reduced mortality risk (Cohen, Bavishi, & Rozanski, 2016).

A variety of potential explanations occur for this wide range of physical and psychological health benefits. Some potential mediators that have been suggested are healthier lifestyles, lower inflammatory markers, lower stress levels, and better psychosocial functioning (Morozink, Friedman, Coe, & Ryff, 2010; Ong & Patterson, 2016). People with a higher sense of purpose might be more concerned about maintaining good health, evidenced by the fact they are more likely to report a healthier and more active lifestyle, such as regular physical activity, better diet and sleep (Hill, Edmonds, & Hampson, 2019), and are less likely to engage in detrimental behaviors such as smoking or drinking (Ong & Patterson, 2016). Moreover, there is indication that the health benefits of purpose on biological markers of inflammation are stronger for those with lower education, suggesting that being able to experience a strong sense of purpose in life could compensate for hurdles earlier in life (Morozink et al., 2010). Finally, people with higher sense of purpose have also been shown to have greater financial success (i.e., income and net worth) (Hill, Turiano, Mroczek, & Burrow, 2016); this pathway might provide evidence of another mediator as financial resources give greater access to, for example, more expensive health care and higher quality food. While there is growing insight into these potential mediators, the specifics of the mechanisms between the experience of purpose and positive aging are poorly understood. Uncovering how these mediators work together and impact on health and mortality remains a challenging question for future research.

The benefits described above demonstrate the potential of purpose as a resource in old age in general but also more specifically for dealing with age-related challenges. One of the particular challenges that many older adults face are changes in cognitive functioning, such as memory loss, diminished processing speed, word finding difficulties, and declined executive functioning (Salthouse, 2004). As such, it is worth noting that studies have promoted the idea that purpose can also be a resource for dealing with such cognitive challenges.

Purpose in life and normal age-related declines in cognition. Sense of purpose seems to protect against normative cognitive decline for older adults without a cognitive disorder. Cross-sectional work has shown that middle aged and older adults with a stronger sense of purpose perform better on cognitive tasks indicative of episodic memory, executive functioning, and processing speed (Lewis, Turiano, Payne, & Hill, 2017; Windsor, Curtis, & Luszcz, 2015). However, these cross-sectional associations could be explained in both directions. Higher levels of purpose could protect against cognitive decline much in a similar way as it supports other aspects of health (e.g., less stress, more physical activity). People who maintain high levels of purpose are also more often exposed to environmental demands that are mentally stimulating, such as being engaged in 'higher-level' social activities, which has been related to white matter preservation of the brain (Köhncke et al., 2016). Similarly, older adults who experience a lower sense of purpose in life might be less engaged in cognitively stimulating activities. This can be framed within theories such as socioemotional selectivity theory (SST; Carstensen, Isaacowitz, & Charles, 1999, Carstensen 2006), which suggest that there are known cognitive and affective shifts as one transitions to older adulthood and begins to face issues related to one's own aging and mortality. According to SST, older adults shift their goal priorities from information and knowledge gathering to more emotionally meaningful goals when they begin to experience their future time as more limited and constrained. Such shifts in cognitive and affective goals towards emotional satisfaction and meaning as one begins to consider their potentially constricted time horizon may help to put the interactions between older adult cognition, emotion, and sense of purpose into context.

On the other hand, changes in cognition might also impact on the experience of purpose in life. Living a purposeful life can be argued to involve complex cognitive skills, such as integrating past, present, and future, reflecting on the self and the world, and planning and coordinating complex sequences of behaviors and activities (McKnight & Kashdan, 2009). Age-related declines in different areas of cognition could compromise the higher cognitive tasks presumed to be involved in experiencing purpose in life, leading to more difficulties in generating and sustaining purpose (McKnight & Kashdan, 2009; Wilson et al., 2013).

Longitudinal investigations of the matter have focused mostly on sense of purpose as predictor of later cognition, rather than on the reversed effect. Taken together, they show growing support for the protective value of sense of purpose for cognition (Boyle, Buchman, Barnes, & Bennett, 2010; Kim, Shin, Scicolone, & Parmelee, 2019; Windsor et al., 2015). Using data from the Rush Memory and Aging Project, Boyle and colleagues found that higher sense of purpose was related to slower general cognitive decline and slower decline in specific areas of cognition (Boyle et al., 2010). In the Australian Longitudinal Study of Ageing, higher levels of purpose predicted slower decline in processing speed (but not episodic memory) (Windsor et al., 2015).

Although more limited, some available longitudinal evidence does suggest a bi-directional relationship between purpose and cognition (Allerhand, Gale, & Deary, 2014; Wilson et al., 2013). Most evidently, in a large sample of older adults of the Rush Memory and Aging Project, sense of purpose in life and a composite measure of cognition predicted each other over time, but the cross-lagged association between sense of purpose and later cognition was stronger than the cross-lagged association between cognition and later sense of purpose. Furthermore, initial level of purpose (intercept) was related to change in cognition (slope), but initial level of cognition was not related to change in purpose (Wilson et al., 2013).

Purpose and cognitive disorder in old age. For most older adults, cognitive changes are limited to small age-related declines (Salthouse, 2010). For a substantial part of our older population, however, these declines can be more severe and interfere with day to day functioning. This is true, for example, for many older adults faced with a diagnosis of mild cognitive impairment or dementia. Unfortunately, no guaranteed preventive measures or treatment are available at the moment for cognitive disorders such as dementia. Supporting a strong sense of purpose in life in older adults could be a promising avenue beyond a purely biomedical approach in protecting against cognitive disorder and supporting cognitive performance.

The strongest evidence for this up to now comes again from the Rush Memory and Aging project. Boyle and colleagues demonstrated that older adults with higher levels of purpose had a smaller risk of developing mild cognitive impairment and Alzheimer's disease (AD), pointing to the potential protective value of purpose in life against neurocognitive disorders (Boyle et al., 2010). They also showed that participants with a certain level of AD related pathological changes in the brain (i.e., amyloid plaques and tau tangles) and high levels of purpose in life, performed better on cognitive tasks than participants with similar AD pathology but lower purpose (Boyle et al., 2012). Moreover, the protective effect of purpose became stronger for higher levels of pathological burden.

4.3   Role-Based Interventions

In sum, research suggests a general trend for a slight decline in purpose in older adulthood (Pinquart, 2002), tied to losses and transitions across different phases of life (Hill & Weston, 2019), although there exists substantial interindividual variability in trajectory of purpose (Hill et al., 2015; Hill & Weston, 2019). Purpose tends to be associated with positive outcomes across the lifespan (Pfund & Hill, 2018), and to outcomes of specific relevance for older adults (Irving et al., 2017). Work then is needed to characterize those who remain engaged and "purpose-driven," which in turn will foster the development of a "purposeful agenda" of interventions to help older adults and reap the benefits that "aging with purpose" may entail. The first step in this process may be to examine different transitions and developmental tasks that occur in adult life. One theory posits that these developmental tasks carry with them "non-normative tasks" that may present challenges for older adults (Hutteman et al., 2014). These challenges may occur in job life (e.g., dealing with changes in employment status), social life (e.g., establishing new social contacts), and family life (e.g., caring for a chronically ill family member). By examining purpose during these non-normative challenges, we may better understand under what conditions and to what extent these different transitions may either hinder or promote a sense of purpose and be better prepared to intervene.

Retirement. The loss of employment, or "job-life transition," is a major life event for many older adults. Often, a job is personally meaningful for the worker and is helpful for structuring their daily life around organized events, both of which are emphasized in the theoretical conception of purpose (McKnight & Kashdan, 2009). As older adults transition from employment to retirement, the loss of this meaningful role and life organization may help to explain the association between retirement and lower sense of purpose. Volunteerism represents one potential avenue to promote purposeful aging among older adults experiencing this transition. First, several individuals may be forced into work that does not provide a sense of purpose due to familial, societal, or financial pressures. For these people, volunteerism later in life represents a second chance to pursue work with passion and which they find personally meaningful. Second, studies suggest that volunteering lends structure to the day-to-day lives of older adults, increases feelings of life engagement, and represents an opportunity to expand their social support networks (Morrow-Howell et al., 2003). Another study using data from the National Survey of Midlife Development in the U.S. (MIDUS) explored the relationships between volunteering, purpose, and affect among those who reported an absence of certain normative roles, such as loss of employment (Greenfield and Marks, 2004). In that study, participants with a greater number of these role-identity absences reported more negative affect, less positive affect, and less sense of purpose. However, formal volunteers exhibited more positive affect and did not display the same decline in purpose in life following these absences. The authors conclude that volunteering may provide older adults a new or extended role-identity which can help bolster or maintain sense of purpose especially in the wake of employment transition. Therefore, it appears that volunteerism may be a pathway by which to promote a sense of purpose in older adults, especially those affected by a role transition. Future research in this area would benefit from focusing specifically on the relationship between volunteering and purpose and identifying the mechanisms by which volunteering may promote purpose. Possible mechanisms include increased social engagement, increased sense of meaning, or renewed daily routine and structure. In addition, interindividual variation in the effect of volunteering on purpose has yet to be fully explored. Identifying individual characteristics that facilitate desire to volunteer and potentially inform the fit between volunteer opportunity and what one finds personally meaningful is paramount. Finally, considering volunteering as a route to purpose, equity in terms of access to volunteering becomes a public health issue. Using volunteering to promote meaningful activities, and therefore purpose, for vulnerable and at-risk older adult populations should be a primary public health intervention target.

Aging in the community. Another transition involves housing, living, and a "social-life transition". For many, the goal is to "age in place" or to remain living in the community, with some level of independence, rather than in residential care (Davey et al., 2004). When asked, older adults cite aging in place as important for reasons related to social connectedness and sense of community (Wiles, Leibing, Guberman, Reeve, & Allen, (2012)); these findings are particularly important given that having positive social relations (Ryff, 1989) and greater social support (Weston, Lewis, & Hill, under review) both appear associated with greater sense of purpose. However, transitions into living communities, or losses of spouses or family can potentially threaten an adult's ability to age in place in a way that may affect purpose. Efforts to promote aging in place and age-friendly community initiatives (AFCIs; Greenfield et al., 2015) are rising in popularity and prevalence and, although they vary in size and scope, are united in their goal to promote older adults' health, well-being, and meaningful engagement (Greenfield, 2015a). They share the common goal of seeing older adults embedded in a community, whether structured (like a retirement community) or naturally occurring where they can both feel supported, support others, and feel as if they are contributing to the overall benefit of the community.

One example of such a program are Naturally Occurring Retirement Community Supportive Service Programs (NORC programs), and research shows that these programs positive influence feelings of neighborly support and sense of community (Greenfield, 2015b). Similarly, The Village program (Poor, Baldwin, & Willett, 2012) emphasizes communities that are designed, built, and governed by older adults and emphasize the social and practical support aspects of a community. There are over 200 Villages across the United States and surveys of Village residents indicate these initiatives promote social connection, with a majority of respondents surveyed reporting that the size of their social circle had increased and they also felt an increased sense of social connection (Graham, Scharlach, & Wolf, 2014). Finally, intergenerational living programs such as students-in-residence in independent living buildings and intergenerational home-shares may also offer aging adults the ability to "age in place" or to create new social connections. These programs, where younger adults (usually university students), share living spaces with older adults and provide services (e.g., companionship, household chores) in exchange for reduced rent. These programs are becoming more and more prevalent in response to the growing older adult demographics combined with the rising cost of housing, especially in metropolitan areas. Research on the benefits of these programs is limited, but likely forthcoming as the number of intergenerational programs increased.

Future research on these programs should attempt to specify which factors, such as companionship, increased activity, or increased agency in these activities may promote purpose in this context. In addition, exploration of whether intergenerational housing programs at all levels of senior housing (e.g., independent vs. assisted living) are feasible, appropriate, and valuable is sorely needed. Finally, as programs designed to promote aging in place expand and proliferate, future research may choose to focus on the training given to the professionals who work in these areas and how best to guide these workers to use their programs in order to promote purpose.

Physical and cognitive changes. Unfortunately, for some older adults, it becomes difficult to stay in their homes or communities because of functional disabilities, chronic disease, or cognitive impairment. When the resilience of an older adult and their support system is exceeded, a move to long term residential care can become necessary. Being removed from the home environment often implies a disruption of previous roles and relationships. Supporting older adults to preserve a sense of purpose in life following the transition to a nursing home is imperative. Although there is widespread recognition on the importance of purposeful activity in nursing homes, recommendations made in this regard are often hard to translate and implement into practice (Smith, Towers, Palmer, Beecham, & Welch, 2017). Not rarely, activities in communities are one-size-fits-all and staff-guided instead of resident-guided, limiting the sense of engagement and purposefulness in the activity (Cook &

Thompson, 2015). To promote purposeful activities, there is a need for motivational policies and leadership from nursing home management, adequate resources, and specialized staff training. These can help to make a shift in overall organizational culture, focused on cultivating purposeful and meaningful day-to-day experiences and interactions, tailored to the interests and qualities of each resident (Cook & Thompson, 2015).

In addition to physical deterioration, a growing number of older adults is dealing with cognitive impairment due to dementia. Research on the experience of purpose in life or related topics for older adults faced with dementia is scarce (Mak, 2010; Stoner, Orrell, & Spector, 2015). More complex psychological phenomena such as purpose are often not addressed in dementia research, partly because of assumptions about the relevance of such concepts for people with dementia and their ability to discuss or even experience them. Nonetheless, some interventions have shown promise for developing programs targeting people with dementia. In an intervention specifically focused on purpose, community residing older adults with dementia who engaged in a goal-directed activity (creating a card for a sick child or soldier) reported higher purpose in the activity than those engaged in a goal-undirected activity (free creative drawing on card) (Mak, 2010). This study demonstrated that it is not only possible to talk about purpose with people with dementia, but also actively support it.

With progressing cognitive decline, many older adults with dementia also have to make the transition to residential care. This group might be especially vulnerable to a loss of sense of meaning and purpose. Promising work in this regard has recently demonstrated the potential of a "spiritual reminiscence" program—a type of life story work that helps older adults with dementia reconnect to what is meaningful and purposeful in their past, present and future lives (MacKinlay & Trevitt, 2010). Wu and Koo (2016) tested the effect of a six-week spiritual reminiscence program in Taiwanese older adults with mild to moderate dementia on outcome measures of hope, life satisfaction, cognitive status (MMSE), and spiritual well-being. The latter was measured with the Spirituality Index of Well-being—a 12-item scale, divided in a self-efficacy and a life scheme subscale. The life scheme subscale consists of items closely related to purpose and meaning (e.g., "I haven't yet found my life's purpose" and "In this world, I don't know where I fit in.") (Daaleman & Frey, 2004). Pre and post program assessments of 53 adults randomly assigned to the spiritual reminiscence program were compared to pre and post assessments of fifty adults randomly assigned to a control group (receiving no extra program or activities). For all outcome measures (hope, life satisfaction, cognitive status, and spiritual well-being), the reminiscence group increased significantly more than the control group.

Existing research regarding purpose in older adults who are dealing with physical and cognitive decline is sparse. Future research should seek to establish foundational understanding of what purpose looks like for people with dementia or with a life-limited illness. It remains an open question in what ways sense of purpose is similar or different to sense of purpose in other older adults dealing with "normative aging changes" and how obstacles to developing or maintaining a sense of purpose may present differently in these two groups. With knowledge of similarities and differences, researchers may begin to tailor interventions to promote purpose in this somewhat marginalized group. In addition, interventions and training for caregivers and nursing staff to promote purpose in these older adults may be an appropriate avenue for translation of research findings to clinical practice.

Caring for someone with dementia. Despite the lack of research on promoting purpose with people with dementia, research does exist regarding the "family-life transition" experienced by the dementia caregiver (whether that be a spouse, family member, or friend). Caring for someone with Alzheimer disease is an undoubtedly difficult and potentially stressful process. Indeed, research highlights negative outcomes for caregivers including depression (Alzheimer's Association, 2017), stress and burden (Ferrara et al., 2008), and adverse physical outcomes including higher blood pressure and mortality (Lovell & Wetherell, 2011). However, caregivers also report positive gains as a result of the caregiving process, such as fulfilling family commitments, mastering new skills, and overcoming challenges (Mackenzie & Greenwood, 2012; Polenick et al., 2018). Sense of purpose has been implicated in caregiving in two ways. First, research shows that a higher sense of purpose in caregivers is associated with offset of caregiver burden and increased caregiving gains (Polenick et al., 2018). The more the caregiver feels like their life has an overall direction, the more likely they are to experience that sense of challenge and mastery, rather than depression and despair. Furthermore, interesting theoretical work by Lang and Fowers suggest, for the AD caregiver, the act of caregiving itself may represent a "constitutive action" (Lang & Fowers, 2019), or an action in which the means cannot be separated from the end because the means embodies or constitutes the end. In this way, it may be theorized that the relationship between caregiving and purpose is more tight-knit and caregiving may not promote purpose, per se, but the act of caregiving may actually *become* the person's purpose (Hill, Wynn, & Carpenter, in press).

Future research needs to focus on inter-individual differences in sense of purpose for AD caregivers and explore the individual differences that may contribute to a person's connection of purpose and caregiving. We typically think of individual differences as factors that affect who selects into a given role, however caregiving is not typically a role we select into, rather it is a role that is thrust upon us. In this sense, the focus of this work is somewhat different, and focuses on identifying individual difference factors that lead someone to integrate their caregiving role into their identity and leverage it to give their life purpose. Potential interventions may leverage these differences in order to help promote purpose in caregivers in the wake of their partner's chronic disease. Classes on caregiving for the newly appointed caregiver may choose to focus on integration of one's identity and purpose in order to ease caregiver stress and burden. Beyond stress and burden, however, research is lacking in terms of what are the necessary conditions for caregiving to be viewed in a positive light. How purpose and caregiving interact with disease-type (dementia vs. life-limiting), caregiver and patient characteristics (personality, sense of social support), as well as formal resources such as support groups and caregiving classes are avenues for potential research.

We focus on discussing purposeful aging with respect to roles and transitions because purpose is often embedded in a social context. Our purpose may be to care for our spouses, our family, and our friends. Our purpose also depends on who is in our life. Unfortunately, as we grow older, the connections we have cultivated throughout our lives can begin to fray. We may lose touch with friends, family members may move away, and everyone grows closer to death. One way to promote purpose may be to promote social connections among and with older adults. This may be accomplished naturally, such as with the birth of a grandchild, or artificially, with programs that promote new social bonds, volunteering activities in-line with a person's values, or encouragement of long-term aims that influence daily behavior. The research so far points to some things that we might be able to do, but future research is sorely needed in order to more directly translate our understanding of sense of purpose in older adults into interventions designed to promote purpose and well-being.

References

Allerhand, M., Gale, C. R., & Deary, I. J. (2014). The dynamic relationship between cognitive function and positive well-being in older people: A prospective study using the English Longitudinal Study of Aging. *Psychology and Aging, 29*(2), 306.

Association, Alzheimer's. (2017). 2017 Alzheimer's disease facts and figures. *Alzheimer's and Dementia, 13*(4), 325–373.

Boyle, P. A., Buchman, A. S., Barnes, L. L., & Bennett, D. A. (2010). Effect of a purpose in life on risk of incident Alzheimer disease and mild cognitive impairment in community-dwelling older persons. *Archives of General Psychiatry, 67*(3), 304.

Boyle, P. A., Buchman, A. S., Wilson, R. S., Lei, Y., Schneider, J. A., & Bennett, D. A. (2012). Effect of purpose in life on the relation between Alzheimer disease pathologic changes on cognitive function in advanced age. *Archives of General Psychiatry, 69*(5), 499.

Bronk, K. C. (2013). *Purpose in life: A critical component of optimal youth development.* New York: Springer Science & Business Media.

Carstensen, L. L. (2006). The influence of a sense of time on human development. *Science, 312*(5782), 1913–1915.

Carstensen, L. L., Isaacowitz, D. M., & Charles, S. T. (1999). Taking time seriously: A theory of socioemotional selectivity. *American Psychologist, 54*(3), 165.

Cohen, R., Bavishi, C., & Rozanski, A. (2016). Purpose in life and its relationship to all-cause mortality and cardiovascular events: A meta-analysis. *Psychosomatic Medicine, 78*(2), 122–133.

Cook, G., & Thompson, J. (2015). Purposeful activity. In M. W. Kazer & K. Murphy (Eds.), *Nursing case studies on improving health-related quality of life in older adults* (pp. 119–130). New York: Springer Publishing Company.

Daaleman, T. P., & Frey, B. B. (2004). The Spirituality Index of Well-Being: A new instrument for health-related quality-of-life research. *The Annals of Family Medicine, 2*(5), 499–503.

Davey, J. A., de Joux, V., Nana, G., & Arcus, M. (2004). *Accommodation options for older people in Aotearoa/New Zealand.* Wellington: New Zealand Institute for Research on Ageing. Centre for Housing Research Aotearoa New Zealand.

Ferrara, M., Langiano, E., Di Brango, T., Di Cioccio, L., Bauco, C., & De Vito, E. (2008). Prevalence of stress, anxiety and depression in with Alzheimer caregivers. *Health and Quality of life Outcomes, 6*(1), 93.

Graham, C. L., Scharlach, A. E., & Price Wolf, J. (2014). The impact of the "village" model on health, well-being, service access, and social engagement of older adults. *Health Education and Behavior, 41*(1), 91S–97S.

Greenfield, E. A. (2015a). Healthy aging and age-friendly community initiatives. *Public Policy and Aging Report, 25*(2), 43–46.

Greenfield, E. A. (2015b). Support from neighbors and aging in place: can NORC programs make a difference? *The Gerontologist, 56*(4), 651–659.

Greenfield, E. A., Oberlink, M., Scharlach, A. E., Neal, M. B., & Stafford, P. B. (2015). Age-friendly community initiatives: Conceptual issues and key questions. *The Gerontologist, 55*(2), 191–198.

Greenfield, E. A., & Marks, N. F. (2004). Formal volunteering as a protective factor for older adults' psychological well-being. *The Journals of Gerontology Series B: Psychological Sciences and Social Sciences, 59*(5), S258–S264.

Havighurst, R. J. (1972). *Developmental tasks and education.* New York: David McKay Company.

Heckhausen, J., Dixon, R. A., & Baltes, P. B. (1989). Gains and losses in development throughout adulthood as perceived by different adult age groups. *Developmental Psychology, 25*(1), 109.

Hill, P. L., Sumner, R., & Burrow, A. L. (2014). Understanding the pathways to purpose: Examining personality and well-being correlates across adulthood. *The Journal of Positive Psychology, 9*(3), 227–234.

Hill, P. L., Edmonds, G. W., & Hampson, S. E. (2019a). A purposeful lifestyle is a healthful lifestyle: Linking sense of purpose to self-rated health through multiple health behaviors. *Journal of health psychology, 24*(10), 1392–1400.

Hill, P. L., Turiano, N. A., Mroczek, D. K., & Burrow, A. L. (2016). The value of a purposeful life: Sense of purpose predicts greater income and net worth. *Journal of Research in Personality, 65,* 38–42.

Hill, P. L., Turiano, N. A., Spiro, A., III, & Mroczek, D. K. (2015). Understanding inter-individual variability in purpose: Longitudinal findings from the VA Normative Aging Study. *Psychology and Aging, 30*(3), 529.

Hill, P. L., & Weston, S. J. (2019). Evaluating eight-year trajectories for sense of purpose in the health and retirement study. *Aging and Mental Health, 23*(2), 233–237.

Hill, P. L., Wynn, M. J., & Carpenter, B. D. (2020). Purposeful engagement as a motivation for dementia caregiving: Comment on Lang and Fowers (2019). *American Psychologist, 75*(1), 113–114.

Hutteman, R., Hennecke, M., Orth, U., Reitz, A. K., & Specht, J. (2014). Developmental tasks as a framework to study personality development in adulthood and old age. *European Journal of Personality, 28*(3), 267–278.

Irving, J., Davis, S., & Collier, A. (2017). Aging with purpose: Systematic search and review of literature pertaining to older adults and purpose. *The International Journal of Aging and Human Development, 85*(4), 403–437.

Kim, G., Shin, S. H., Scicolone, M. A., & Parmelee, P. (2019). Purpose in life protects against cognitive decline among older adults. *The American Journal of Geriatric Psychiatry, 27*(6), 593–601.

Köhncke, Y., Laukka, E. J., Brehmer, Y., Kalpouzos, G., Li, T.-Q., Fratiglioni, L., et al. (2016). Three-year changes in leisure activities are associated with concurrent changes in white matter microstructure and perceptual speed in individuals aged 80 years and older. *Neurobiology of Aging, 41,* 173–186.

Lang, S. F., & Fowers, B. J. (2019). An expanded theory of Alzheimer's caregiving. *American Psychologist, 74*(2), 194.

Lewis, N. A., Reesor, N., & Hill, P. L. (Under review). Perceived barriers and contributors to sense of purpose in life in retirement community residents.

Lewis, N. A., Turiano, N. A., Payne, B. R., & Hill, P. L. (2017). Purpose in life and cognitive functioning in adulthood. *Aging, Neuropsychology, and Cognition, 24*(6), 662–671.

Lovell, B., & Wetherell, M. A. (2011). The cost of caregiving: Endocrine and immune implications in elderly and non elderly caregivers. *Neuroscience and Biobehavioral Reviews, 35*(6), 1342–1352.

Mackenzie, A., & Greenwood, N. (2012). Positive experiences of caregiving in stroke: A systematic review. *Disability and Rehabilitation, 34*(17), 1413–1422.

MacKinlay, E., & Trevitt, C. (2010). Living in aged care: Using spiritual reminiscence to enhance meaning in life for those with dementia. *International journal of mental health nursing, 19*(6), 394–401.

Mak, W. (2010). Self-reported goal pursuit and purpose in life among people with dementia. *Journals of Gerontology. Series B, Psychological Sciences and Social Sciences, 66*(2), 177–184.

McKnight, P. E., & Kashdan, T. B. (2009). Purpose in life as a system that creates and sustains health and well-being: An integrative, testable theory. *Review of General Psychology, 13*(3), 242–251.

Morozink, J. A., Friedman, E. M., Coe, C. L., & Ryff, C. D. (2010). Socioeconomic and psychosocial predictors of interleukin-6 in the MIDUS national sample. *Health Psychology, 29*(6), 626.

Morrow-Howell, N., Hinterlong, J., Rozario, P. A., & Tang, F. (2003). Effects of volunteering on the well-being of older adults. *The Journals of Gerontology Series B: Psychological Sciences and Social Sciences, 58*(3), S137–S145.

Ong, A. D., & Patterson, A. (2016). Eudaimonia, aging, and health: A review of underlying mechanisms. In J. Vittersø (Ed.), *Handbook of eudaimonic well-being* (pp. 371–378). Cham: Springer.

Pinquart, M. (2001). Correlates of subjective health in older adults: A meta-analysis. *Psychology and Aging, 16*(3), 414.

Pinquart, M. (2002). Creating and maintaining purpose in life in old age: A meta-analysis. *Ageing international, 27*(2), 90–114.

Pfund, G. N., & Hill, P. L. (2018). The multifaceted benefits of purpose in life. *The International Forum for Logotherapy, 41,* 27–37.

Polenick, C. A., Sherman, C. W., Birditt, K. S., Zarit, S. H., & Kales, H. C. (2018). Purpose in life among family care partners managing dementia: Links to caregiving gains. *The Gerontologist, 59*(5), 424–432.

Poor, S., Baldwin, C., & Willet, J. (2012). The Village movement empowers older adults to stay connected to home and community. *Generations, 36*(1), 112–117.

Riley, M. W., & Riley, J. W., Jr. (2000). Age integration: Conceptual and historical background. *The Gerontologist, 40*(3), 266–270.

Rowe, J. W., & Kahn, R. L. (2015). Successful aging 2.0: Conceptual expansions for the 21st century. *The Journals of Gerontology: Series B, 70*(4), 593–596.

Ryff, C. D. (1989). In the eye of the beholder: Views of psychological well-being among middle-aged and older adults. *Psychology and Aging, 4*(2), 195.

Ryff, C. D., & Keyes, C. L. M. (1995). The structure of psychological well-being revisited. *Journal of Personality and Social Psychology, 69*(4), 719.

Salthouse, T. A. (2004). What and when of cognitive aging. *Current Directions in Psychological Science, 13*(4), 140–144.

Salthouse, T. A. (2010). Selective review of cognitive aging. *Journal of the International Neuropsychological Society, 16*(5), 754–760.

Scheier, M. F., Wrosch, C., Baum, A., Cohen, S., Martire, L. M., Matthews, K. A., ... & Zdaniuk, B. (2006). The life engagement test: Assessing purpose in life. *Journal of behavioral medicine, 29*(3), 291.

Smith, N., Towers, A.-M., Palmer, S., Beecham, J., & Welch, E. (2017). Being occupied: supporting 'meaningful activity' in care homes for older people in England. *Ageing and Society,* 1–23.

Steptoe, A. (2019). Happiness and health. *Annual Review of Public Health, 40,* 339–359.

Stoner, C. R., Orrell, M., & Spector, A. (2015). Review of positive psychology outcome measures for chronic illness, traumatic brain injury and older adults: adaptability in dementia? *Dementia and Geriatric Cognitive Disorders, 40*(5–6), 340–357.

United Nations, Department of Economic and Social Affairs, Population Division. (2017). *World population ageing 2017—Highlights.* New York: United Nations.

Weston, S. J., Lewis, N. A., & Hill, P. L. (2020). Building sense of purpose in older adulthood: Examining the role of supportive relationships. *The Journal of Positive Psychology,* in press.

World Health Organization. (2018). *Life expectancy and healthy life expectancy: Data by country.* Retrieved from https://apps.who.int/gho/data/node.main.688.

Wiles, J. L., Leibing, A., Guberman, N., Reeve, J., & Allen, R. E. (2012). The meaning of "aging in place" to older people. *The Gerontologist, 52*(3), 357–366.

Wilson, R. S., Boyle, P. A., Segawa, E., Yu, L., Begeny, C. T., Anagnos, S. E., et al. (2013). The influence of cognitive decline on well-being in old age. *Psychology and Aging, 28*(2), 304.

Windsor, T. D., Curtis, R. G., & Luszcz, M. A. (2015). Sense of purpose as a psychological resource for aging well. *Developmental Psychology, 51*(7), 975.

Wu, L. F., & Koo, M. (2016). Randomized controlled trial of a six-week spiritual reminiscence intervention on hope, life satisfaction, and spiritual well-being in elderly with mild and moderate dementia. *International Journal of Geriatric Psychiatry, 31*(2), 120–127.

Chapter 5
Discovering the Possible: How Youth Programs Provide Apprenticeships in Purpose

Reed W. Larson

Abstract Youth development programs are rich contexts in which teenagers build competencies and begin to gain direction for purpose. Youth in these programs work on projects over weeks or months to achieve meaningful goals (e.g., creating films, painting murals, lobbying public officials). Their high investment in this work helps them learn skills for navigating real-world challenges, achieving goals, and managing the strong emotions that accompany purposeful work. The roles youth hold in programs provide opportunities to enact a moral identity as someone who is responsible to others. These experiences awaken the possibility of purposeful action.

Keywords Youth development programs · Purpose development · Moral development · Development of emotion-regulation · Youth practice

I've learned skills here; and it makes me feel better about life beyond high school: the life that makes us all freak out. I've realized that even small projects, our projects, can mean a big deal to other people. I realized that I just want to make a difference.

Liliana, Member of Unified Youth[1]

To develop purpose young people need to discover they can influence the future. Many teens live in the present. The possibility of achieving long-term goals can be unimaginable (Damon, 2008). As described by Liliana, the adult world can be frightening and overwhelming. Society seems rigged against them, and it *is* for youth who experience marginalization (Furstenberg, 2006). To develop purpose, teens must believe they can overcome obstacles to their goals—and must develop competencies and dispositions to do so (Hill, Burrow, & Sumner, 2013).

Youth development programs (including school extra-curricular and community programs) are a context in which many teens discover they can make a difference and build competencies for purpose. My research team has focused on project-based arts, technology, and leadership programs in which high-school-age teens

---

[1] Names of youth, staff, and programs are pseudonyms.

R. W. Larson (✉)
University of Illinois at Urbana-Champaign, Urbana, IL, USA
e-mail: larsonr@illinois.edu

work over time to plan, create, or achieve something meaningful. The ethnically diverse low-to-middle class youth in our studies created films, planned events, and lobbied public officials, among other projects. Liliana organized community events for Latinx families; and through these experiences she developed planning skills and became invested in serving her community. These programs and projects, as I describe, provide a rich apprenticeship in purpose building.

Several authors have recognized the role of youth programs in purpose development (Bronk, 2014; Damon & Malin, 2020; Sumner, Burrow, & Hill, 2018), but little research has examined *how* this occurs: What are the processes? Studying this question can help illuminate professional practices and youth processes that support purpose development across organizational settings (including schools and faith-based organizations). But it is a complex question. We know that adults cannot directly *teach* or *impose* purpose on youth. The development of purpose and competencies for purpose need to be youth-driven (Damon, 2008). Adults' role requires skilled, soft-touch transactions that serve youth's self-creation processes.

This question is also complex because many of the youth processes my team has identified involve struggle. As I discuss, youth like Liliana build competencies for purpose through episodes of grappling with difficult, ill-structured challenges in their projects. These include the challenges of pursuing real-world goals (e.g., navigating the unknown, confronting injustices, creating art that impacts others) and challenges with their own emotions (e.g., frustration, experiences of failure). Because these processes are complex and are played out within the nuanced dynamic context of program activities, we have studied them with qualitative methods. My goal here is to illuminate processes of purpose development in context, as supported by staff and enacted by youth.

5.1 Background

5.1.1 Purpose Development in Adolescence

Before introducing our research, let me situate it within the purpose literature. Studies indicate that few teens develop a lasting life purpose—that is more likely in early adulthood (Malin, Reilly, Quinn, & Moran, 2014). However research suggests that adolescence can be an important period to develop competencies and dispositions that contribute to purpose (sometimes called "precursors"). These include skills for planning, self-regulation, interpersonal skills, and moral character strengths (Bronk, 2014; Damon & Malin, 2020; Koshy & Mariano, 2011; Linver et al., 2018). Teens in our research reported gains in these competencies in youth programs.

The literature also identifies some of the experiences that can contribute to purpose development in adolescence. One is experiences of pursuing and successfully achieving meaningful goals (Bronk, 2014; Sumner et al., 2018). I will describe how project-based programs excel in providing these. Other experiences that can contribute to purpose-building include: exploring interests, discovering talents, having a mentoring relationship (Bronk, 2014), and developing a social network of people with shared goals (Sumner et al., 2018). Our studies show how programs afford youth these purpose-building opportunities.

5.1.2 Our Research on Development in Youth Programs

A context of high engagement. My interest in programs as developmental contexts was sparked decades ago, when I was conducting experience sampling studies of adolescents' daily lives. Teens reported on their psychological states when signaled at random times across the day. My attention was captured by the repeated finding that programs were a unique context in teens' lives where they experienced much higher than average levels of feeling challenged, intrinsic motivation, and concentration, *simultaneously* (Larson & Klieber, 1993; Csikszentmihalyi, Rathunde, & Whalen, 1993; Larson, 2011). *Whatever challenges they were working on in programs appeared to be really engaging!* This is a state that is optimal for leaning. The high motivation suggested that youth were energized; and the high concentration suggested youth had the cognitive bandwidth to devote their minds fully to new and complex challenges in their projects (Larson & Rusk, 2011).

I became especially interested in project-based programs because Heath (1998) found that conducting a project over an *arc of work* provides special affordances for youth's learning. I suspected that being highly engaged across this arc of challenging work could be a driver of powerful developmental processes (Larson, 2000), which could include developing purpose. This hunch led me to drop what I was doing and change the purpose driving *my* research life. I devoted myself fully to the idea that youth in project-based programs might be voluntarily and intensely engaged in powerful processes of self-creation.

Now, 20 years later, my team has completed qualitative interview studies with hundreds of youth in dozens of high-quality project-based programs. We confirmed that these youth were often "super-motivated" (as one said) and deeply engaged. We discovered that this was partly because they became *personally invested* in their projects (Dawes & Larson, 2011). When my collaborator Nickki Dawes asked our youth what motivated them, they said their projects had become connected to personal goals, including to future school and work goals, experiencing competency, and Damon's (2008) noble goals that are "beyond the self" (these included goals like teaching children and working to keep teens out of gangs). An additional discovery was that youth were invested not just as individuals, but often as members of teams working toward shared project goals (Larson, McGovern, & Orson, 2019).

Because they were so motivated they dived deeply into their projects: they took on difficult challenges and roles; they learned to work together and developed competencies for purpose. Before discussing these findings, however, let me describe our research.

Research methods for studying processes in youth programs. Our studies obtained youth's and staff's accounts of their program experiences. We interviewed youth about ongoing progress and challenges in their projects, how challenges were resolved, what they learned, how they learned it, and the roles of leaders and peers in supporting this learning. We interviewed adult staff (henceforth "leaders") about why, when, and how they provided supports for youth's work and learning. For both, we repeatedly asked for examples of specific experiences, actions and interactions that were related to youth's projects and learning processes. Although we did not ask about development of purpose, much of the data we obtained were directly related.

The findings I report come from three studies with a total of 29 project-based programs that served high-school-aged youth. We selected programs that had features of high quality: they were youth-centered, had experienced staff, and high rates of youth retention (Larson, McGovern, & Orson, 2019). The net sample included 259 youth and 84 experienced program leaders, most interviewed at multiple points over the course of the program.[2] The interviewed youth were about equally African American, Latinx, and European American. Because they represent two-thirds of the sample, most of the examples I feature here are youth of color.

In the chapter, I first present a case study of one youth's program experiences that shaped her purpose development. Then I describe how programs and staff create an environment that supports youth's purpose building. The next two sections report findings on how youth develop competencies and direction for purpose. In the conclusion, I then provided an integrated picture of how program supports and youth processes together facilitate purpose development.

5.2   A Case Example: Imani's Development of Purpose in a Mural Arts Program

Sponsored by a local Mexican art museum, Toltecat Muralists has been a neighborhood institution for years. Youth learn graffiti and mural skills, meet local artists, and have created over 30 community murals. Photos of some were on the walls of the studio, along with art by current members. Toltecat exemplifies key elements we found in other high-quality programs. The program members (all Latinx and African American) described a positive interpersonal environment. The two Mexican-American leaders cultivated high standards for youth's work, at the same time they supported youth's artistic expression and ownership.

Joining the program. During her year in Toltecat, Imani Marks reported a chain of meaningful experiences that contributed to her active processes of purpose development. Imani was an African American 10th grader from a Westside Chicago neighborhood. Asked what her life would have been like if she hadn't participated, she said: "Before I joined, I wasn't doing a lot and I felt tired. Me and my friend would

---

[2]Results from these studies have been reported in numerous publications (www.youthdev.illino is.edu).

hang out after school and do nothing." Imani was shy and quiet, but she was interested in art. So she decided to try it.

On the first day Imani found the group environment welcoming, "I liked how all the other students greeted me and I was real comfortable." They shared her interest in art, and she quickly became friends, as they worked side-by-side on initial training activities, like learning to spray-paint block letters. As their projects became bigger, the group bonded around their shared investment in the Toltecat tradition of doing good murals.

Imani also progressively opened up and developed a trusting relationship with the adult program leader, Desiree Bustamante:

> She would help with some of my strokes that I got wrong, with critical advice. That really helped me a lot. It made me respect her more too. She never really insulted me at all – other adults they just want to hit it into your head. She's just so fun and laid back that it makes me comfortable around her… Things she does inspire me.

Many youth distrust adults because of encounters in which teachers, public officials and others were domineering and disrespectful toward them, an experience especially frequent for youth of color (Jarrett, Sullivan, & Watkins, 2005; Yeager, Purdie-Vaughns, Garcia, Apfel, Brzustoski, Master, Hessert, Williams, & Cohen, 2014). But Desiree was like a friend. She supported Imani's agency as a learner and artist; she provided straightforward feedback that helped her develop new skills and take on more ambitious artistic goals.

Much to Imani surprise, she emerged as a group leader. Although shy, she was highly self-motivated (an asset confirmed by her mother). Imani explained, "I motivate myself, usually just by thoughts in my head like, 'I can do this.'" Desiree described how other youth started to turn to Imani for advice, and Imani began to recognize that she had an important role in the group: "When I said something and everyone agreed with me, I felt I should speak my mind more often." Imani took responsibility within the group. She said it was a new experience to be a leader, "with other people depending on me; before, it was always just me."

Creating a community mural. The climax of the year was students' creation of a mural on the front of the program building. Imani described how the group planned the mural. "Usually it would start as a conversation about bad things [in the city] and, then, how we can turn that into something good." They were particular concerned about the negative attitudes Chicago adults had toward them. (Earlier in the year, the group had been racially profiled and followed when they visited a downtown art store; Gutiérrez, Raffaelli, Fernandez, & Guzman, 2017). Imani said, "We wanted to show the community something different." They decided: "We're going to put a Hispanic [girl] on one side and an African American girl on the other side and they would have inspiring words around them to show that there is good out there." This was a "beyond-the-self" purpose.

As they got into the painting, Imani said: "It was really starting to build up. It was getting fun and intense." The mural caught the attention of passersby, who stopped to talk with them and complement them on it. Youth saw that it was meaningful to community members.

But they also encountered challenges. Imani was responsible for spray-painting the African American girl, and she painted her over and over again trying to get her to look "natural." There were other challenges in the work they had to resolve (color scheme, choosing inspiring words). I'll discuss later how grappling with these challenges in projects builds real-world strategic skills that are important to purpose.

Youth also encountered emotional-motivational challenges that interfered with their work. Imani described getting frustrated with painting the girl for the mural and with having to stand in the hot sun for a long time: "Sometimes I felt like, 'I'm done! I quit!' I put the cans down and I just walk in and sit there pouting." But the group helped her re-motivate herself: "They would just make me laugh, and then I noticed I was laughing. I would forget the frustration and start doing what I was doing." Because the youth were highly invested in the mural, they developed strategies for being resilient to emotional setbacks. Desiree coached youth on some of these strategies.

When it was finished Imani and others reported being proud of their mural. It was meaningful to have it represent them on a major Chicago street. Toltecat held an end-of-year showcase event that helped youth celebrate. These showcase events serve important functions in validating youth's hard work and success in overcoming challenges (Smith, McGovern, Larson, Hilltaker, & Peck, 2016).

Gaining purpose. At the end Imani reported how her experiences at Toltecat had made her into a different more purposeful person:

> Before I thought I was less than I was, and then when people started telling me what I could do, it was like 'I didn't know that!' They were telling me something about myself that I didn't know, and that *changed how I view myself completely* (emphasis added).

Her cumulative experiences—close bonds with peers and Desiree, her emergence as a leader, overcoming challenges, the success of the mural—all added up to give Imani greater confidence and self-efficacy. As was common among youth we studied, she discovered she could do remarkable things she never imagined she could do. She discovered the possible.

Interrelated with this increased self-efficacy, Imani developed multiple new competencies. She described acquiring a toolkit of new artistic skills. She had become less shy: "Now I feel like I can just walk up to somebody and have a conversation with them." She learned new "leadership skills, before I didn't really take charge of anyone, but I was given the opportunity, and that's what I did." She also gained skills for persevering through frustration, and for pushing herself to higher standards: "That was good, but you could do so much better." In addition, Desiree reported that Imani developed greater responsibility, and Imani said that the program had made her more responsible at home: taking care of her brothers and sisters. These are all competencies for acting deliberately in the world and likely contributors to purpose.

Indeed, Imani said her Toltecat experiences had given her more direction and purpose in life:

> Since being here, I am focusing more... It made me want to do something with my future. I don't want to be another girl that dropped out of high school and is sitting around doing nothing with her life... It made me want to do more

We did not follow youth in this study, so we do not know Imani's subsequent life trajectory. But at the end of the program she described wanting to pursue a career in the arts. Overall, she said: "Being in Toltecat gave me the experience that I need and want for my future career."

5.3 Youth Programs as Intentional Environments for Purpose Building

I now examine how youth programs provide structures and supports that allow teens to have experiences like Imani's: How do they engender high motivation and support youth's active engagement in purpose-building processes? The short answer is that high quality programs are designed and intentionally cultivated by staff to facilitate members' engagement in youth-driven learning experiences (Walker, Marczak, Blyth, & Borden, 2005; Smith et al., 2016).

To go deeper, let's start with youth's answer to this question. When we asked them what motivated and engaged them in program activities, they attributed it to programs being "different," "new" and "more fun" than other parts of their lives. When they walked in the door they experienced an environment with distinct ways of being—new ways of thinking, relating to others, and acting that were shared norms among members (Larson, McGovern, & Orson, 2019).

We found that this new and motivating shared environment consisted of both an interpersonal environment and work environment. I describe both, including how they were supported by program leaders.

A constructive high-functioning community. Across programs we studied, the interpersonal environment was that of a mutually-respectful and caring community. Youth said their programs were a place where anger was rare and "people won't make fun of me." As at Toltecat, members were committed to relating to each other in principled, high-functioning ways: "people stay positive," communicate honestly, and everyone was viewed as equal, different and important (Larson, McGovern, & Orson, 2019; Smith et al., 2016).[3] As a result, youth reported feeling safe, included, and cared for. They also experienced strong bonds to the group, to the "we." The adult leaders were participants in these positive norms and bonds. As happened with, Imani, youth experienced leaders as atypical adults whom they came to trust as both friends (i.e., as equals and partners in the "we") and as program mentors (Griffith & Larson, 2016; Walker, 2011). This contributed to youth's motivation.

These collective norms and bonds among youth—and with leaders—resemble those of learning communities that support moral development (Snarey & Samuelson, 2014). We found that they also served as powerful catalysts for youth's active developmental processes, including building purpose. Because youth felt safe and respected, they were able to share new ideas, be honest about feelings, construct meaning, and

---

[3]There were times youth had conflicts. But the positive norms included expectations that conflicts be resolved.

learn collaboratively (Larson, McGovern, & Orson, 2019; Larson, Raffaelli, Guzman, Salusky, Orson, & Kenzer, 2019). This kind of support network can be valuable to purpose development (Sumner et al., 2018).

In high quality programs, this positive principled community is cultivated by staff, following shared professional practices (Smith et al., 2016). Leaders do not impose community norms on youth. On the first day many leaders ask youth to decide on norms *they* want to follow, which inevitably lead to the positive interpersonal norms just described. Leaders also use icebreakers and group activities to help youth build positive group norms and relationships (Orson, McGovern, & Larson, submitted). Then as needed later, they remind youth of these norms and ensure they are maintained.[4] In short, staff facilitate youth's ownership of this new and different interpersonal environment, which helps catalyze youth's purpose building.

A work environment that supports successful projects. Damon and Malin (2020) suggest that programs contribute to purpose development by providing "integrated supports" that help youth engage in purposeful activities. High-quality programs, like Toltecat, provide an intentional work environment that does this (Larson, McGovern, & Orson, 2019). To begin with, programs draw on the norms for positive high-functioning relationship just discussed. Youth describe these relationships as contributing to their motivation and to their doing high-quality work. Projects are often done collaboratively and youth report benefiting from working in an effective, principled team: They are able to pool ideas, grapple with challenges, and learn together. Even when youth work separately, they often exchange feedback and support each other's projects (Larson et al., 2012; Orson et al., submitted).

The long-term arc of project work is often the vehicle for youth-driven learning processes (as discussed in next sections). Our research identified consistent norms across programs that supported youth's learning over this arc. Like other norms, these are cultivated by leaders and embraced by youth. First, leaders in all programs we studied supported youth's agency in their projects (Larson, Izenstrak, Rodriguez, & Perry, 2016). As at Toltecat, it was recognized that youth had input and make decisions. Youth said that experiencing this agency contributed to their motivation and experience of responsibility for their projects. A second frequent shared norm was that people took their work seriously ("we do good work"), which seems valuable to building purpose. A third norm was that mistakes and setbacks are viewed as normal and as valuable opportunities for learning (Smith et al., 2016). Episodes of ups and downs are expected in pursuing goals.

But although setbacks were expected, the ultimate success of projects appeared to be important to validating youth's developing capacities for long-term work. As with Imani, we found that experiencing success and pride helps build youth's confidence; and it provides confirmation of skills they are developing for purposeful action (Larson & Angus, 2011a; Smith et al., 2016). Success helps transform a youth's arc of hard work and grappling with challenges into a narrative of successful struggle that achieved meaningful goals. But how do programs make it possible for youth—often novices in the project work—to experience success?

---

[4]Leaders also modeled these norms in their relationships with youth.

This is another domain where experienced staff play a skilled role in providing structures and supports (Larson et al, 2016). As I have said, the professional goals of staff put a high priority on supporting youth's agency. However, leaders' provide this support within an intentional framework of short and longer-term goals: they try to maximize youth's agency over decisions, but they also provide supports for the long-term success of youth's work. How do they do this? They have a partnership of mutual respect with youth, in which their greater experience and knowledge is valued, but is used sparingly. For example, they may use their experience to set realistic initial limits on projects and to coach youth on reachable goals. When youth want assistance with a challenge they can't solve, leaders are available to help them think it through, so that youth regain the experiences of control over their work. Youth in our research gratefully reported that leaders provided this assistance in situations where they needed it: "when ideas wouldn't work" or "if we get stuck." The delicate skill here is that staff provide help in restrained ways that support youth's ongoing ownership of their work and learning processes. This can include soft-touch assistance that keeps their projects on track, helps youth finish on time (no small thing, even for adults!), and that allows youth to experience success and learn from the affirmation that success provides. This limited assistance (we called it "the art of restraint") both supports youth's ongoing experience of agency and contributes to youth's development of competencies for agency (Larson et al., 2016).

To summarize, staff in high-quality programs do many things, from cultivating positive group norms to providing guard rails for youth's work and ongoing coaching. Youth report that these practices support their motivation and learning. As a whole the program and staff curate a social and work environment that, as we'll see next, provides favorable conditions for developing purpose.

5.4 Youth's Processes Building Competencies for Purpose

We found that youth's experiences in these high-quality environments generates a cascade of social-emotional learning processes. Youth's intense investment in their projects drives learning in many social and emotional domains [including teamwork, empathy, problem-solving, time-management; also project-specific skills, e.g., arts skills; Larson, 2011; Smith et al., 2016)].

In this Sect. 5.1 focus on youth's development of two competencies for pursuing purpose: strategic skills and skills for regulation of emotion and motivation. In the next section, I will describe processes that influenced the direction of purpose.

5.4.1   Developing Strategic Skills for Achieving Real-World Goals

Purpose often involves pursuing goals. But achieving goals in real-world contexts is hard. Whether your aim is excelling in a career, creative achievement, or community service, the pathway is not likely to be linear. Numerous unruly challenges and obstacles are likely to stand in the way or emerge unexpectedly (Hill et al., 2013). Pursuing purpose can require figuring out how other people think, navigating the contradictions and complexity of human systems, and anticipating unintended consequences (Larson, 2011).

We found that program projects provide youth valuable learning experiences grappling with these kinds of unruly real-world challenges. Imani discovered that painting a girl who looks "natural" to others was more difficult than she thought. Youth who were lobbying officials, teaching children, and planning events encountered challenges that involved ill-structured multi-dimensional problems, catch 22 s, and "adults who tell you yes, and later say no" (Larson & Angus, 2011a, p.283; Larson & Hansen, 2005).

How did youth learn from these unruly real-world challenges? Often youth's learning process started with brainstorming to figure out what the challenge or "problem" was that they needed to solve. Then they developed plans, experimented with different solutions, and learned from their mistakes and successes. Throughout these steps, new youth learned partly from observing peers with experiences from prior projects. Adult leaders sometimes suggested new ways of viewing situations and provided coaching, but in restrained ways that supported youth's agency (e.g., by posing questions rather than solving the challenge). Over the arc of projects, youth learned through repeated cycles of brainstorming, trying out strategies, and evaluating what works (Heath, 1998; Larson & Angus, 2011a, b).

Xavier (an African American) in a media program illustrates this processes of learning through cycles of challenges. He and a friend wanted to make a film that communicated the passion of a Chicago folk singer they liked. An early challenge they grappled with was how to get their viewers' full attention. To do this, they decided to start the film with a gunshot. But the program leader asked if gunshot effectively drew attention *to the singer*. Their next idea was to use footage of the singer talking about his passion. But they tried it and discovered that film clips of him saying "making music makes me happy" were not convincing. They decided they needed to "show" his passion. So they picked out footage of him playing where: "You can see how emotional he gets. He's making hand gestures, you can tell it's what he loves." This worked somewhat better. But in a next iteration, they discovered that interweaving shots of the singer talking and singing with passion worked best: it synthesized the power of his personality and his music. From addressing these challenges, Xavier reported: "We learned how to say things without actually saying it: to get at the meaning under it." Through this arc of interactive cycles, Xavier and his friend had an impactful experience of becoming more creative and purposeful artists.

What competencies did youth learn from this process? In analyses of accounts from 108 youth, we identified a skill set we called "strategic thinking." It included three components: active anticipation of future scenarios, using knowledge of how people think, and flexible if-then planning (Table 5.1). These are not rote skills that can be directly taught, they need to be (at least partly) learned from experience. They are "process skills" for navigating the diverse, unpredictable challenges encountered in pursuing real-world goals. Some of youth's learning was specific to the domain of youth's projects (e.g., learning to think like a child you are teaching or an official you are trying to influence), but many had more generalizable applicability. Youth in this study described transferring these strategic skills to goal pursuits in other domains of their lives; and when we interviewed them two years later, many reported that they were applying strategic skills learned from the program to pursuing educational, career and civic goals (Larson & Angus, 2011a). The programs had provided an apprenticeship in purpose.

Table 5.1 Skills for strategic pursuit of goals that youth report learning through experiences in program projects

1. Active anticipation. Forecasting how different scenarios might unfold. Imagining and critiquing the risks and possible payoffs with each

- A member of Youth Action, an activism program, reported learning: *"to be more critical and really understand your situation, "Well this can work; this might not"*

- In a 4-H leadership program, where youth led activities for younger 4-H members, a youth learned: *"to visualize being a kid and what they would like"*

2. Using knowledge of how people think and act. Understand others' perspectives and shaping communications and courses of action accordingly

- At Nutrition Rocks where youth developed learning games for children, a youth learned that with younger children: *"You have to make it so they'll understand and want to keep playing, so not too hard. But with older kids, you have to make it to where it's a challenge... We had to change the way we do the games for different age groups"*

- In a leadership program where youth dealt with school officials, store owners, police, a youth learned: *"how [these] people act about being who they are"*

3. Flexible planning: Monitoring work, adjusting, and incrementally improving your strategies. Use of if-then thinking

- At Youth Action, members learned that, at the same time you are holding rallies protesting officials' policies, you should cultivate back-channel relationships with them

- Nutrition Rocks: *"Even though everything is structured, things can get out of hand and then you need to know how to deal with it"*

- Learned skills for dealing with Murphy's Law: *"Allow extra time," "Always have a backup plan," "Just go overboard with it"*

Note These findings are reported in: Heath, 1998; Larson & Angus, 2011a, b; Larson & Hansen, 2005)

5.4.2 Building Competencies for Dealing
with Emotional-Motivational Downturns

Exceptional people who pursued noble life purposes (e.g., Abraham Lincoln, Nelson Mandela, Ruth Bader Ginsberg) had to overcome intense experiences of frustration, disappointment, and self-doubt. Less ambitious forms of life purpose can also require competencies for overcoming these internal emotional-motivational obstacles. We found that youth's projects helped them learn skills for dealing with these downturns. Even though staff encouraged them to see setbacks as normal, many encountered at least one episode of negative emotions accompanied by self-doubt and reduced motivation (Larson, McGovern, & Orson, 2019). For Imani it was triggered by frustration with not getting her painting of the girl right. For others it happened when they performed poorly in a theater rehearsal or realized that the work required was much greater than they could handle.

How did youth learn to manage these strong emotions? Some youth learned through experimentation or analyzing the situation: They tried out different strategies for self-talk and reframing the cause of their distress. Many benefited from others' help. Like Imani youth got help from peers to distract themselves, laugh off their distress, and try different coping strategies. Leaders were also valuable sources of modeling and coaching on self-regulation of emotions (Rusk et al., 2013; Smith et al., 2016). In instances when youth showed signs of spiraling distress, leaders helped them better understand the emotions and learn strategies for managing them. They helped youth turn emotional setbacks into learning experiences (Orson & Larson, in press).

Across multiple studies, youth described developing a range of knowledge and strategies for regulation of emotions and motivation in goal pursuits (Table 5.2). These include not just learning to manage these downturns, but also learning to use emotions constructively (e.g., for motivation, as sources of information, Rusk et al., 2013). Program members describe gaining psychological knowledge for recognizing emotions and understanding their causes and effects. They also described learning problem- and emotion-focused coping strategies and strategies for managing emotions in groups. Some also described learning skills for managing their motivation. These skills are important to purpose (Livner et al., 2018).

Further research is needed. But these findings suggest how projects and the supports provide by staff can help youth develop competencies for dealing with both the external real-world challenges and internal emotional challenges that can accompany a life purpose.

Table 5.2 Knowledge and skills for managing emotions and motivation that youth report learning through experiences with projects

1. Knowledge of Emotions (Larson, 2011; Larson & Brown, 2007)
• Causes of emotions, e.g., personalities, physical states (like tiredness), different types of situations
• Effects of emotions, e.g., frustration "blocks out ideas," anger is contagious, emotions can provide useful information (Rusk et al., 2013)
2. Strategies for managing negative emotions (Larson & Brown, 2007; Rusk et al., 2013)
• Use of problem and emotion focused strategies
• Learning to limit expression of negative emotion to avoid emotional contagion in a group
• Learning to seek support and advice from others (Orson, McGovern, & Larson, submitted)
3. Strategies for managing motivation (Larson, McGovern, & Orson, 2019)
• Self-encouragements. Using self-talk to counteract self-doubt.
• Maintaining a balance between the challenges of the work and ones skills
• Learning that good work leads to authentic pride (Rusk et al., in process)
• Using emotions for motivation (Rusk et al., 2013)

5.5 Developing Direction

Youth in programs also reported developing direction (or aims) for purpose. They described how programs helped them shape ideas about what they wanted to do for their career—for their life's work. Some also reported developing moral direction.

5.5.1 Career Direction: Finding Fit

"Wow, this is something I would love to do," this is what Maria reported after a program experience in industrial design, "It has everything I'm looking for: the business aspect, people interaction, painting, being an innovator, and a different challenge every week." My former student, Aimee Rickman (2009), found that many youth like Maria, used program experiences to discover, explore, and narrow down the work they wanted to do as adults. They described benefiting from real-world experiences enacting roles within a profession. This helped them see how the daily work of an occupation fit (or did not fit) their personal interests and sensibilities.

Many had doubted their abilities to succeed in a desired profession; but program experiences addressed their doubts. For example, Jake was interested in ministry, but was unsure he had the needed interpersonal skills. In a theater program he had experiences practicing those skills and developing confidence in using them. As a result, he said: "Theater's definitely made [ministry] a viable option for me." Rickman reported that program experiences helped youth get beyond idealized and glamorous images of a career, and provided them a more realistic understanding of the day-to-day challenges and rewards of an occupation. It helped them align their occupational choice with their emerging purpose.

5.5.2 Moral Direction: Embracing Responsibilities Beyond the Self

Malin et al.'s (2014) suggested that the *roles* youth hold in programs can contribute to formation of purpose that is meaningful beyond the self—a significant moral function. Youth in our studies described the process through which this occurs. We found that many youth in programs take on roles (e.g., cameraperson, dance captain, teacher) in which they experienced moral accountability to others. Holding these roles (like conducting a project) appears to be a powerful vehicle for learning and self-change (Larson, et al., 2019; Salusky et al., 2014). These roles entailed substantial and challenging responsibilities to peers and sometimes to people outside the program (e.g., community members, youth they were mentoring).

An important finding, from a sample of 73 youth with roles, was that they chose or voluntarily accepted these positions and were committed to carrying out the role's responsibilities (Larson, et al., 2019). Even when youth discovered that these responsibilities were more demanding than they expected (which happened often), they remained faithful to fulfilling them. As with projects, program leaders provided coaching when youth asked for it; and peers were helpful with support—including giving them a nudge when needed to complete the role obligations.

The most important finding was that many teens not only embraced their role, they internalized it. They reported transferring the responsible ways of acting they had learned from their role to relationships outside the program. In other parts of their lives they were now more proactive in "thinking about, anticipating, and responding to situational needs of others" (Larson, et al., 2019). But why? Aren't teenagers supposed to abhor responsibility? The answer is no. Like Imani, they were proud of what they contributed to the group and to others through their role. They also liked the mature, responsible, and ethical self they experienced in the role. Riley, an African American, who was mentoring middle school students, discovered that: "Helping people feels good. You can help yourself while you're helping someone else." This fits Damon's (2008) definition of purpose as an aim that is "meaningful to the self and consequential beyond the self" (p. 33). Through their role experiences, youth appeared to develop a moral identity, as someone who is responsible to others.

In programs focused on service, youth also developed a sense of responsibility to the community. We studied two youth activism programs (whose members were youth of color), and some described developing a long-term commitment to working for social justice. These youth were following a path to purpose that is catalyzed by reactions to injustice and discrimination (Sumner et al., 2018). Xiamara, an African

American, described how the program had opened her to seeing the injustices experienced by different groups (e.g., Latinx, GLBT youth), and she became interested in becoming a community activist to fight injustice. Two other teens in this program wanted to become lawyers and defend people's rights (Watkins, Larson, & Sullivan, 2007).

Again, we did not follow these youth into adulthood, so we don't know whether these aims became life purposes. Nonetheless, the findings illuminate how youth's experiences in programs can provide opportunities for youth to work on and develop moral direction.

5.6 Conclusion: Purpose Development in Youth Programs

I think it can be very difficult growing to adulthood in the complex and disorderly world of the twenty-first century (Larson, 2011); and developing purpose can be even more daunting. The world we live in is incredibly heterogeneous, often chaotic and unjust, and mostly outside our control. No wonder teens tune out. It can take a lot of mental bandwidth and support from others for them to develop an empowered self to pursue purpose, especially goals "beyond the self."

Project-based youth programs are intentional settings designed to provide conditions for teens to experience empowerment. Viktor Frankl (1959) describes how WWII concentration camps were radically *inhospitable* to prisoners' experience of meaning and purpose. Youth programs provide what might be seen as mirror-opposite *hospitable* conditions for purpose-building experiences. These include:

1. A culture of safety, inclusion, and principled relationships—caring bonds among youth and staff that provide a positive learning community.
2. Opportunities to undertake projects—time-limited experiences of purpose that require grappling with real-world challenges, but that ultimately allow youth experiences of success.
3. Norms that support serious, high-functioning collaboration with peers, which allows youth to provide mutual support, pool resources, learn to together, and develop purpose through collective meaning-making.
4. Opportunities to hold meaningful roles in which they have substantive responsibilities and experience moral accountability to others.
5. Staff who are skilled in practices that sustain these conditions for youth, including practices for cultivating positive relationships, facilitating youth-driven projects, and providing restrained assistance in ways that supports youth's agency while also helping them succeed and develop their skills for agency (see also Smith et al., 2016).

In providing these conditions, programs deliberately accommodate teens who are tuned out, wary of adulthood, and doubt their capacity to influence the future.

When youth have these opportunities and supports, we find, they come alive pursuing project goals, in ways that are outside many adults' conception of teens. The mostly African-American and Latinx youth in our study became actively engaged in processes that built foundations for purpose. To be supportive of youth, it is essential that we understand and respect these processes—as teens experience and enact them. Let me postulate three processes that I think are central, based on findings from youth programs:

1. A key is that youth become highly invested in their projects, as individuals and collectively. Because they have support, feel connected, and their projects have meaningful goals, youth experience a high level of intrinsic motivation and cognitive engagement. This state creates energy and cognitive bandwidth for youth to engage with complex problems (Larson & Rusk, 2011). For some it may be the first time they have thrown themselves into a long-term purposeful venture.

2. This high investment and bandwidth enables youth to take on the difficult challenges inherent in pursuing goals. These include multidimensional real-world challenges and periodic internal emotional challenges created by setbacks or being overwhelmed. Youth learn through repeated episodes of grappling with complex tasks and situations: through brainstorming, experimenting, and assessing solutions. Through these processes they develop strategic skills and self-regulation skills that I suggest are vital to purpose.

3. Another important process occurs when youth voluntarily take on substantive program roles. Having a position of responsibility to (and for) others is an opportunity to be in charge of something that matters—that is meaningful to both the self and to others. Through embracing these roles, youth have positive experience of enacting a moral identity and purpose, which they find powerful. Many report transferring this new responsible way of thinking and acting to other life contexts.

I have described the outcomes of youth's learning as "competencies and dispositions." But it may be that what youth most carry forward and use in the future is the narratives they obtain of successful struggle: narratives of working toward goals, solving challenges, holding consequential roles, collaborating effectively, and succeeding in their goals. Such narratives are tangible evidence to oneself (and to others) that you can pursue a purpose and succeed.

5.6.1 Taking Stock: Limits and Future Research

Our research leaves a lot of gaps to fill. Let me highlight just a few. First, I have described processes as experienced by staff and youth, but I have not tested their impact. Second, youth who join programs are not a representative sample of all youth. It is possible that youth who don't join may not be as ready to become motivated and throw themselves into purpose-building projects as these youth. Third, it is important to conduct longitudinal studies, and examine how teenagers' program experiences influence further purpose development as they get older. What happens when they attempt to pursue purpose *without* the structures and supports described here? Do programs provide a valuable stepping stone to successful engagement in purposeful projects in contexts that are less accommodating?

Fourth, it is critical that we ensure that these experiences are available to all youth. Teens from different backgrounds may bring to programs different assets, assumptions, and experiences with challenges, which, for example, could affect how they respond to and learn from project challenges (see: Rose & Paisley, 2012). The pathways to purpose and the components of purpose development (e.g., competencies, aims) may differ for youth with different lived experiences and cultural backgrounds (Sumner et al., 2018). These questions are critical to helping programs provide equity in purpose development (Simpkins, Riggs, Ettekal, Ngo& Okamoto, 2017).

5.6.2 Implications for Practice

Despite incompleteness, these grounded-theory findings, based on many hundreds of interviews suggest practices that support purpose in youth programs, and possibly in other youth serving organizations. They indicate that purpose development can be facilitated when adults help create a positive culture, support teens' engagement in meaningful youth-driven projects, and support youth's ownership of their work while helping them succeed. Youth's accounts show us the importance of understanding their learning process, for example, understanding how they develop investment and sustain motivation in projects, recognizing the importance of their experiences grappling with and solving challenges, and supporting youth's experience of responsibility, pride, and purpose in taking on substantive roles. All youth need opportunities for apprenticeships purpose: for discovering the possible.

Acknowledgements This research was supported by generous grants from the William T. Grant Foundation. I would also like to thank Vanessa Gutiérrez, Aimee Rickman, Gina McGovern, Carolyn Orson, and Marcela Raffaelli for contributions to this research. We also thank Yollocalli Arts Reach for their excellent arts program.

References

Bronk, K. C. (2014). *Purpose in life: A critical component of optimal youth development.* New York: Springer.

Csikszentmihalyi, M., Rathunde, K., & Whalen, S. (1993). *Talented teenagers: The roots of success and failure.* Cambridge, England: University Press.

Damon, W. (2008). *The path to purpose: Helping our children find their calling in life.* New York: Free Press.

Damon, W., & Malin, H. (2020). The development of purpose: An international perspective. In L. A. Jensen (Ed.), *Handbook of moral development: An interdisciplinary perspective.* NYC: Oxford Press.

Dawes, N. P., & Larson, R. W. (2011). How youth get engaged: Grounded-theory research on motivational development in organized youth programs. *Developmental Psychology, 47*(1), 259–269.

Frankl, V. E. (1959). *Man's search for meaning: An introduction to logotherapy.* Boston, MA: Beacon.

Furstenberg, F. (2006). *Diverging development: The not-so-invisible hand of social class in the United States.* Paper presented at the biennial meetings of the Society for Research on Adolescence, San Francisco, CA, March.

Griffith, A. N., & Larson, R. W. (2016). Why trust matters: How confidence in leaders transforms what adolescents gain from youth programs. *Journal of Research on Adolescence, 26*(4), 790–804. https://doi.org/10.1111/jora.12230.

Gutiérrez, V., Larson, R. W., Raffaelli, M., Fernandez, M., & Guzman, S. (2017). How staff of youth programs respond to culture-related incidents: Non-engagement vs. going 'full-right-in'. *Journal of Adolescent Research. 32*(1), 64–93. https://doi.org/10.1177/0743558416664028.

Heath, S. B. (1998). Working through language. In S. M. Hoyle & C. T. Adger (Eds.), *Kids talk: Strategic language use in later childhood* (pp. 217–240). New York, NY: Oxford University Press.

Hill, P. L., Burrow, A. L., & Sumner, R. (2013). Addressing important questions in the field of adolescent purpose. *Child Development Perspectives, 7*(4), 232–236. https://doi.org/10.1111/cdep.12048.

Jarrett, R., Sullivan, P., & Watkins, N. (2005). Developing social capital through participation in organized youth programs: Qualitative insights from three programs. *Journal of Community Psychology, 33*(1), 1–15. https://doi.org/10.1002/jcop.20038.

Koshy, S. I. & Mariano, J. M. (2011). Promoting youth purpose: A review of the literature. In *New Directions for Youth Development, 2001*(132), 13–29. https://doi.org/10.1002/yd.425. SF: Jossey-Bass.

Larson, R. W. (2000). Towards a psychology of positive youth development. *American Psychologist, 55*(1), 170–183.

Larson, R. W. (2011). Positive development in a disorderly world: SRA presidential address. *Journal of Research on Adolescence, 21,* 317–334.

Larson, R. W., & Angus, R. M. (2011a). adolescents' development of skills for agency in youth programs: Learning to think strategically. *Child Development, 82,* 277–294.

Larson, R. W., & Angus, R. (2011b). Pursuing paradox: The role of adults in creating empowering settings for youth. In M. Aber, K. Maton, & E. Seidman (Eds.), *Empowering settings and voices for social change* (pp. 65–93). New York: Oxford Press.

Larson, R. W., & Brown, J. R. (2007). Emotional development in adolescence: What can be learned from a high school theater program. *Child Development, 78,* 1083–1099.

Larson, R., & Hansen, D. (2005). The development of strategic thinking: Learning to impact human systems in a youth activism program. *Human Development, 48,* 327–349.

Larson, R. W., Izenstrak, D., Rodriguez, G., & Perry, S. C. (2016). The art of restraint: How experienced program leaders use their authority to support youth agency. *Journal of Research on Adolescence, 20*(4), 845–863. https://doi.org/10.1111/jora.12234.

Larson, R. W., Jensen, L., Kang, H., Griffith, A., & Rompala, V. (2012). Peer groups as a crucible of positive value development in a global world. In G. Trommsdorff & X. Chen (Eds.), *Values, religion, and culture in adolescent development* (pp. 164–187). New York: Cambridge University Press.

Larson, R., & Kleiber, D. (1993). Daily experience of adolescents. In P. Tolan & B. Cohler (Eds.), *Handbook of clinical research and practice with adolescents* (pp. 125–145). NY: Wiley.

Larson, R. W., McGovern, G., & Orson, C. (2019a). How adolescents develop self-motivation in complex learning environments: Processes and practices in afterschool programs. In A. Renninger & S. Hidi (Eds.), *The Cambridge handbook of motivation and learning* (pp. 111–138). NYC: Cambridge Press.

Larson, R. W., Raffaelli, M., Guzman, S., Salusky, I., Orson, C. N., & Kenzer, A. (2019b). The important (but neglected) developmental value of roles: Findings from youth programs. *Developmental Psychology, 55*(5), 1019–1033. https://doi.org/10.1037/dev0000674.

Larson, R. W., & Rusk, N. (2011). Intrinsic motivation and positive development. In R. M. Lerner, J. V. Lerner, & J. B. Benson (Eds.), *Advances in child development and behavior: Positive youth development* (Vol. 41, pp. 89–130). Oxford, UK: Elsevier.

Linver, M. R., Urban, J. B., MacDonnell, M., Roberts, E. D., Quinn, J., Samtani, S., … Morgan, D. (2018). Mixed methods in youth purpose: An examination of adolescent self-regulation and purpose. *Research on Human Development, 15*(2), 118–138. https://doi.org/10.1080/15427609. 2018.1445925.

Malin, H., Reilly, T. S., Quinn, B., & Moran, S. (2014). Adolescent purpose development: Exploring empathy, discovering roles, shifting priorities, and creating pathways. *Journal of Research on Adolescence, 24*(1), 186–199. https://doi.org/10.1111/jora.12051.

Orson, C. and Larson, R. (in press). Helping teens overcome anxiety episodes in project work: The power of reframing. *Journal of Adolescent Research.*

Orson, C., McGovern, G., & Larson, R. W. (Revise & Resubmit). How challenges and peers contribute to social-emotional learning in outdoor adventure education programs. *Journal of Adolescence.*

Rickman, A. N. (2009). *A challenge to the notion of youth passivity: Adolescents' development of career direction through youth programs. Unpublished masters equivalency paper.* Urbana-Champaign: University of Illinois.

Rose, J., & Paisley, K. (2012). White privilege in experiential education: A critical reflection. *Leisure Sciences, 34*(2), 136–154. https://doi.org/10.1080/01490400.2012.652505.

Rusk, N., Izenstark, D. & Larson, R. (in process). Youth earning and learning from authentic pride in project-based work.

Rusk, N., Larson, R., Raffaelli, M., Walker, K., Washington, L., Gutierrez, V., et al. (2013). Positive youth development in organized programs: How teens learn to manage emotions. In C. Proctor & P. A. Linley (Eds.), *Positive psychology: Research, applications and interventions for children and adolescents* (pp. 247–261). New York: Springer.

Salusky, I., Larson, R. W., Griffith, A., Wu, J., Raffaelli, M., Sugimura, N., et al. (2014). How youth develop responsibility: What can be learned from youth programs. *Journal of Research on Adolescence, 24*(3), 417–430.

Simpkins, S., Riggs, N., Ettekal, A., Ngo, B., & Okamoto, D. (2017). Designing culturally responsive organized after-school activities. *Journal of Adolescent Research, 32*(1), 11–36. https://doi.org/ 10.1177/0743558416666169.

Smith, C., McGovern, G., Larson, R. W., Hilltaker, B., & Peck, S. C. (2016). *Preparing youth to thrive: Promising practices for social emotional learning.* Washington, D.C.: Forum for Youth Investment. www.SELPractices.org.

Snarey, J., & Samuelson, P. L. (2014). Lawrence Kohlberg's revolutionary ideas: Moral education in the cognitive-developmental tradition. In L. Nucci, D. Narvaez, & T. Krettenauer (Eds.), *Handbook of moral and character education* (2nd ed.). New York, NY: Routledge.

Sumner, R., Burrow, A. L., & Hill, P. L. (2018). The development of purpose in life among adolescents who experience marginalization: Potential opportunities and obstacles. *American Psychologist, 73*(6), 740–752. https://doi.org/10.1037/amp0000249.

Walker, J., Marczak, M., Blyth, D., & Borden, L. (2005). Designing youth development programs: Toward a theory of developmental intentionality. In J. L. Mahoney, R. W. Larson, & J. S. Eccles (Eds.), *Organized activities as contexts of development: Extracurricular activities, after-school and community programs* (pp. 399–418). Mahwah, NJ: Erlbaum.

Walker, K. C. (2011). The multiple roles that youth development program leaders adopt with youth. *Youth and Society, 43*(2), 635–655. https://doi.org/10.1177/0044118X10364346.

Watkins, N., Larson, R., & Sullivan, P. (2007). Learning to bridge difference: Community youth programs as contexts for developing multicultural competencies. *American Behavioral Scientist, 51,* 380–402.

Yeager, D. S., Purdie-Vaughns, V., Garcia, J., Apfel, N., Brzustoski, P., Master, A., et al. (2014). Breaking the cycle of mistrust: Wise interventions to provide critical feedback across the racial divide. *Journal of Experimental Psychology: General, 143*(2), 804–824. https://doi.org/10.1037/a0033906.

Chapter 6
Discovering Identity and Purpose in the Classroom: Theoretical, Empirical, and Applied Perspectives

Lisa Kiang, Heather Malin, and Amy Sandoz

Abstract Identity formation has long been considered a crucial developmental task that evolves into a deep sense of purpose. As many adolescents spend the majority of their waking hours within the school context, there is great potential to boost both identity and purpose through the educational setting—via curriculum and instruction, extracurricular opportunities, school climate and culture, purpose development classes, and guidance from teachers. This chapter reviews the theoretical foundations and empirical evidence for expecting links between identity and purpose. The challenges, opportunities, and benefits of addressing identity and purpose within the school context are also discussed. An innovative charter school program is unpacked as an illustration of how identity and purpose might be effectively fostered in the classroom. Conclusions and implications are examined in light of cultural sensitivity, diversity, and inclusion.

Keywords Identity · Purpose · Schools · Education · Purpose Learning

Identity formation has long been considered a quintessential life aim and developmental task that is particularly relevant to adolescents, largely because of the deep sense of purpose that theoretically evolves out of a strong understanding of self-identity (Erikson, 1968). Purpose itself is also a fundamental aspect of youth development and well-being (Damon, 2008; Ryff, 1989), dovetailing with other important changes in adolescence such as greater sophistication in diverse socioemotional and cognitive competencies (e.g., empathy, moral reasoning, self-regulation, autonomy) that enable and are linked with various characteristics that reflect both a sense of purpose as well as identity (e.g., volunteering, community involvement, civic engagement) (Metzgeret al., 2018). Practically speaking, given that many adolescents spend

L. Kiang (✉)
Wake Forest University, Winston-Salem, NC, USA
e-mail: kiangl@wfu.edu

H. Malin
Stanford University, Stanford, CA, USA

A. Sandoz
Marshall Street at Summit Public Schools, Redwood City, CA, USA

© Springer Nature Switzerland AG 2020
A. L. Burrow and P. Hill (eds.), *The Ecology of Purposeful Living Across the Lifespan*,
https://doi.org/10.1007/978-3-030-52078-6_6

the majority of their waking hours within the school context (Stepick & Stepick, 2002), there is great potential to tap into this crucial developmental period and boost identity and purpose through the educational setting—via curriculum and instruction, extracurricular opportunities, changes to school climate and culture, purpose development classes, and relationships and guidance from teachers and school staff.

The present chapter discusses opportunities to promote youth development by unpacking the critical convergence of identity, purpose, and school. We begin by building an understanding of developmentally-relevant processes by briefly reviewing the theoretical foundations for expecting close links between identity and purpose among youth. The potential challenges and opportunities in addressing identity and purpose within the school context, including basic and applied research evidence that supports the benefits of doing so, will be next discussed. An innovative in-school program will be provided as an illustration of how identity and purpose can be intentionally and effectively fostered in the classroom and within the educational system. We conclude by discussing implications, as well as further opportunities to move forward. Our overall approach incorporates the importance of considering cultural sensitivity and inclusion, as well as the unique processes and mechanisms that might be found among youth from ethnically diverse groups and immigrant backgrounds.

6.1 Defining the Construct of Purpose

Many scholars and practitioners acknowledge purpose as a key developmental virtue and character strength that encompasses a deep sense of self-actualization, flourishing, and a solid understanding of what individuals would like to accomplish with their lives (Kiang & Witkow, 2015; Malin, Reilly, Quinn, & Moran, 2014; Seligman, 2002). However, precise conceptualizations of purpose have varied in the psychological literature. For example, some researchers have focused on its role as a unique dimension of subjective well-being (Deci & Ryan, 2008; Ryff & Keyes, 1995). Others have employed definitions that view purpose as interchangeable with meaning in life (Steger, Oishi, & Kashdan, 2009). Notable approaches have also attempted to delineate different aspects of purpose, such as its presence versus search (Steger, Frazier, Oishi, & Kaler, 2006), or in terms of the content of an individual's purpose in addition to an individual's purpose commitment (Hill, Burrow, & Sumner, 2013; Burrow, O'Dell, & Hill, 2010). Some conceptual perspectives, especially among those that focus on adolescents, argue that purpose involves intentions and goals that are both personal and of consequence to the world outside of the self (Damon, Menon, & Bronk, 2003). Scholars have increasingly rallied around framing purpose as both a future-directed goal that is personally meaningful and aimed at contributing to something larger than the self (e.g., Malin et al., 2014). The current chapter largely adopts this latter perspective and considers purpose as both an inward and outward facing motivational driving force that shapes well-being and behavior.

Consistent with this view, purpose must clearly be personally meaningful and central to one's identity (Hill et al., 2013), given its powerful role in directing and organizing life goals, activities, and actions (Damon, 2008; Emmons, 1999; McKnight & Kashdan, 2009; Moran, 2017; Ryff, 1989). Indeed, all conceptualizations of purpose, however diverse, point to the developmental importance of its existence, especially for adolescents who are often forming foundations of purpose while also maturing in both self-views and in other important physical, social, and cognitive ways. For example, among cross-sectional and longitudinal samples, and among youth from ethnically diverse and immigrant backgrounds, greater purpose in life has been associated with a host of positive outcomes including lower depressive symptoms and negative affect, and higher self-esteem, personal agency, life satisfaction, positive affect, and academic adjustment (Bronk, Hill, Lapsley, Talib, & Finch, 2009; Burrow, O'Dell, & Hill, 2010; Kiang & Witkow, 2015). Purpose has also been shown to be protective, perhaps boosting resilience to help individuals cope with stressors and life challenges (Brassai, Piko, & Steger, 2011; Frankl, 1959). In light of these empirically-validated links, one understudied question is how youth purpose can be cultivated. Theoretically, identity formation appears to be one promising pathway to consider.

6.2 Theoretical Perspectives Linking Identity and Purpose

Theoretical perspectives have long linked identity and purpose. The current chapter centers on two major models proposed in the psychological literature, Eriksonian and Social Identity Theory, each of which establish these links and are particularly relevant in terms of youth development.

Erikson's psychosocial theory with identity crisis leading to self/purpose. Erikson's (1959) psychosocial theory of human development puts forth eight stages or conflicts that are developmentally-relevant across different periods of the lifespan. During the period of adolescence, the relevant conflict or crisis focuses on the struggle between Identity versus Role Diffusion (Erikson, 1968). According to the model, adolescents are challenged with finding ways in which their identities are unique and distinct from other people around them or risk failing to establish a firm understanding of oneself. A successful resolution to this conflict is characterized by a strong sense of identity, from which evolves a commitment to the self and the development of life purpose as a virtue. Once adolescents develop a sense of who they are, they can then use their sense of identity to live a more agentic or purposeful life. In Erikson's words, "We are what we love". Drawing on his model, who we are is what we love and what we love is what drives us and gives our life meaning and purpose.

The theoretical premise that identity development precedes purpose has been empirically supported. For example, among a sample of Asian American adolescents, ethnic identity has been longitudinally associated with self-reported purpose one year later, and not the other way around, providing support for Erikson's model (Kiang & Fuligni, 2010). Drawing on both Eriksonian ideas and Côte's (1997) identity capital model, Burrow and Hill (2011) similarly found that purpose in life manifests from a sense of identity and, together, both purpose and identity contribute to well-being and positive youth development.

Although adolescence is one developmental period that is most directly relevant to purpose, it is important to recognize that identity is a constantly evolving process and there is always the possibility of encountering experiences that shape one's sense of self at all developmental periods (Ethier & Deaux, 1994; Phinney, 2003). Hence, to the extent that identity is intricately tied to purpose, there are chances for growth and further differentiation beyond adolescence and across the entire lifespan and in ways that Erikson did not originally address. For example, much of the literature in this area has focused on older adolescents, college students, and the period of emerging or young adulthood more generally (Damon, 2008). As illustrated through a study on emerging adults (Bundick, 2011), reflecting on and discussing one's purpose in life was longitudinally related to greater levels of purpose as defined by goal directedness which, in turn, contributed to greater life satisfaction. Moreover, in directly addressing the limitation that much of the field's understanding of purpose post-adolescence has relied on college student and well-educated adult samples, Sumner (2017) found that overall levels of purpose did not significantly vary according to the reported education levels of adults; however, some corollaries of purpose (e.g., agency) were significantly higher among adults who reported attaining higher levels of education. Beyond adolescence, opportunities therefore abound in terms of better understanding why and how identity and purpose can continue to evolve and flourish, whether through exploratory experiences in higher education, and/or real-world experiences such as in work or community settings.

Theoretically, the collective experiences that culminate from adolescence through adulthood could come to a head in later stages in Erikson's model, which also implicate salient links between identity and purpose. For example, the Generativity versus Stagnation stage points to the importance of laying the foundation for role fulfillment and of committing to personally meaningful and outward facing goals. Particularly relevant among older adults, individuals must evaluate whether they have sufficiently made their mark on the world (e.g., caring for others, accomplishing goals, engaging with the community, creating a better world) or whether they have failed to find a way to contribute to something outside of the self (Ehlman & Ligon, 2012). Again, such processes invoke the idea that a deep sense of purpose remains a vital component of overall life satisfaction and well-being that is relevant across the entire lifespan and, as such, is highly interdependent with one's continually developing sense of self and identity (Erikson, 1950; Hill & Burrow, 2012; McAdams & de St. Aubin, 1992).

Tajfel's social identity theory with group identity leading to purpose, commitment, and group maintenance. Social identity refers to the knowledge, value, and emotional significance attributed to group membership (Tajfel & Turner, 2001). Having a strong sense of social identity, or perceiving oneself as tied to a group, can contribute to a psychological sense of togetherness, we-ness, or belongingness (Turner, 1982). In turn, the group membership and affiliation that come from feeling closely connected to one's group can provide youth with a sense of purpose and meaning (Fuligni, 2010), and manifest through behavioral goals and attitudes that are purposeful (e.g., imbued with personal meaning) and supportive of the group (e.g., outward-facing).

Using the family as an example of one specific group that is highly salient to many adolescents, theoretical and empirical work suggests that family identity can operate in ways that promote a sense of purpose (Fuligni & Flook, 2005). Indeed, culturally-relevant constructs stemming broadly from principles of familism suggest that purpose can be embodied through family obligation, or attitudes and behaviors that endorse the importance of assisting, supporting, and respecting the family in the interest of maintaining one's family stability and well-being (Fuligni & Pedersen, 2002). In a daily diary study, day-to-day activities related to family connectedness, for example, helping take care of siblings or running errands for the family, as compared to purely hedonic or leisure activities, such as watching television or playing video games, were associated with higher levels of daily reported purpose (Kiang, 2012).

More broadly, a social identity perspective would also suggest that social group membership can contribute to a sense of group solidarity and collective action, perhaps paving the way towards not only meaningful action in support of one's specific group, but also for more general social movements and political engagement (Watts, Diemer, & Voight, 2011). Such pathways are also consistent with the Rejection-Identification Model (RIM; Branscombe, Schmitt, & Harvey, 1999) which argues that experiences of rejection or group threat (e.g., discrimination based on one's social group membership) could promote identification with the rejected group(s). In turn, the strengthening of group identity can ultimately enhance psychological adjustment by allowing individuals to maintain self-esteem and sense of belonging (e.g., Brittian et al., 2015; Cronin et al., 2012; Tabbah et al., 2016), perhaps through the means of developing a sense of purpose and engagement to directly combat such initial threat. Empirical links between ethnic identity and civic engagement have been indeed found among U.S. adults from immigrant backgrounds (Stepick & Stepick, 2002). Flanagan, Syvertsen, Gill, Gallay, and Cumsille (2009) found similar evidence among adolescents in that greater ethnic awareness, which can be seen as a marker of social identity, is associated with greater civic commitments, such as the reported importance of improving race relations and of advocating for or supporting one's ethnic group. Hence, both conceptual models and emerging empirical work support the idea that identity and purpose, as reflected through collective action and social and civic engagement, can be bolstered in the face of marginalization and ultimately serve to promote youth development as well as potentially buffer against the negative impact of such socially challenging experiences.

From theory to application. Taken together, classic developmental mechanisms that suggest that a sense of purpose emerges from identity formation, and views from social identity theory arguing that group connectedness can initiate positive attitudes and purposeful action in support of one's group, reflect just two conceptual reasons for why we might expect identity and purpose to be intricately linked. Given that adolescence is a prime time for the simultaneous formation of both identity and purpose (Damon et al., 2003; Hill et al., 2013), it is important to think about the primary influences within this period and specific ways that both constructs can be promoted. Purpose can be shaped by social context (Liang, White, Mousseau,

Hasse, Knight, Berado, & Lund, 2017); hence, opportunities and benefits abound in terms of exploring how parents, teachers, practitioners, and adolescents' broader community and educational settings might contribute to youth purpose and identity development.

Notably, while early socialization experiences take place in the microenvironment of the home, adolescents spend intensive and prolonged periods of engagement within the educational context, which is one of the most important factors that shape the lives of youth (Stepick & Stepick, 2002). For example, academics aside, schools constitute key settings that provide adolescents with the opportunity to engage in socioemotional learning as well as identity exploration and development (Tseng & Seidman, 2007). Moreover, within the school context, adolescents learn formally and programmatically, but also informally through peer relations, extracurriculars, and out-of-classroom experiences (Hughes, Watford, & Del Toro, 2016). Adolescents' engagement within the school context can therefore occur not only within the scope of academic activities and actual school hours, but also in light of structured experiences within the school (e.g., student clubs, sports) (Fredricks & Eccles, 2006). Research has increasingly highlighted the importance of organized activities among out-of-school contexts in also shaping adolescent development (e.g. Bohnert, Fredricks, & Randall, 2010; Larson, 2000). That said, we next turn to a more focused and applied discussion on how a broad conceptualization of the school setting can play an impactful role in youth purpose and identity formation before providing one concrete example of an innovative school curriculum that aims to foster these constructs among students.

6.3   Sociocontextual Promoters of Purpose and Applied Empirical Evidence

The theoretical background indicating that purpose develops according to the social contexts a young person experiences is increasingly supported by empirical evidence. Some constructs that can be seen as indicators or correlates of purpose (e.g., moral identity, meaning in life are clearly influenced by contextual factors such as family environment, community, and institutional settings (e.g., Hardy, Walker, Olsen, Woodbury, & Hickman, 2014; Steger, Bundick, & Yeager, 2011). For example, prosocial and civic development—indicated by prosocial attitudes and behaviors and suggestive of adolescents' developing moral identity—are predicted by family, community, and peer socialization (e.g., Atkins & Hart, 2003; Carlo, Knight, McGinley, & Hayes, 2011; da Silva, Sanson, Smart, & Toumbourou, 2004; Rossi, Lenzi, Sharkey, Vieno, & Santinello, 2016). Meaning in life, similarly, can vary according to parental factors, religious affiliation and support, and support from non-family significant others (Brassai, Piko, & Steger, 2013; Dunn & O'Brien, 2009; Newton & McIntosh, 2013).

There are fewer studies demonstrating the influence of the developmental ecology on purpose specifically, but the research in this area is growing. Findings from youth purpose research about the ways that adults structure developmental contexts to nurture purpose can directly inform our understanding of the role that schools might play in supporting adolescent purpose development. There are likely multiple pathways and mechanisms involved, which have yet to be firmly established, but the literature suggests that schools (e.g., teachers and other purpose role models within the school setting, programs within the school that motivate critical thinking and personal engagement and growth, peer influences through friendships and organized activities) can provide the scaffolding for youth to both discover and build new purposes, as well as refine an already existing sense of purpose (e.g., Gutowski, White, Liang, Diamonti, & Berado, 2018; Liang et al., 2017; Malin, Ballard, & Damon, 2015; Malin, Liauw, & Remington, 2019; Moran, Bundick, Malin, & Reilly, 2013).

The affective context that adults create for young people at school might be an important factor in whether and how school serves as a setting that supports purpose development. The potential relevance of affective environment to purpose development is suggested in at least two studies, which show that parent/child relationships characterized by positive attachment and trust are associated with a greater sense of purpose and purpose commitment among their adolescent children, whereas relationships characterized by alienation are associated with lower purpose commitment (Blattner, Liang, Lund, & Spencer, 2013; Hill, Burrow, & Sumner, 2016). These studies suggest that providing young people a school environment where they can trust adults and feel a sense of belonging may be most conducive to purpose development.

Adults can further provide a purpose-supporting context for adolescents by acting as purpose role models and mentors, suggesting that schools can foster student purpose by preparing adults in the school to take on these roles. "People" was one of the essential elements of purpose development that emerged in a qualitative study with highly purposeful adolescents, with important support coming from adults who provided purpose affirmation and guidance (Liang et al., 2017). Another study found that it was not just the presence or quantity of mentors that predicted purpose development among college students, but the quality of mentorship they experienced, indicated by the students' perception of the mentor relationship as mutual, empathic, authentic, and empowering (Lund, Liang, Konowitz, White, & Mousseau, 2019). Finally, among adolescents in an interview study of purpose development, some of those who described being strongly committed to a beyond-the-self purpose said that they had teachers who mentored them in their purpose by responding to, encouraging, and suggesting pathways they could take to pursue their personal interests (Moran et al., 2013). In the same study, adult and peer role models of prosocial activity and purpose appeared to support adolescents in developing their own purpose.

Of particular relevance to school-based purpose development efforts is research suggesting that institutional settings can provide integrated sources of purpose support. Moran et al. (2012) found that some highly purposeful adolescents received multiple, integrated forms of support for their purpose in community-based or church-based youth groups. These young people described the emotional encouragement and social network that youth organizations provided, the training and material resources needed for pursuing purpose, and opportunities to act on purpose goals. Schools are similarly positioned to provide an integrated web of support for purpose. Although this web of school-based support has not been directly investigated, at least one other study with young adolescents suggests that some schools might provide a more purpose-conducive culture or ecology than others (Malin et al., 2019). In that study, certain resources that middle school students reported having access to in the school environment (e.g., classroom activities related to purpose goals and adult role models at school) correlated with purpose, measured as beyond-the-self life goal orientation (i.e., selecting beyond-the-self oriented life goals over self-oriented life goals) and purpose goal commitment (i.e., engagement in pursuing selected goals). In particular, purpose goal commitment was associated with students' perception that their school assignments helped them pursue their important goals. However, the effects of those specific perceived resources were small compared to the differences in purpose scores across the seven school sites (Malin, Liauw, & Remington, 2019). For example, students at one school scored significantly higher on beyond-the-self goal orientation and on goal commitment compared to students from all other schools, while at another school students scored significantly lower on these measures than their counterparts in all of the other schools. This suggests that a more holistic approach to supporting purpose development at school—for example, by creating an environment of trust, providing purpose mentors, engaging students in identity and purpose exploration, and providing opportunities for students to act on their purpose—might be more effective than small interventions that target just one aspect of purpose support. Indeed, research has yet to systematically isolate specific predictors of purpose, and perhaps a more whole, integrated approach would be particularly worthwhile in understanding what mechanisms and resources might be involved.

6.4   School-Based Interventions to Support Purpose Development

Although it may be that comprehensive sources of support are more effective than targeted interventions for developing student purpose, there are a few school-based interventions that have been evaluated and shown to have modest success. These interventions offer insight into the outcomes that might be expected to result from targeted efforts to encourage purpose development. Engaging students in a semi-structured interview about the things that matter most to them, their life goals, and the motivations driving their most important goals and activities—that is, the aspects of life that would indicate purpose—resulted in gains in life satisfaction and goal-directedness, but did not directly influence sense of purpose (Bundick, 2011). Another intervention sought to foster purpose among high school students by engaging them in bimonthly discussions about their aspirations, followed by sessions dedicated to planning and acting on their postsecondary purpose (Pizzolato, Brown, & Kanny, 2011). The evaluation showed that it had a positive effect on purpose in life as well as internal locus of control for academic achievement.

One important potential contributor to students' purpose and identity development is the school culture and climate they experience. As was noted above, students benefit from an environment where they experience trusting relationships with adults and a sense of belonging. A similar effect was seen specifically in students' school experiences in a study showing that a sense of feeling connected at school was associated with stronger future-orientation (Crespo, Jose, Kielpikowski, & Prior, 2013). In another series of studies, greater sense of belonging was associated with higher sense of meaning in life and better ability to articulate a meaning for life, and experiments designed to enhance sense of belonging predicted an increase in the sense that life has meaning (Lambert et al., 2013).

6.5 School-Based Purpose Learning Programs

A number of purpose learning programs have emerged in recent years that are grounded in the research on adolescent purpose development (Malin, 2018). These programs, most of which are created by external organizations (e.g., non-profits), provide curricula and teacher professional development designed in part to support student purpose development. Recognizing that purpose does not develop in isolation but requires a foundation of social and emotional capacities, these programs aim to develop self-awareness, empathy, civic engagement, innovation, and future-mindedness, among other strengths, along with purpose. For example, Mastering Our Skills and Inspiring Character (MOSAIC), a program created for middle school students by the Social-Emotional and Character Development Lab at Rutgers, aims to build the virtue of noble purpose by helping students learn skills such as effective communication and emotion regulation (Hatchimonji, Linsky, & Elias, 2017). In the MOSAIC model, noble purpose is theorized as a superordinate goal that organizes subordinate goals, and those subordinate goals are supported through the socioemotional skills and character traits developed through MOSAIC lessons and activities. Using an entirely different approach, Quaglia Institute builds purpose by supporting teachers to develop a sense of leadership and the confidence to take action, thereby preparing teachers to share these capacities with their students and model purpose in their classrooms (Quaglia Institute for School Voice and Aspirations, 2016).

These programs, though diverse in their approaches, suggest a curriculum framework for schools that want to support student identity and purpose development (Malin, 2018). This framework is made up of the following four components: (1) values exploration and self-awareness, (2) social awareness and beyond-the-self thinking, (3) future-oriented goal setting and planning, and (4) taking action. Notably, growth in self and identity are inexorably threaded within all of the following components of the purpose learning framework.

The first part of the purpose learning framework is self-awareness. In this component, students (and in some cases, teachers) engage in activities such as values reflection, identity exploration, discussion of deep and meaningful questions, and sharing their voice in the classroom. Trust is an essential precursor to any of these activities, and a critical element of this component is building a sense of safety and belonging for all students prior to and through self-awareness activities in the classroom. By exploring values, meaning, and identity openly in a classroom environment that is psychologically safe, the expectation is that students and teachers together can develop confidence, compassion, and human connection that provides a foundation for exploring purpose.

The second part of the purpose learning framework is social awareness, or an awareness and understanding of self in the world. Social awareness is developed through activities that engage students in looking outward and reflecting on their role in the community, society, and the world. Students might discuss social responsibility or explore issues in their community that cause them to feel concerned. Some purpose learning programs engage students in thinking about the people in their lives who are resources for their own development, especially those people who can support them as they pursue their life goals. Other programs ask students to teach or mentor each other, explore personal values together, or collaborate on social projects. In all of these ways, it is hoped that students can build their awareness of and connection to the social world and gain the capacity to make meaningful contributions to that social world. In answering these questions, students begin to articulate goals that might give them a sense of purpose.

The third part of the framework is goal setting and planning. In these purpose learning programs, students practice thinking about higher level goals that they want to pursue and plotting the steps they need to take to pursue these goals. They are asked to reflect on questions such as: What kind of person do I want to be? What do I want my life to contribute? And, how do I want to make a difference in my community or in the world? The answers to these questions can provide the seeds of shorter-term purposeful projects as well as future-oriented purposeful life goals. Goal setting in a purpose learning program includes developing the capacity to plan and act on higher-order goals, such as self-regulation skills and the ability to set small-step short term goals.

Finally, this purpose learning framework includes a component on taking action to accomplish goals. Typically, the action component follows from goal setting and builds on self-awareness and social-awareness, and has the student identifying a concern or interest that is personally meaningful and a need in the world that they can act on. However, it is also possible for self-awareness and social-awareness to follow from action, as students are given opportunities to pursue meaningful projects and asked to reflect on the experience. The actions that students take in purpose learning programs are generally age-appropriate, and might include collaborative school-improvement projects, civic action in the student's community, an internship at a local business, or any other opportunity that results in real-world participation that integrates what matters to the student with a need in the world.

Specific classrooms, schools, and school systems have been gravitating towards adopting essential elements of a purpose learning framework and towards educating the whole child more generally (Stafford-Brizard, 2016). We provide a glimpse into one school system's efforts to intentionally foster youth purpose through a comprehensive, systematic curriculum and innovative student learning experiences to illustrate the promise and effectiveness of implementing such purpose learning approaches to adolescents' educational contexts.

6.6   A Case Example of Purpose Learning: Summit Public Schools

Since inception in 2003, Summit Public Schools has been interested in facilitating identity and purpose development with students, as senses of purpose and identity are recognized as foundational precursors of college readiness. In 2018–19, Summit piloted a new identity and purpose development curriculum with more than 100 students in the 10th and 12th grades in an opt-in electives class. As described in greater detail shortly, students who completed the curriculum reported substantial increases in their sense of purpose and identity over time.

About Summit Public Schools. Summit Public Schools (Summit) is a public charter school network with schools located in California and Washington. Summit serves approximately 4650 students annually at 15 middle and high schools. The student populations at Summit schools reflect the diversity of the communities in which they are located: 45% of Summit students receive free and reduced-price lunch, 14% have an Individualized Education Plan, and 14% are English Learners. Approximately 46% of students are Hispanic, 17% White, 14% Asian, 9% two or more races, 11% African American, and 12% who indicated another race not specified here.

Purpose and identity development at Summit Public Schools. To intentionally foster identity and purpose development in students, Summit has implemented several identity and purpose development strategies network-wide: (1) trusting relationships between students and adults, and (2) dedicated class time to explore identity and purpose.

Summit's strategies to build trusting relationships within the school environment are grounded in empirical work establishing that purpose development is enabled when students have a trusting relationship with an adult (e.g., Liang et al., 2016; Lund et al., 2019; Moran et al., 2012). To help facilitate close student-adult relationships, Summit schools are designed intentionally to be small so that every student is known. This approach is consistent with theory and research implicating the crucial role that feelings of belonging have on purpose development (e.g., Blattner et al., 2013; Hill et al., 2016; Crespo et al., 2013). Additionally, each student at Summit has a designated Mentor, an adult on campus who loops with the student throughout their time at the school, and counsels the student on not only academic development but also identity and purpose development on a highly individualized basis.

Summit's commitment to fostering students' identity and purpose is also reflected through protected class-time to explore these constructs. On a weekly basis, students engage in dedicated development of social-emotional skills and identity via specific projects. In addition, students explore their own interests and passions via a robust electives program called Expeditions, which represents eight weeks of annual class-time.

Purpose and Identity Course Pilot at Summit Public Schools. Above and beyond these two network-wide strategies, in 2017–18 and 2018–19, Summit piloted elective courses designed to help students go even deeper on identity and purpose development. The focus of the courses was to provide a more holistic approach to purpose and identity development in school. These yearlong courses were opt-in for 10th and 12th graders, and students spent time reflecting on their identity and emerging sense of purpose, prototyping their purpose through a variety of strategies, and, finally, setting a long-term goal for their life based on their purpose and building a corresponding roadmap towards that goal. The process that students piloted was adapted from the process outlined in "Designing Your Life" (Burnett & Evans, 2016).

In brief, the curriculum of these year-long electives courses was divided into the following four projects. (1) The first project was a reflection of identity and exploration of what lives that consist of well-being and purpose could look like. The project culminated in students building a draft purpose statement for themselves. (2) The second project was an exploration of either careers (for 10th graders) or an exploration of and support in applying to concrete next step options for after high school (for 12th graders), such as four-year college, vocational school, gap years, etc. This project culminated in students setting a long-term career or college goal for themselves related to their purpose. (3) The third project was an opportunity to prototype their emerging purpose and life goals. Students were able to choose a variety of strategies to prototype such as doing a project consultancy in a career of interest, exploring a purpose-related research question of their own design such as what success means to them or what is important in managing money. This third project culminated in students refining their emerging sense of purpose and life goals. (4) The final project was for students to build a plan to reach their life goals and to solicit feedback on their plans from a group of advisors they trust. Students mapped out several possible five-year plans for themselves that would move them towards their purpose and life goals, and then defended those plans and asked for feedback, such as authenticity of their plans to their purpose, practicality of their plans, or reflections on unanticipated obstacles, from their Personal Advisory Board. At a minimum, their Personal Advisory Boards consisted of their parents/guardians, their Summit mentor teacher, and a peer. The project culminated in students making a decision about which life plan to embark upon.

Evaluation of Purpose and Identity Pilot Course. To evaluate the efficacy of Summit's pilot course, we utilized a pre- and post- survey as well as ongoing student feedback surveys. We focused on understanding if there had been a change in purpose as a result of engaging in the courses. For the context of the pilot, Summit defined purpose as, "A process by which students seek, identify, pursue, and refine a central life aim that is both meaningful to the student and consequential to the world." Survey questions were designed in collaboration with a team of both researchers and practitioners and built upon purpose survey questions found in the literature (e.g., Steger et al., 2006). For example, students were asked to rank the degree to which they agreed with such statements as: "I have a good sense of what makes my life meaningful," "I have discovered a satisfying life purpose," and "My life has a clear sense of purpose."

Overall, an increase in sense of purpose as a result of the courses was found, with students reporting that the experience, particularly the final project of the year, was helpful to them. For example, students enrolled in the courses reported an increase in having a good sense of what makes their lives meaningful from 66% at the beginning of the school year to 76% at the end of the school year. An increase in discovering a satisfying life purpose, from 50% at the beginning of the year to 66% at the end of the school year, was also reported. There was also evidence of an increase in students believing that their life has a clear sense of purpose, from 52% at the beginning of the year to 65% at the end of the year. While these patterns suggest that the Summit program increased average levels of purpose among students, it is also important to note that many students (half or more), did not start the year with a completely blank state of purpose. That is, consistent with the overall themes of this chapter, it appears that schools could play a role in not only igniting the development of youth purpose if it does not already exist, but also in helping to expand, refine, and concretize the seeds of purpose that have already been planted.

Students' open-ended feedback corroborates these results and perhaps provides more in-depth information on the effectiveness of the program. For example, with respect to the developmentally salient conflict of identity versus role diffusion (Erikson, 1968), Summit's course was set up in such a way for a student to explore their identity and purpose and then frame and present back their conclusions to their family and friends. The intention is to give students agency in their identity versus role diffusion conflict and students appeared to find the program's experience, particularly of building their life plans and soliciting feedback on their life plans, to be useful. As one student noted, "It gave me a chance to clearly understand for myself and explain to those close to me what I plan for my life to look like." Another interesting feedback point was how many students appreciated the opportunity to plan for their futures, something that is of key concern, especially in the 12th grade year and in terms of developmental needs for autonomy and future-orientation (Metzger et al., 2018). A student shared, "I liked that I had to thoroughly plan my future for the next 5 years. This forced me to plan for any issue that can possibly go wrong and it helped me make the best possible plan for myself. I also liked that I got feedback on my plan which improved it overall."

The learnings from these innovative pilot courses suggests that there could be great promise for schools to implement effective purpose learning curricula to foster youth development. Notably, more detailed results and conclusions can be found in the following report: *Clearing the Path: How Schools Can Improve College Access and Persistence for Every Student*, which can be found on Summit's website at https://

summitps.org/the-summit-model/the-science-of-summit/ or directly online at https://
summitps.org/wp-content/uploads/2019/09/CNS-whitepaper-092419.pdf.

6.7 Implications and Challenges to School-Based Purpose Learning Programs

From a theoretical, empirical, and applied perspective, the importance of both identity and purpose, as well as their inextricable links, are abundantly clear (Hill &
Burrow, 2012). Particularly for adolescents, for whom processes of identity and
purpose formation are highly salient (Erikson, 1968), the school setting is thick with
great opportunities to cultivate these crucial developmental assets (Malin, 2018).
Researchers and practitioners alike have called for greater attention towards clarifying the diverse pathways that might lead to purpose development (e.g., Hill et al.,
2013; Liang et al., 2017), and our work offers several specific suggestions and related
implications as well.

However, as school-based purpose learning programs are spreading and currently
in demand, there are challenges that need to be addressed as the field grows. One
significant challenge can be posed as a question: What is the impact on students
when they are asked to explore personal values, identity, meaning, and purpose at
school? This question is particularly important given the number of students who
experience marginalization both in society and at school, and the likely impact that
marginalization can have on purpose development (Sumner, Burrow, & Hill, 2018).
It raises follow-up questions about cultural differences in attitudes about sharing and
discussing personal and family values at school, about possible conflicts between
family and school values, about the vulnerability of some students who do not feel
safe at school or who have aspects of their identity that may not be safely explored
at school, and about the risk for students who have experienced trauma and may not
be provided the psychological resources in the classroom to be safe discussing their
personal lives. For example, students may feel threatened or vigilant if they perceive
that aspects of their identity could result in negative treatment in a setting such as
a classroom (Cohen & Garcia, 2008). These are issues that need to be a central
consideration when proposing that schools implement a purpose learning program.

Although these are clear challenges to school-based purpose learning initiatives,
there is theory and research evidence suggesting that classroom activities such as
personal values exploration can have a positive impact on students. Self-affirmation
theory, for example, proposes that people can recover from the psychological damage
of identity threats by reflecting on and asserting the aspects of themselves that
they value most (Sherman & Cohen, 2006; Steele, 1988). Experiments with self-
affirmation interventions with students have had positive results. For example, ethnic
minority middle school students who reflected on a value that was important to them
at the start of the year experienced a greater sense of trust and fairness in school
throughout the year compared to classmates who did not reflect on an important

value (Cohen, Garcia, Apfel, & Masters, 2006). In another experiment, middle school students who were in racial groups most susceptible to identity threat at school (Black and Hispanic students) had a positive impact on their academic performance if they completed a self-affirmation activity, whereas White and Asian students did not experience the same effect (Hanselman, Bruch, Gamoran, & Borman, 2014). The results of these studies suggest that exploring and expressing important personal values at school may benefit students who are most vulnerable to identity threat, though considerably more research should be done to examine the possible differential impacts of school-based purpose learning experiences on heterogeneous students.

The importance of considering a more individualized and culturally-sensitive approach can be more broadly reflected in light of Erikson's (1968) original references to the adolescent period as being characterized by a "crisis." There are likely key individual differences in terms of how stressful or conflictual these explorative processes might be, but some research indeed suggests that the search for purpose (e.g., as measured through a survey that assesses both purpose and meaning) can be negatively associated with well-being (Kiang & Witkow, 2015; Steger et al., 2006). Burrow et al. (2010) applied an identity status framework (e.g., Marcia, 1966) to the construct of purpose itself and found that positive outcomes and emotional well-being tended to be linked to individuals who have established a clear sense of purpose, as compared to their counterparts who have not yet committed and might still be in "crisis" or engaging in purpose exploration. However, other work points to the search for purpose as having positive implications, and linked to both hope and life satisfaction, especially among samples of youth and adolescents (Bronk et al., 2009). Given these competing views, one important area for future research is to better understand the specific processes of purpose development, with the understanding that precise pathways might look different for adolescents from different backgrounds (Liang et al., 2017). More systematic attention towards understanding identity and purpose development with the use of longitudinal data and person-centered approaches, such as cluster analyses or profile approaches as described by Burrow et al. (2010), could be helpful in delineating heterogeneity in developmental pathways.

Purpose researchers and school-based purpose learning programs also face challenges in measuring and reporting their outcomes. As described earlier, purpose is defined in different ways in the literature, with some shared understanding of the core elements of the purpose construct but significant disagreement about whether, for example, purpose is necessarily beyond-the-self oriented or whether it is a "sense" that someone experiences or demonstrates in their actions in the world. Numerous measures of purpose have been used in the research, with no conclusion about which are best to measure growth in purpose resulting from an intervention. The working definition that we attempted to focus on in the current chapter is one that views purpose as both inward and outward facing, but it is important to note that the literature that we reviewed varied in specific operationalizations. It remains an empirical question whether certain measures of purpose, for example, those that rely on beyond-the-self perspectives versus those that focus more on goal orientation versus those that simply assess the presence of purpose more broadly speaking, are more or less strongly linked to either identity constructs and/or adjustment. Consequently, although the use of the purpose learning framework is increasing across the U.S., there is still a lack of clarity on how to precisely target and assess purpose, and limited evidence to demonstrate whether and how these programs impact students' purpose development and positive identity formation. Early efforts to evaluate these programs are underway, including our described evaluation work at Summit Public Schools, but far more work needs to be done.

In light of broader implications, we should explicitly note that the adjustment indicators we have focused on in this chapter have been largely based on students' and teachers' subjective self-reports. Moreover, one of our goals with this chapter is to promote the argument that purpose is an important outcome of education in its own right. However, the current policy context emphasizes that the primary target of school is a narrower index of academic achievement and more objective measures of success. Although there is little and inconsistent support for any direct links between purpose development and academic achievement, and although it is not our intention to argue for academic-instrumental motivations for focusing on purpose development at school, there is some evidence suggesting that promoting purpose at school might benefit academic engagement and actual performance. For example, students who had a self-transcendent purpose for learning showed greater academic diligence and academic performance compared with those who did not (Yeager et al., 2014). Research also suggests that academic performance might be enhanced when students perceive that what they are learning has useful purpose in their lives, or when they have an internal purpose for what they are learning as opposed to an externally imposed purpose for learning (Hulleman, Godes, Hendricks, & Harackiewicz, 2010; Niemiec & Ryan, 2009). While having a purpose for learning is not the same thing as having a purpose in life, these studies suggest that the internal drive that purpose in life provides might be a source of motivation for academic engagement and performance. Consistent with these perspectives, Kiang and Witkow (2015) found that adolescents' presence and search for purpose were both associated with academic motivation and the perception that academic success has real-world utility, which could arguably serve as mediators for subsequent indictors of achievement and success.

That said, there is also the possibility that the pursuit of purpose and academic performance (e.g., grades, test scores) might not align. For example, if purpose is not inherently related to the school context (e.g., wanting to become an NBA basketball player), then it is possible that any purpose-related activities might take time away from school and hinder academic success. However, if one's purpose is tied to academics (e.g., wanting to become a doctor to help people with cancer), then we might see positive links between purpose and doing well in school, knowing that this is needed to achieve one's goals. Emerging work similarly suggests that interventions that boost both purpose and internal feeling of control over academic success could improve actual grades (Pizzolato et al., 2011). Further empirical work could more systematically examine such possible individual differences and unpack specific longitudinal and mediating pathways to better pinpoint diverse adjustment implications including more objective, markers of success within the academic realm.

6.8 Summary and Conclusions

Purpose and identity development are foundational and complementary activities of adolescence. As adolescents spend a large portion of time at school, both students and school personnel can benefit from giving dedicated class-time to the exploration of purpose and identity and its impacts both inside and outside of the classroom. If designed carefully with cultural, social, and emotional considerations in mind, schools can offer the unique opportunity of allowing students to explore their purpose and identity development in ways that students may or may not receive outside of the classroom. Additionally, intentional and culturally sensitive reflection on purpose and identity can increase a student's sense of belonging in school, resulting in a host of positive impacts within a classroom environment as well as in terms of youth socioemotional well-being more generally. Key factors to consider when designing school-based purpose and identity programs include selecting the definition of purpose that most resonates for the school's context, selecting the framework for identity and purpose development, and implementing activities and experiences that acknowledge manifold paths to purpose that are ideally tailored to each adolescent's background and needs. Ultimately, by capitalizing on school contexts to help build adolescent identity and purpose, youth could be better poised to strengthen their sense of self, face and overcome challenges, and contribute in meaningful and highly personal ways to their family and social groups, community, and the broader world around them.

References

Atkins, R., & Hart, D. (2003). Neighborhoods, adults, and the development of civic identity in urban youth. *Applied Developmental Science, 7,* 156–164.

Blattner, M. C. C., Liang, B., Lund, T., & Spencer, R. (2013). Searching for a sense of purpose: The role of parents and effects on self-esteem among female adolescents. *Journal of Adolescence, 36*(5), 839–848.

Bohnert, A., Fredricks, J., & Randall, E. (2010). Capturing unique dimensions of youth organized activity involvement: Theoretical and methodological considerations. *Review of Educational Research, 80,* 576–610.

Branscombe, N. R., Schmitt, M. T., & Harvey, R. D. (1999). Perceiving pervasive discrimination among African Americans: Implications for group identification and well-being. *Journal of Personality and Social Psychology, 77,* 135–149.

Brassai, L., Piko, B. F., & Steger, M. F. (2011). Meaning in life: Is it a protective factor for adolescents' psychological health? *International Journal of Behavioral Medicine, 18,* 44–51.

Brassai, L., Piko, B. F., & Steger, M. F. (2013). Individual and parental factors related to meaning in life among Hungarian minority adolescents from Romania. *International Journal of Psychology, 48*(3), 308–315.

Brittian, A. S., Kim, S. Y., Armenta, B. E., Lee, R. M., Umaña-Taylor, A. J., Schwartz, S. J. … Castillo, L. G. (2015). Do dimensions of ethnic identity mediate the association between perceived ethnic group discrimination and depressive symptoms? *Cultural Diversity and Ethnic Minority Psychology, 21,* 41–53.

Bronk, K., Hill, P. L., Lapsley, D. K., Talib, T. L., & Finch, H. (2009). Purpose, hope, and life satisfaction in three age groups. *The Journal of Positive Psychology, 4,* 500–510.

Bundick, M. J. (2011). The benefits of reflecting on and discussing purpose in life in emerging adulthood. *New Directions for Youth Development, 132,* 89–103.

Burnett, W., & Evans, D. J. (2016). *Designing your life: How to build a well-lived, joyful life.* New York: Alfred A. Knopf.

Burrow, A. L., & Hill, P. L. (2011). Purpose as a form of identity capital for positive youth adjustment. *Developmental Psychology, 47,* 1196–1206.

Burrow, A. L., O'Dell, A. C., & Hill, P. L. (2010). Profiles of a developmental asset: Youth purpose as a context for hope and well-being. *Journal of Youth and Adolescence, 39,* 1265–1273.

Carlo, G., Knight, G. P., McGinley, M., & Hayes, R. (2011). The roles of parental inductions, moral emotions, and moral cognitions in prosocial tendencies among Mexican American and European American early adolescents. *Journal of Early Adolescence, 31,* 757–781.

Cohen, G. L., & Garcia, J. (2008). Identity, belonging, and achievement: A model, interventions, implications. *Current Directions in Psychological Science, 17*(6), 365–369.

Cohen, G. L., Garcia, J., Apfel, N., & Master, A. (2006). Reducing the racial achievement gap: A social-psychological intervention. *Science, 313,* 1307–1310.

Côté, J. E. (1997). An empirical test of the identity capital model. *Journal of Adolescence, 20,* 577–597.

Crespo, C., Jose, P. E., Kielpikowski, M., & Pryor, J. (2013). "On solid ground": Family and school connectedness promotes adolescents' future orientation. *Journal of Adolescence, 36,* 993–1002.

Cronin, T. J., Levin, S., Branscombe, N. R., van Laar, C., & Tropp, L. R. (2012). Ethnic identification in response to perceived discrimination protects well-being and promotes activism: A longitudinal study of Latino college students. *Group Processes & Intergroup Relations, 15,* 393–407.

Damon, W. (2008). *The path to purpose: How young people find their calling in life.* New York: The Free Press.

Damon, W., Menon, J., & Bronk, K. (2003). The development of purpose during adolescence. *Applied Developmental Science, 7,* 119–128.

Da Silva, L., Sanson, A., Smart, D., & Toumbourou, J. (2004). Civic responsibility among Australian adolescents: Testing two competing models. *Journal of Community Psychology, 32,* 229–255. https://doi.org/10.1002/jcop.20004.

Deci, E. L., & Ryan, R. M. (2008). Hedonia, eudaimonia, and well-being: An introduction. *Journal of Happiness Studies, 9,* 1–11.

Dunn, M. G., & O'Brien, K. M. (2009). Psychological health and meaning in life: Stress, social support, and religious coping in Latina/Latino immigrants. *Hispanic Journal of Behavioral Sciences, 31,* 204–227.

Ehlman, K., & Ligon, M. (2012). The application of a generativity model for older adults. *The International Journal of Aging and Human Development, 74,* 331–344.

Emmons, R. A. (1999). *The psychology of ultimate concerns: Motivation and spirituality in personality.* New York: Guilford Press.

Erikson, E. H. (1950). *Childhood and society.* New York: Norton.

Erikson, E. H. (1959). *Identity and the life cycle: Selected papers.* Oxford, England: International Universities Press.

Erikson, E. H. (1968). *Identity: Youth and crisis.* New York: Norton.

Ethier, K. A., & Deaux, K. (1994). Negotiating social identity when contexts change: Maintaining identification and responding to threat. *Journal of Personality and Social Psychology, 67,* 243–251.

Flanagan, C. A., Syvertsen, A. K., Gill, S., Gallay, L. S., & Cumsille, P. (2009). Ethnic awareness, prejudice, and civic commitments in four ethnic groups of American adolescents. *Journal of Youth and Adolescence, 38,* 500–518.

Frankl, V. (1959). *Man's search for meaning.* New York: Simon & Schuster.

Fredricks, J. A., & Eccles, J. S. (2006). Is extracurricular participation associated with beneficial outcomes? Concurrent and longitudinal relations. *Developmental Psychology, 42,* 698–713.

Fuligni, A. J. (2010). Social identity, motivation, and well-being among adolescents from Asian and Latin American backgrounds. In G. Carlo, L. J. Crockett, & M. A. Carranza (Eds.), *Health disparities in youth and families* (pp. 97–120). New York: Springer.

Fuligni, A. J., & Flook, L. (2005). A social identity approach to ethnic differences in family relationships during adolescence. In R. Kail (Ed.), *Advances in child development and behavior* (pp. 125–152). New York: Academic Press.

Fuligni, A. J., & Pedersen, S. (2002). Family obligation and the transition to young adulthood. *Developmental Psychology, 38,* 856–868.

Gutowski, E., White, A. E., Liang, B., Diamonti, A. J., & Berado, D. (2018). How stress influences purpose development: The importance of social support. *Journal of Adolescent Research, 33,* 571–597.

Hanselman, P., Bruch, S. K., Gamoran, A., & Borman, G. D. (2014). Threat in context: School moderation of the impact of social identity threat on racial/ethnic achievement gaps. *Sociology of Education, 87*(2), 106–124.

Hardy, S. A., Walker, L. J., Olsen, J. A., Woodbury, R. D., & Hickman, J. R. (2014). Moral identity as moral ideal self: Links to adolescent outcomes. *Developmental Psychology, 50,* 45–57.

Hatchimonji, D. R., Linsky, A. V., & Elias, M. J. (2017). Cultivating noble purpose in urban middle schools: A missing piece in school transformation. *Education, 138*(2), 162–178.

Hill, P. L., & Burrow, A. L. (2012). Viewing purpose through an Eriksonian lens. *Identity, 12,* 74–91.

Hill, P. L., Burrow, A. L., & Sumner, R. (2013). Addressing important questions in the field of adolescent purpose. *Child Development Perspectives, 7,* 232–236.

Hill, P. L., Burrow, A. L., & Sumner, R. (2016). Sense of purpose and parent–child relationships in emerging adulthood. *Emerging Adulthood, 4*(6), 436–439.

Hughes, D. L., Watford, J. A., & Del Toro, J. (2016). A transactional/ecological perspective on ethnic-racial identity, socialization, and discrimination. *Advances in Child Development and Behavior, 51,* 1–41.

Hulleman, C. S., Godes, O., Hendricks, B. L., & Harackiewicz, J. M. (2010). Enhancing interest and performance with a utility value intervention. *Journal of Educational Psychology, 102,* 880–895.

Kiang, L. (2012). Deriving daily purpose through daily events and role fulfillment among Asian American youth. *Journal of Research on Adolescence, 22,* 185–198.

Kiang, L., & Fuligni, A. J. (2010). Meaning in life as a mediator of ethnic identity and adjustment among adolescents from Latin American, Asian, and European American backgrounds. *Journal of Youth and Adolescence, 39,* 1253–1264.

Kiang, L., & Witkow, M. R. (2015). Normative changes in meaning in life and links to adjustment in adolescents from Asian American backgrounds. *Asian American Journal of Psychology, 6,* 164–173.

Lambert, N. M., Stillman, T. F., Hicks, J. A., Kamble, S., Baumeister, R. F., & Fincham, F. D. (2013). To belong is to matter: Sense of belonging enhances meaning in life. *Personality and Social Psychology Bulletin, 39*(11), 1418–1427.

Larson, R. W. (2000). Toward a psychology of positive youth development. *American Psychologist, 55,* 170–183.

Liang, B., White, A., Mousseau, A. M. D., Hasse, A., Knight, L., Berado, D., et al. (2017). The four P's of purpose among college bound students: People, propensity, passion, prosocial benefits. *The Journal of Positive Psychology, 12,* 281–294.

Lund, T. J., Liang, B., Konowitz, L., White, A. E., & Mousseau, A. D. (2019). Quality over quantity? Mentoring relationships and purpose development among college students. *Psychology in the Schools, 56,* 1472–1481. https://doi.org/10.1002/pits.22284.

Malin, H. (2018). *Teaching for purpose: Preparing students for lives of meaning.* Cambridge, MA: Harvard Education Press.

Malin, H., Ballard, P. J., & Damon, W. (2015). Civic purpose: An integrated construct for understanding civic development in adolescence. *Human Development, 58,* 103–130.

Malin, H., Liauw, I., & Remington, K. (2019). Early adolescent purpose development and perceived supports for purpose at school. *Journal of Character Education, 15*(2).

Malin, H., Reilly, T. S., Quinn, B., & Moran, S. (2014). Adolescent purpose development: Exploring empathy, discovering roles, shifting priorities, and creating pathways. *Journal of Research on Adolescence, 24*(1), 186–199. https://doi.org/10.1111/jora.12051.

Marcia, J. E. (1966). Development and validation of ego-identity status. *Journal of Personality and Social Psychology, 3,* 551–558.

McAdams, D. P., & de St Aubin, E. D. (1992). A theory of generativity and its assessment through self-report, behavioral acts, and narrative themes in autobiography. *Journal of Personality and Social Psychology, 62,* 1003–1015.

McKnight, P. E., & Kashdan, T. B. (2009). Purpose in life as a system that creates and sustains health and well-being: An integrative, testable theory. *Review of General Psychology, 13,* 242–251.

Metzger, A., Alvis, L. M., Oosterhoff, B., Babskie, E., Syvertsen, A., & Wray-Lake, L. (2018). The intersection of emotional and sociocognitive competencies with civic engagement in middle childhood and adolescence. *Journal of Youth and Adolescence, 47,* 1663–1683.

Moran, S. (2017). Youth purpose worldwide: A tapestry of possibilities. *Journal of Moral Education, 46,* 231–244.

Moran, S., Bundick, M., Malin, H., & Reilly, T. (2013). How supportive of their specific purposes do youth believe their family and friends are? *Journal of Adolescent Research, 28*(3), 348–377. https://doi.org/10.1177/0743558412457816.

Newton, T., & McIntosh, D. N. (2013). Unique contributions of religion to meaning. In J. A. Hicks (Ed.), *The experience of meaning in life: Classical perspectives, emerging themes, and controversies* (pp. 257–269). New York: Springer.

Niemiec, C. P., & Ryan, R. M. (2009). Autonomy, competence, and relatedness in the classroom: Applying self-determination theory to educational practice. *Theory and Research in Education, 7,* 133–144.

Phinney, J. S. (2003). Ethnic identity and acculturation. In K. M. Chun, P. B. Organista, & G. Marin (Eds.), *Acculturation: Advances in theory, measurement, and applied research* (pp. 63–81). Washington, DC: American Psychological Association.

Pizzolato, J. E., Brown, E. L., & Kanny, M. A. (2011). Purpose plus: Supporting youth purpose, control, and academic achievement. *New Directions for Youth Development, 132,* 75–88.

Quaglia Institute for School Voice and Aspirations. (2016). *School voice report.* Portland, ME: Quaglia Institute for School Voice and Aspirations.

Rossi, G., Lenzi, M., Sharkey, J. D., Vieno, A., & Santinello, M. (2016). Factors associated with civic engagement in adolescence: The effects of neighborhood, school, family, and peer contexts. *Journal of Community Psychology, 44*(8), 1040–1058.

Ryff, C. D. (1989). Happiness is everything, or is it? Explorations on the meaning of psychological well-being. *Journal of Personality and Social Psychology, 57,* 1069–1081.

Ryff, C. D., & Keyes, C. L. M. (1995). The structure of psychological well-being revisited. *Journal of Personality and Social Psychology, 69,* 719–727.

Seligman, M. E. P. (2002). *Authentic happiness: Using the new positive psychology to realize your potential for lasting fulfillment.* New York: Free Press.

Sherman, D. K., & Cohen, G. L. (2006). The psychology of self-defense: Self-affirmation theory. In M. P. Zanna (Ed.), *Advances in experimental social psychology* (Vol. 38, pp. 183–242). San Diego, CA: Academic Press.

Stafford-Brizard, K. B. (2016). *Building blocks for learning: A framework for comprehensive student development.* New York: Turnaround for Children.

Steele, C. M. (1988). The psychology of self-affirmation: Sustaining the integrity of the self. In L. Berkowitz (Ed.), *Advances in experimental social psychology* (Vol. 21, pp. 261–302). New York: Academic Press.

Steger, M. F., Bundick, M. J., & Yeager, D. (2011). Meaning in life. *Encyclopedia of Adolescence,* 1666–1677.

Steger, M. F., Frazier, P., Oishi, S., & Kaler, M. (2006). The meaning in life questionnaire: Assessing the presence of and search for meaning in life. *Journal of Counseling Psychology, 53,* 80–93.

Steger, M. F., Oishi, S., & Kashdan, T. B. (2009). Meaning in life across the life span: Levels and correlates of meaning in life from emerging adulthood to older adulthood. *The Journal of Positive Psychology, 4,* 43–52.

Stepick, A., & Stepick, C. D. (2002). Becoming American, constructing ethnicity: Immigrant youth and civic engagement. *Applied Developmental Science, 6,* 246–257.

Sumner, R. (2017). More education, more purpose in life? A comparison of purpose across adults with different levels of education. *Applied Research in Quality of Life, 12,* 17–34.

Sumner, R., Burrow, A. L., & Hill, P. L. (2018). The development of purpose in life among adolescents who experience marginalization: Potential opportunities and obstacles. *American Psychologist, 73,* 740–752.

Tabbah, R., Chung, J. J., & Miranda, A. H. (2016). Ethnic identity and discrimination: An exploration of the rejection-identification model in Arab American adolescents. *Identity, 16,* 319–334.

Tajfel, H., & Turner, J. C. (2001). An integrative theory of intergroup conflict. In M. A. Hogg & D. Adrams (Eds.), *Relations: Essential readings. Key readings in social psychology* (pp. 94–109). New York: Psychology Press.

Tseng, V., & Seidman, E. (2007). A systems framework for understanding social settings. *American Journal of Community Psychology, 39,* 217–228.

Turner, J. C. (1982). Towards a cognitive redefinition of the social group. In H. Tajfel (Ed.), *Social identity and intergroup relations* (pp. 15–40). Cambridge, England: Cambridge University Press.

Watts, R. J., Diemer, M. A., & Voight, A. M. (2011). Critical consciousness: Current status and future directions. *New Directions for Child and Adolescent Development, 134,* 43–57.

Yeager, D. S., Henderson, M. D., Paunesku, D., Walton, G. M., D'Mello, S., Spitzer, B. J., et al. (2014). Boring but important: A self-transcendent purpose for learning fosters academic self-regulation. *Journal of Personality and Social Psychology, 107,* 559–580.

Chapter 7
Supporting Youth Purpose in Adolescence: Youth-Adult Relationships as Ecological Assets

Mark Vincent B. Yu and Nancy L. Deutsch

Abstract Having or developing a sense of purpose is an important component of positive adolescent development. However, there is limited empirical understanding of how youth purpose develops and what aspects of youth's ecologies best support purpose development during adolescence. This chapter seeks to provide insight into how significant adults, both parents and non-parental adults, serve as ecological assets that may support purpose development for youth during adolescence. We begin by discussing how developmental and ecological theories can inform the broader literature on youth purpose. We then present findings from a study examining the development, characteristics, and influence of youth–adult relationships across multiple contexts and over key transition points across adolescence, focusing on the ways in which relationships with parents and other significant adults can play a key role in cultivating and nurturing purpose development during adolescence. We close by discussing implications for understanding effective ways of supporting purpose development during adolescence and the benefits of mixed methods research for those aims.

7.1 Introduction

Having purpose in life is linked to positive youth development and youth thriving (Mariano & Going, 2011; Scales, Benson, & Roehlkepartain, 2011). Yet currently, there is limited empirical understanding of how youth purpose develops and what aspects of youth's ecologies best support and scaffold purpose development during adolescence (Hill, Burrow, & Sumner, 2013). This chapter seeks to provide insight into how significant adults, both parents and non-parental adults, serve as ecological assets (Theokas & Lerner, 2006; Scales et al., 2011) that may support purpose

M. V. B. Yu (✉)
University of California—Irvine, Irvine, USA
e-mail: markv.yu@uci.edu

N. L. Deutsch
University of Virginia, Charlottesville, USA

© Springer Nature Switzerland AG 2020 115
A. L. Burrow and P. Hill (eds.), *The Ecology of Purposeful Living Across the Lifespan*,
https://doi.org/10.1007/978-3-030-52078-6_7

development for youth during adolescence. In addition, we consider how youth-adult relationships may serve as settings in and of themselves, and the ways in which different developmental needs across adolescence may shape what youth seek from relationships and settings in relation to their purpose development as they move through this developmental period. In doing so, we discuss findings from a study of youth-adult relationships that highlights the benefits of mixed methods research for understanding the processes of purpose development.

7.1.1 Benefits of Purpose in Adolescence

Purpose has been generally defined as "a stable and generalized intention to accomplish something that is at once meaningful to the self and of consequence to the world beyond the self" (Damon, Menon, & Bronk, 2003, p. 121). Whereas different specific definitions of purpose exist, our aim here is not to distinguish between definitions of purpose, but to consider why purpose in general is important during adolescence and the ways in which it may be fostered during this time period. A large body of research suggests having purpose is beneficial for youth. Youth who report having a sense of purpose are happier, less susceptible to risky behaviors, and more academically engaged, (e.g., Brassai, Piko, & Steger, 2011; Sumner, Burrow, & Hill, 2015; Yeager & Bundick, 2009). Moreover, there is evidence to suggest that purpose is associated with key indicators of positive youth development including connection, confidence, competence, caring, and character, in addition to being associated with prosocial outcomes that reflect engagement with and contribution to community and society (Johnson, Tirrell, Callina, & Weiner, 2018; Malin, Ballard, & Damon, 2015; Scales et al., 2011). Although we know a great deal about the outcomes associated with purpose, we know less about the developmental and relational processes that support its development during adolescence (Hill et al., 2013).

7.1.2 Purpose and Stage-Environment Fit in Adolescence

Adolescence can be a formative period for cultivating a sense of purpose, in part because of the overlap between the developmental tasks of adolescence and the characteristics and mechanisms of purpose development. During adolescence, young people are actively exploring their identities and developing a sense of who they are now, as well as who they hope to be in the future (NASEM, 2019). Thus, identity formation is a key developmental task of this period. Purpose is inherently related to identity, as it encompasses a sense of commitment to personally meaningful goals. Indeed, prior research has identified a link between having a sense of purpose and identity exploration and commitment during adolescence (Bronk, 2011; Hill & Burrow, 2012). Further, engaging in activities that cultivate a sense of purpose has been linked to self-esteem, another construct that comes to the fore during adolescence (Liang, Lund, Mousseau, & Spencer, 2016).

Yet adolescence is not a uniform developmental period; developmental needs and tasks shift across early, middle, and late adolescence, and there are significant inter-individual differences within stages in terms of developmental needs and statuses (NASEM, 2019). As researchers have focused more on the contexts of adolescent development (Steinberg & Morris, 2001), the features of settings which promote or inhibit development are of increasing importance to both researchers and practitioners. Importantly, those features are not necessarily uniform across *adolescence* or across *adolescents*. According to stage-environment fit theories, optimal development occurs in environments in which the structures and processes map onto and meet the needs of the people in the setting (Eccles & Midgley, 1989). Eccles and colleagues suggest their idea could be a useful lens for adolescent researchers, pointing to the "mismatch" between the developmental needs of youth and the "opportunities afforded them by their environments (Eccles et al., 1993, p. 90)" as a potential origin for negative outcomes during adolescence. Given the variance in needs between as well as within youth over time, across early to late adolescence, different youth may need different things from different environments at different ages. This is true for how youth develop purpose across adolescence as well, including what aspects of youth's environments may support purpose development across different stages in adolescence.

Developmentally appropriate and regressive shifts in the social environments of youth can influence purpose development during adolescence. Importantly, youth's perceptions of the fit between themselves and their social environments depend highly on the supportive relationships available to them in their various settings (Zimmer-Gembeck, Chipuer, Hanisch, Creed, & McGregor, 2006). During early adolescence, the school context can have considerable influence on youth's purpose development (Koshy & Mariano, 2011). Unfortunately, the goals for learning emphasized through school policies and practices become more tightly controlled and scheduled as youth move into middle school, limiting youth access to and time with supportive adults, and opportunities for healthy individuation and meaningful challenges (Pianta, Hamre, & Allen, 2012). These regressive changes may hinder young adolescents' abilities to meet their needs for connection, autonomy, and competence-building experiences, needs which undergird youth's motivations to pursue goals that are personally meaningful and beneficial to others (Dawes & Larson, 2011; Deci & Ryan, 2000).

Across adolescence, the social dynamics of youth's family and peer relationships change as well. Research suggests that the most salient sources of social support shift across adolescence, with younger adolescents reporting higher levels of support from parents and older youth reporting greater support from peers (Bokhorst, Sumter, & Westenberg, 2010). Thus, parents may play a particularly influential role in youth's purpose development during early adolescence (Malin, Reilly, Quinn, & Moran, 2014). As youth continue to age, youth's relationships with supportive nonparental adults—adults who have been noted as often operating in a space somewhere between

that of parents and peers—become increasingly salient, in part because these relationships complement the structure and support provided by parents while providing
the companionship that is typical of peer relationships (Hirsch, 2005).

Older adolescents also begin to explore the possibilities of intimate relationships
and options for higher education and/or career, and thus move gradually toward
making enduring choices (Arnett, 2004). Therefore, this developmental period facilitates great personal growth. However, as late adolescents navigate transitions (e.g.,
high school to college/career) and forge pathways towards their purpose in life, they
are also taking in information about the obstacles and supports that they encounter
along the way, information that can shape their perceptions of meaningful and achievable options moving forward (Malin et al., 2014). As adolescents transition from high
school, they are likely to distance themselves (e.g., either physically or through less
contact) from their immediate family members (Lindell & Campione-Barr, 2017). In
the process, they access a broader network of relationships for support, including
peers and nonparental youth-adult relationships, through the various contexts to
which they become exposed (e.g., work, college). These changes in youth's social
environments are highly relevant to thinking about how youth develop purpose during
different stages in adolescence and the potential relationships they may turn to for
support along the way.

In addition to changes in social environments during adolescence, there are significant changes that occur within the brain related to the development of executive function and social cognition (e.g., self-regulation, self-awareness, perspective-taking;
Blakemore & Choudhury, 2006), changes that relate to their development of a sense
of purpose. As adolescents develop, they continue to refine their capacity for abstract
thought processes, increasing their ability to understand, reason, and make independent decisions towards their purpose in life (Moran, Bundick, Malin, & Reilly, 2013).
Younger adolescents may have a broader sense of purpose but be less able to act on it
(Malin, Liauw & Damon, 2017). Older youth, on the other hand, may have a narrower
sense of purpose and have a wider set of supports and opportunities to be able to
enact it (e.g., Clydesdale, 2015; Johnson et al., 2018; Malin et al., 2014).

Taken together, as youth develop a sense of purpose during adolescence, they are
confronted with myriad changes including physical, socio-emotional and cognitive
changes (Steinberg, 2016). As described above, these changes have strong implications for how to structure developmentally appropriate supports for youth within and
across different stages in adolescence to facilitate the development of purpose.

In addition to considering youth's shifting needs during adolescence, it is also
important to consider larger societal and structural changes at play. For example,
adolescents become subject to a variety of influences and choices that can introduce stress and confusion as they work towards their purpose in life. In the United
States today, adolescents, compared to previous generations, face more economic,
institutional, and social disparities (NASEM, 2019), and greater pressure to achieve
"success" and "perfection" in pursuit of purposeful goals (e.g. Spencer, Walsh,
Liang, Mousseau, & Lund, 2018). These disparities and pressures may impact youth
from different social positions in different ways. For example, youth from historically marginalized racial or ethnic groups may be thinking about their sense of

purpose in the context of daily, racialized microaggressions that impact their well-being (e.g., Keels, Durkee, & Hope, 2017; Wong, Derthick, David, Saw, & Okazaki, 2014). Strong racial and ethnic identity, which can be a protective factor for racially minoritized youth (e.g., Sellers, Copeland-Linder, Martin, & Lewis, 2006), also has developmental trajectories across adolescence (Umana-Taylor et al., 2014) as well as intersections with other social identities (Williams, Tolan, Durkee, Francois, & Anderson, 2012) and implications for how young people think about their sense of purpose in relation to these identities. Thus, understanding the supports and opportunities that exist within youth's environments to help them develop a sense of purpose is important. This process involves understanding key developmental differences across stages in adolescence as well as considering the larger societal and structural changes that confront youth today.

7.1.3 An Ecological View of Youth Development of Purpose: Internal and External Assets

We take an ecological view of youth development (Bronfenbrenner, 1979), considering the ways in which development is nested within layers of environments that together influence, and are influenced by, individuals. Within this frame, youth's developmental processes are supported by a set of internal and ecological assets which interactively influence each other and the developmental pathways along with youth proceed (Benson, Mannes, Pittman, & Ferber, 2004). Internal assets are characteristics that are considered to reside within the young person, such as skills and competencies, values, and a positive identity. External assets are characteristics of an adolescent's environments, such as the presence of supportive relationships, opportunities for constructively using one's time, clear boundaries and high expectations, and norms that empower and value youth (Benson et al., 2004). Within our framing, relationships with adults are both an asset within youth's ecosystem, and settings in and of themselves, which have their own processes and influences on youth's developmental pathways.

Youth-Adult Relationships as Ecological Assets. Although we often stereotype teens as caring only about their peers, adults in fact serve an important role in adolescents' lives, and adolescents are especially attuned to the actions and reactions of the adults around them, who can serve as sources of support and models of adulthood (NASEM, 2019). These adults may span a variety of roles and contexts, including parents but also non-parental adults such as teachers, coaches, and extended kin among others. These naturally occurring non-parental adult relationships, often called natural mentoring relationships, typically arise within youth's existing social networks and are characterized by bonds between older, more experienced adults and youth (Dubois & Silverthorn, 2005). These relationships serve as important ecological assets in the lives of youth by providing different yet distinct supports that help to meet youth's varying developmental needs during different stages in adolescence

(Yu & Deutsch, 2019). In this chapter, we refer to youth-adult relationships, or YARs, as ecological or "external" developmental assets because they have the potential to cultivate and support youth's sense of purpose (often considered an internal asset) and positive developmental trajectories across adolescence (Liang et al., 2017; Lund, Liang, Konowitz, White & Mousseau, 2019; Robinson & Glanzer, 2017; Theokas & Lerner, 2006). YARs can serve multiple functional roles in the lives of youth based on youth's evolving academic and socioemotional needs (Arbeit, Grabowska, Mauer & Deutsch, 2019; Hamilton, Hamilton, DuBois & Sellers, 2016). In line with this perspective, previous research has found that one of the functional roles of YARs is providing support for purpose development across adolescence (Koshy & Mariano, 2011; Mariano & Going, 2011). During early and mid-adolescence, adults, particularly parents, can help youth identify "sparks" and "hidden strengths" related to purpose by providing support and opportunities for empowerment during what can be a particularly challenging period of transition (Benson, 2008; Scales et al., 2011). During late adolescence, youth's social networks expand and can include significant relationships with more supportive adults as well as peers which can further aid purpose questing and development (Clydesdale, 2015; Hurd, Stoddard, Sarah, Bauermeister, & Zimmerman, 2014; Robinson & Glanzer, 2017).

YARs cultivate and nurture youth's purpose development through several mechanisms, including the provision of different types of social support and role modeling. YARs provide different types of social support which are associated with increases in youth's academic functioning and self-esteem as well as decreases in youth's behavioral and emotional difficulties (Sterrett, Jones, McKee, & Kincaid, 2011). Specific to youth purpose, Liang et al. (2017) found that adult mentors provide youth with social support including guidance, opportunities, and affirmation for youth's purpose-related decisions and goals. Additional research has found that positive feedback coupled with high expectations from adults help to sustain youth's commitment to their purpose-related goals (Bronk, 2011; Gutowski, White, Liang, Diamonti, & Berado, 2018). In addition to providing different types of social support, adults can influence youth purpose development through role-modeling and serving as exemplars for purpose (e.g., Bronk, 2011; Hamilton et al., 2016; Liang et al., 2017). To provide further insight into the role of YARs in supporting purpose development during adolescence, in the following sections we discuss findings from a study examining the development, characteristics, and influence of youth–adult relationships across multiple contexts and over key transition points across adolescence. Our aim was to explore: (1) in what ways significant non-parental YARs support youth purpose during adolescence, and; (2) how processes of YARs (with both parents and non-parental adults) that relate to purpose development differ between younger and older adolescents.

7.2 The Youth-Adult Relationship Study

As part of the youth-adult relationship study, adolescents (ages 12–17; N = 289) were recruited from a mid-sized Atlantic city through local youth programs, schools, and community settings to participate in a screening survey. A sub-sample of 40 youth (half middle schoolers and half high schoolers) was purposively recruited to participate in five in-depth interviews and surveys over 3.5 years (see Futch Ehrlich, Deutsch, Fox, Johnson, & Varga, 2016 for details). The sample was balanced by gender and criteria used in the purposeful selection process included youth's relational styles (i.e., anxious, avoidant), number of after-school activities youth participated in, number of significant nonparental adults youth reported having in their lives, and youth's socioeconomic background and racial and ethnic identification. We deliberately combined quantitative measures of a variety of internal and external assets and youth outcomes with qualitative exploration of youth's experiences and perceptions and creative methods such as social network mapping and relational graphing. Together, these different data sources provided us with opportunity to explore both outcomes and processes within and across youth, providing a more complete picture of not just the "what" but the "how" of the processes we were studying.

7.2.1 Interview Protocol and Procedures

During each interview time point, youth were asked to nominate a significant nonparental adult (herein referred to as Very Important Adult or "VIP"), which we defined as a "person you count on and that are there for you, believe in and care deeply about you, inspire you to do your best, and influence what you do and the choices that you make" (adapted from Hirsch, Deutsch, & DuBois, 2011). Of the VIPs youth nominated throughout the study, 40.5% were from school settings (mostly teachers and coaches), 26.7% from family settings (extended kin), 6.9% from work settings, 3.9% from community settings (e.g., church, afterschool programs), and 21.7% from other settings (e.g., family friends).

The present study focused on data collected at the end of the study when we asked youth to reflect on their sense of purpose. Youth completed a survey that included the Categories of Identified Purpose scale (Bundick et al., 2006). This scale is intended to provide information about how individuals find purpose in life. The scale includes 17 categories/goals that represent the many possible ways that individuals might find purpose in life (e.g., help others, fulfill my obligations, have a good career). Youth rated the importance of each category/goals to their "purpose in life." Some of the categories (e.g., help others, make the world a better place) in the scale can be used to indicate beyond-the-self (BTS) oriented purpose (purpose motivated by a desire to contribute something to the world). We used this scale as a way for youth to think about their purpose in life prior to their interviews.

During interviews with youth, we showed the list of 17 categories and asked them if there were any particular goals on the list that guide how they think about their purpose in life. To facilitate deeper discussion, we asked youth to choose and describe three that they felt were most core to their purpose in life. Additionally, to help us understand youth's sense of purpose more broadly, we asked about their current goals and dreams and their definition of success. Based on their responses, we asked a series of follow-up questions including their perceptions of purpose-related support from adults in their lives (including parents and VIPs) and their biggest adult influences or role models for their purpose in life over the past few years.

By studying purpose, we in some ways are assuming that the youth in our study are "purposeful." Various definitions of purpose exist in the youth development literature which vary in emphasis on intentional goals that are personally meaningful and/or beneficial to others (i.e., "beyond the self" goals) (Damon, Menon, & Cotton Bronk, 2003; Mariano & Going, 2011). In our study, we consider both dimensions of purpose (i.e., personal and beyond-the-self goals) critical to understanding how adults can best support youth purpose development during adolescence. However, because purpose comes from within and is formed by youth's experiences, interests, and worldview (Bronk, 2014), separate dimensions of purpose may be more salient to youth during different adolescent stages (e.g., Malin et al., 2014). Thus, while we consider both dimensions as important components of youth purpose, we focus more on the mechanisms of support in YARs that help to promote purpose as a general developmental asset in adolescence. By using a common quantitative measure of purpose and following up with qualitative exploration of the content of that measure, we are able to draw on the strengths of quantitative data for assessing magnitude and making comparisons in patterns of magnitude across youth while also understanding the context of those patterns and the processes behind them.

A total of 31 youth participated in this phase of study (n = 18 females, 13 males; ages ranged from 15 to 20). In order to identify differences between youth in mid- and late adolescence, the sample was split into two adolescent age groups: a younger adolescent group (age 16 or below; n = 13) and an older adolescent group (age 17 or above; n = 18). Eighty-one percent of youth reported their racial/ethnic background as White, 14% Hispanic, 6% African American, and 3% multiethnic. Less than 15% were eligible for free or reduced-lunch at school.

We used a process of thematic analysis (Braun & Clarke, 2012) involving multiple researchers to analyze the interview data. First, three researchers individually read each interview transcript. Each researcher then focused on the section of the transcripts related to youth purpose and developed initial codes that appeared interesting and meaningful, while also memoing to begin developing overarching themes within the data. The three researchers then met to discuss initial codes and memos across all the transcripts followed by a more targeted discussion of differences between the mid and late adolescent transcripts. Based on these discussions, a codebook of themes was then applied to each transcript. Researchers met to discuss transcripts and themes where they did not have agreement and came to consensus (Hill et al., 2005). To further illustrate the role of youth-adult relationships, exemplary case studies were selected for each adolescent group. Analysis of case studies involved an examination of data from previous interview time points for the core purpose-related relational processes identified.

7.2.2 Youth's Purpose-Related Goals

Analysis of youth's quantitative ratings of the 17 purpose categories show that overall, youth in our sample gave the highest ratings to personal goals such as "Have fun", "Live my life to the fullest"' and "Be successful." However, youth also rated some BTS oriented goals, such as "Do the right thing" and "Supporting my family and friends" as being important. The latter goal (supporting my family and friends) can be described as a hybrid, spanning "personal" and BTS goals; supporting family and friends goes beyond the youth themselves, but also remains rooted in the youth's microsystem (Bronfenbrenner, 1979) referencing relationships in the individual's immediate settings.

Older adolescents tended to rate all categories of purpose as more important to their overall sense of purpose than younger adolescents did. This likely reflects a developmental difference in how salient purpose is across middle to later adolescence. It may also be related to the broader tasks of goal setting and planning, which have their own developmental processes across adolescence as youth identify, plan for, and narrow down the goals that they pursue and seek to attain in their lives (Massey, Gebhardt, & Garnefski, 2008).

Although during their interviews 29 of the 31 youth named at least one BTS goal as part of their top three goals, older adolescents were more likely than younger adolescents to name multiple BTS goals (11/14 or 79% of older adolescents compared to 9/17 or 53% younger adolescents). Here again, this may reflect developmental differences in the ways in which identity is construed across middle and late adolescence and the increasing importance of thinking about one's self more abstractly and in relation to the larger world as one moves across the stages of adolescence (NASEM, 2019).

7.2.3 The Role of Youth-Adult Relationships in Youth Purpose Development

The following sections present findings focused on the ways in which youth reported the adults in their lives supported their development of purpose. Results regarding themes specific to the role of VIPs in youth purpose are presented first, followed by a section on thematic differences that emerged between the younger and older adolescents in our sample with regards to support from both VIPs and parents.

Support from VIPs. Two overarching themes emerged related to the role of VIPs in supporting or influencing youth purpose development during adolescence:

(1) supporting youth's interests and goals, and; (2) providing social support during key moments in youth's lives.

Across the sample, youth reported that the nonparental adults in their lives provided them with various types of social support, including informational, emotional, instrumental, validation, and companionship. It was common for this support to facilitate youth's personal interests and goals in ways that often related to their sense of purpose. For example, one youth, who wants to be a mechanic in the future, said, "[my VIP] teaches me a lot of stuff. He always answers my questions about cars." For this youth, it was significant that his VIP provided information support (e.g., advice, guidance) for his interest in cars. This interest was a major part of both his current passions and his future life goals, both in terms of a career and how he saw himself as being able to help other people. The fact that youth and VIPs often had shared or similar interests helped youth see their VIPs as sources of informational support related to their goals and sense of purpose.

Youth also talked about receiving instrumental support (e.g. tangible or practical assistance) from their VIPs for their purpose-related goals. This included key opportunities for skill-advancement (e.g., leadership roles) and other education (e.g., college and service-learning activities) and career-related (e.g. internships) opportunities and supports. Youth described VIPs as making intentional efforts to provide these growth opportunities. In some cases, VIPs connected youth with others who were better positioned to support youth's goals and aspirations.

Another way in which VIPs supported youth's interests and goals was through providing youth with validation support (e.g., positive feedback). This could be specifically related to the youth's purpose-related interests and goals. Yet it was also sometimes more general, reminding youth of their strengths and supporting their overall sense of confidence and competence. For example, one youth said "[my VIP] reminds me of what I am good at." We hypothesize that this kind of validation, via its links to self-competence, may potentially foster purpose-related intention and engagement.

An additional aspect of validation support from VIPs involved having "high expectations" for youth. When we asked youth why this was important to them one said, "If you set high standards for people, then they're gonna try to push themselves and push others to do their best as well." It is important to note that setting high expectations for youth doesn't necessarily mean wanting them to be perfect or never make mistakes. Instead, youth described the significance of their VIPs providing them with growth-inducing challenges to practice their skills and at the same time being consistent in reminding them of their strengths and their potential to achieve their goals regardless of how small or big they are. Overall, youth appreciated advice, guidance, opportunities and positive feedback from their VIPs that helped them to better meet their purpose-related interests and goals.

A common theme that emerged from the data, and that we see as providing evidence for the potential of VIPs to support youth's purpose development, is the ways in which VIPs support youth during critical moments in their lives. Youth reported that VIPs provided critical social support during school transitions (from middle to high school, high school to college or to work) and personal hardships such as parent divorces and other times of family conflict (e.g., between youth and parents) and personal distress such as feeling depressed. VIPs were also reported as "being there" during key moments of identity development when youth were pursuing new hobbies or interests, joining new activities, or taking on new roles such as being the lead for a school play or becoming a leader in a school organization. Thus, these adults were present during times when youth were grappling with key developmental tasks. They were available to support youth as they considered the ways in which these transitions fit into and/or shaped their overall life goals, identity, and sense of purpose.

Differences Between Youth in Mid- and Late Adolescence. Given the distinct developmental needs and tasks of youth across adolescence (NASEM, 2019), we were interested to see whether differences emerged between the younger and older adolescents in our sample in terms of how they discussed the role of YARs in their life and sense of purpose. As we analyzed the youth interviews, two areas of difference emerged between middle and later adolescents in relation to: (1) adult sources of support and influence, and; (2) views of adults as role models for purpose.

Younger youth (age 16 and below) as compared to older youth (age 17 and above), were more likely to indicate the significant role of parents as sources of support and influence for purpose development. For example, when discussing who had influenced their goals and sense of purpose and why, younger adolescents made statements such as "My parents have strong expectations" and "I care because of my parents." Living with and consistently being around their parents appeared to influence younger adolescents' perception of their parents' role in the process of purpose development. This is reflected by a youth who said: "I'm around [my parents] every day...there's no one else who would be more influential than them."

Compared to younger adolescents, older adolescents were more likely to emphasize a larger network of support for their purpose in life, including parents but also VIPs and peers. One older youth, for example, said "I get support from bits of different people—not just one person." Similarly, another older youth said, "I think about all the people in my network [as being key influences for my purpose in life], I respect them for what they've chosen to do with their lives and take pieces from each of them."

In line with previous research (e.g., Bronk, 2011), we found that parents and VIPs serve as role models and exemplars for adolescents' sense and development of purpose. Youth reported that the adults in their lives modeled behaviors that they saw as entwined with their own goals and purpose. This included "leading by example" and "practicing what you preach." Indeed, youth often referenced their VIPs and parents as individuals who not only "help and teach others" but also as adults who "walk the talk" with regard to other aspects of their lives such as contributing to their communities and "being happy" and "being content" with their careers and life choices.

There were some differences between younger and older adolescents in our sample, however, in terms of how they described these adult roles. Some younger youth had a more superficial view of adults as role models for purpose. They said things like "because he's the boss of people" and "she makes a lot of money" as key reasons for choosing specific adults as role models for purpose. Older youth, on the other hand, had a more abstract view of adults as role models for purpose. For example, one older youth said, "she is doing something that she feels called to do, her passion." Related to this sentiment, another older youth said, "he seems really happy with what he's doing and he's doing what he loves." In general, younger youth seem to rely on more "material" markers such as the social roles the adults had in their lives and their externally validated accomplishments. Older youth, on the other hand, seem to rely more on "affective" markers, based on feelings and emotion such as "being passionate and happy."

7.2.4   Case Studies of Youth-Adult Relationships in Mid- and Late Adolescence

"Carrie",[1] *female, age 15*. Carrie, a white cis-gender female, identified her top three purpose-related goals as "serve God", "help others" and "be successful." During the interview, Carrie identified "Christine", her Church youth group leader, as a VIP. At the time of her first interview (3.5 years prior), Carrie reported that she had joined the youth-group led by Christine because her parents encouraged her to go to it. With each passing interview Carrie reported feeling closer with Christine. This sense of closeness was facilitated through a series of events that provided a context for their relationship to develop: two mission trips and Carrie taking on leadership roles within the church with Christine's help. As time went on Carrie reported that she wanted to become a youth minister when she grew up. She noted her parents and Christine as being influential in this decision. For Carrie, Christine and her parents all served as ecological assets that facilitated opportunities within settings (e.g., youth-group activities, mission trips, church leadership opportunities) and supportive mechanisms (advice-giving and role modeling behaviors from the adults) which supported Carrie in setting her intention (to become a youth minister) and engage in activities to support that sense of purpose.

"Bodos", *male*, age 19. Bodos, a Black cis-gender male, listed his top three purpose related goals as: "support my family and friends," "make the world a better place," and "be successful". His goals are similar to Carrie's, and other youth in the study, as they combine personal and beyond-the-self goals. Bodos is somewhat unique in our study, however, for his large network of social support; he is well-connected to many adults that he considers VIPs. When discussing the ways in which adults in his life have influenced his sense of purpose, he said "I've learned a lot from a lot of different adults, useful information that I could just absorb to make myself a well-rounded person." The nature of Bodos' relationship with one of his VIP's, Ms. Michael, who was his teacher and theater director, reflected key themes that emerged across youth in the study. At the beginning of our study Bodos described his participation in school plays as playing a key role in his life because

---

[1]All names used in this paper are pseudonyms that were selected by the participants.

it helped to initiate a VIP relationship with Ms. Michael. Importantly, this activity was prompted by Ms. Michael who had Bodos in class, recognized his potential talent, and encouraged him to try theater. Thus, she sparked his interest in theater, which became a large part of his life and identity in high school. Bodos described Ms. Michael as having high expectations and consistently being a large impact on his direction in life. She was instrumental in helping Bodos land lead roles for school plays, attend a prestigious summer high school program, and get into college. Aside from providing these growth opportunities, Ms. Michael supported Bodos' various interests including engaging in conversations about politics and race, which further supported Bodos' future career interest in global affairs. Bodos described Ms. Michael as a great model for purpose because she leads by example and practices what she preaches: "She really cares about the minorities. She supports them and lifts them up." Bodos' relationship with Ms. Michael highlights the role that nonparental adults can play in late adolescence in terms of supporting youth's purpose-related growth and development. Similarly, to Christine for Carrie, Ms. Michael provided Bodos with opportunities to engage in activities (e.g., school play) that allowed him to explore new interests and identities and set and meet goals. Further, their relationship was characterized by a number of mechanisms (e.g., high expectations, educational support, support for interests, and role modeling behaviors) through which Ms. Michael supported Bodos' development of a sense of purpose over time.

7.3 Discussion

The aim of this chapter was to provide insight into how YARs, as ecological assets, support youth purpose during adolescence. In line with previous literature, we found that significant non-parental adults (VIPs) provide opportunities for youth to engage in activities and conversations that foster purpose development during adolescence. Further, these adults can serve as role models for youth. Youth identified different types of social support that they received from these adults, including informational, instrumental, and validation support, that appear to cultivate and nurture youth's purpose-related interests and goals. Further, we found VIPs provide support during key moments in youth's lives (e.g., during school transitions, personal hardships, and key moments of identity development), making them well-positioned to provide purpose-related support during adolescence. Additionally, we found key differences related to the nature of YARs (with both parents and VIPs) between youth in mid and late adolescence including differences in (1) adult sources of support and influence and (2) view of adults as role models for purpose.

7.3.1 Stage-Environment Fit: Youth-Adult Relationships as Ecological Assets for Adolescent Purpose

Stage-environment fit theory asserts that adolescents' socio-emotional and cognitive needs shift as they age (Eccles & Midgley, 1989). Consistent with an ecological view (e.g., Bronfenbrenner, 1979), this theory views developmental contexts as a synergy of multiple, interdependent levels of organization (Eccles & Midgley, 1989). This dynamic process influences adolescent development through their impact on the daily experiences that adolescents encounter as they move through the various contexts of their lives. With regard to youth's purpose development, this perspective provides an important lens for understanding the salience of YARs during different stages in adolescence.

In line with stage-environment fit theory and previous research, we found that youth's relationships with adults (both parents and VIPs) supported youth purpose in a way that "fit" youth's changing social environments in adolescence. For instance, for the younger adolescents in our sample, we found that parents served as an important source of support for purpose. Early in adolescence, parents are very influential, and in many ways still dictate the activities that youth pursue and participate in (Bokhorst et al., 2010). They serve as models of possible roles that youth could take in society and provide youth with opportunities to realize purposeful roles (Malin et al., 2014). On the other hand, older adolescents in our sample reported a larger network of support for their purpose in life which may reflect social changes associated with late adolescence—a time when youth's social worlds broaden and they shift from family embeddedness to greater independence (Arnett, 2004). Youth in our study perceived support from VIPs as being complementary to the support provided from other individuals in their social network. Importantly, VIPs used their unique positions within youth's social network to provide support and opportunities that aligned with youth's purpose in life. This was evident in Bodos' description of his relationship with his VIP, Ms. Michael, who provided him with several growth opportunities throughout high school based on her position in the Bodos' school (i.e., school theater director) and her broader connections in the community.

Social Support in Youth-Adult Relationships. In line with previous research, we found that social support was a key mechanism through which YARs influenced purpose development during adolescence. In previous research (Yu & Deutsch, 2019), we found key differences between younger and older youth with regard to the general processes of these types of social support. For example, compared to older youth, younger youth tend to emphasize the "process" rather than the "content" of informational support from their VIPs. In the case of instrumental support, whereas younger youth noted concrete, practical assistance with "present" tasks (e.g., homework, school projects) or during specific times of hardship (e.g., needing money), older youth noted the importance of support that helped them to "get ahead" (e.g., internships, college recommendation letters). These differences reflect the unique needs of youth during key stages in adolescence including, for example, the importance and need for scaffolding opportunities during early and mid-adolescence and the increasing significance of future-oriented support during late adolescence (Yu & Deutsch, 2019).

These factors may affect the ways in which adult support for and influence on youth purpose shifts across adolescence and what relational mechanisms may be most effective at supporting youth purpose across different developmental stages. For example, adult support may be most effective when they involve scaffolding opportunities to help younger youth identify their "sparks" (Benson, 2008) or specific guidance to older youth as they navigate life transitions and create pathways to adult purpose (Malin et al., 2014). Adult support that takes into account the types and configurations of purpose-related goals across and within adolescent stages may also be helpful. In our study, while all of the youth identified a range of goals, we found that older adolescents tended to endorse more beyond-the-self goals. More specific research on age trends and goal configurations by Johnson et al., (2018) found that while consistent typologies of life goals across adolescent stages (i.e., low endorsement of goals, prominence of helping others and contributing to community goals, prominence of goals related to a good life, and endorsement of most life goals), they identified additional typologies that were only prominent in their older adolescent/young adult samples: a religiously focused group and a social entrepreneurship-focused group. These findings suggest that adults can play multiple functional roles (Hamilton et al., 2016) in youth's lives and that effective support for purpose development during late adolescence might be better served by focusing on youth's narrowing sense of purpose. Further understanding these differences (with regard to adolescents' changing needs and goals) is an important step in providing developmentally appropriate support for youth purpose during adolescence.

Youth-Adult Relationships in Schools and Organized Out-of-School Activities. As youth transition across adolescence, they spend a considerable amount of time in schools and organized out-of-school time activities. In our study, more than 40% of the adults nominated as VIPs by youth were from these settings. As such, a discussion of stage-environment fit is incomplete without considering the role of these settings for YARs and the development of youth purpose. While schools create meaningful opportunities for youth that can support the development of purpose, factors such as lack of adult support, ineffective curriculum, and limited resources impact the quality of these settings and their subsequent engagement of youth (Bronk, 2014; Yeager & Bundick, 2009). This can lead to poor environment fit which can constrain academics, as youth lose access to the resources necessary for success, as well as the ability to construct positive future selves (Clemens & Seidman, 2002). Despite these challenges, a growing body of research suggests that schools serve as important settings that can help cultivate and support youth purpose (see Koshy & Mariano, 2011 for a review). Moreover, research on out-of-school time activities suggests that these settings provide additional opportunities to learn and build important skills and resources, including purpose (e.g., Burrow, Agans & Rainone, 2018; Dawes & Larson, 2011). What is currently lacking in the literature, however, is how to best develop appropriate educational practices to support youth purpose in these settings that align with youth's needs in adolescence. Mariano, Going, Schrock, and Sweeting (2011) found that adolescents whose purpose formation was with either partial ("dreamer" and "dabbler" forms) or nonexistent reported significantly greater support from school and their teachers than did youth with clear purpose ("self-oriented purpose" or "beyond-self purpose" forms). In a study of 4-H youth programs, Burrow et al. (2018) found that intentional activities such as writing about purpose were more beneficial to older youth compared to younger youth. Younger youth had difficulty articulating their purpose while older youth were much more able to describe their intentions, engaging activities, and reasons (beyond-the-self or self-oriented) for their purpose in life. The findings of these studies point to the importance of considering how educational practices designed to support purpose might best align with the varied needs and developmental stage of adolescents. These efforts should take into account different forms of youth purpose during adolescence and youth's readiness to meaningfully engage in educational activities designed to support purpose development. Importantly, it should also take into account youth's relationships with adults in these settings. For many adolescents, adults in these settings signify a stable source of nonparental support. They provide critical support outside of prescriptive curricula including guiding and affirming youth and providing information and key opportunities for youth to reflect and act on their goals and aspirations.

The Important Positions of VIPs in Youth's Ecologies. The finding that VIPs provide support during key moments in youth's lives, when put in the context of previous research on the origins of purpose in life (Kashdan & McKnight, 2009), suggests that VIPs may be well-positioned to foster youth's exploration of purpose. For example, one study by Hill, Sumner, and Burrow (2014) found that, similar to the process of identity development during adolescence, purpose may develop as the result of an exploration process. This process usually follows one of three pathways: proactive, reactive, or social learning. The first pathway, proactive exploration, involves actively seeking out experiences and information related to one's potential purpose. The VIPs that youth talked about in our study often provided support to youth in times when they were taking on new roles and/or joining new activities, thus making it possible for them to support youth's proactive exploration of purpose. The second pathway, reactive exploration, involves youth considering a particular purpose after having a formative experience, such as a parental divorce, or the transition to college, after which the youth begins thinking more strongly about their goals and future directions. Here again, these naturally occurring VIP relationships were often drawn on by youth during transition periods in their lives, which would allow for VIPs to support reactive exploration of purpose. The third pathway is social learning, wherein another person serves as a model for how to live purposefully. In our study, VIPs and parents both served as role models and exemplars for purpose, and youth spoke about the ways in which both observing and speaking with their VIPs and parents taught them about different ways to live out their goals and sense of purpose.

Bi-directional Influences and a Network of Support. Taking an ecological approach to development involves the consideration of complex bi-directional influences between youth purpose and YARs. In this view, both youth characteristics (e.g., needs, goals) and adult characteristics (e.g., roles, attitudes) can influence the quality of YARs and their overall effects. Further, while adults "provide" support for youth purpose, youth seek out and make sense of supportive YARs in light of their budding sense of purpose and may refine their engagement with adults and their sense of purpose in turn. For example, purposeful adolescents who have adults within their families who provide support for purpose, may be less dependent on the resources and support from school-based adults (Mariano et al., 2011). At the same time, youth who have a caring adult outside the home are more likely to talk with their parents about "things that really matter" (Murphey, Brandy, Schmitz & Moore, 2013). In our study, we found that parents initiated and complemented VIP support, and vice versa, in several ways. This was apparent in Carrie's case study where her parents encouraged her to attend a church group which in turn helped Carrie form a relationship with Christine, her VIP, which influenced her sense of purpose. Further, for some youth, VIP support became relevant during critical moments of youth-parent conflict, which at times involved support to help youth mend their relationships.

As youth's sense of purpose becomes more refined, they become more likely to seek out specific individuals who can support the development of that more specified purpose (Moran et al., 2013). This was evident in older adolescents' narratives of "multiple sources of support" in our study which included youth leveraging support from parents, VIPs and peers. Taken together, previous studies and our findings imply that YARs are integrated into a network of social and institutional foundations (Moran et al., 2013) wherein multiple adults serve as connected sources of social support for purpose (Varga & Zaff, 2018). It also suggests that youth themselves are capable of creating environments that enable their own positive development (Benson et al., 2004). Such capabilities can be constrained, however, by structural and systemic issues that create inequities in access to resources across different environments. Additional research is needed to determine how different relationships optimally operate together to provide youth with the developmental supports they need (Varga & Zaff, 2018). Further, because youth are not just passive recipients of support, but active participants in their own development (Koshy & Mariano, 2011), future research should examine how youth's individual needs shape their relationships with significant adults across adolescence (e.g., Arbeit et al., 2019).

7.3.2 Strengths, Limitations, and Directions for the Future

A strength of this study is that we utilized mixed-methods and longitudinal data, and multiple ways of examining the role of adolescent purpose and YARs (e.g., through surveys, interviews, case studies). Further, we examined relational processes of purpose development in two different adolescent periods. Because our study is made up of mostly White and affluent adolescents, and has a small sample size, our findings cannot be generalized to more heterogeneous and less privileged populations. Purpose development and the supports that youth need may vary according to youth's social position factors (e.g., Gutowski, White, Liang, Diamonti, & Berado, 2018; Sumner, Burrow, & Hill, 2018) and thus such factors are important to consider.

However, in the context of the body of research on purpose in adolescence, this study is an example of the ways in which qualitative and mixed methods can be leveraged to deepen our understanding of the processes of purpose development across adolescence and the ecological assets that support those processes. Whereas developmental research has relied heavily on quantitative methods to examine patterns of inter- and intra-individual change over time, combining qualitative and quantitative methods provides unique opportunities to examine those developmental patterns and processes as they occur in context (Tolan & Deutsch, 2015). Further, they provide more nuanced understanding of how youth themselves make meaning of purpose and purpose-related activities and relationships. This is crucial for practitioners who wish to support youth purpose development. Using mixed methods in a longitudinal study provides important opportunities for unpacking both within and between person outcomes and processes over time as both youth's developmental needs, and the contexts in which they are developing, shift. Better understanding of the development of purpose across the span of adolescence for youth from diverse backgrounds will be enhanced by in-depth studies framed by ecological approaches and utilizing multiple methods.

7.4 Conclusion

As the field of positive youth development increases in significance, so too does identifying and understanding the factors that promote thriving in the everyday lives of youth. Among these factors, having a sense of purpose has been considered a developmental asset for youth, one that is predictive of both individuals' outcomes and engagement within the broader community and society. Thus, purpose is a key developmental strength. The potential for positive youth development is promoted during adolescence through the interplay of intrapersonal strengths such as purpose and ecological assets. Utilizing developmental and ecological theories to frame our study's findings and the broader literature on youth purpose, we demonstrate ways in which relationships with parents and other significant adults can play a key role in cultivating and nurturing purpose development during adolescence.

References

Arbeit, M. R., Johnson, H. E., Grabowska, A. A., Mauer, V. A., & Deutsch, N. L. (2019). Leveraging relational metaphors: An analysis of non-parental adult roles in response to youth needs. *Youth & Society*.

Arnett, J. J. (2004). *Emerging adulthood: The winding road from the late teens through the twenties*. Oxford: Oxford University Press.

Benson, P. L. (2008). *Sparks: How parents can ignite the hidden strengths of teenagers*. New York: Wiley.

Benson, P. L., Mannes, M., Pittman, K., & Ferber, T. (2004). Youth development, developmental assets, and public policy. In R. M. Lerner & L. Steinberg (Eds.), *Handbook of adolescent psychology* (2nd ed., pp. 781–814). Hoboken, New Jersey: Wiley.

Bokhorst, C. L., Sumter, S. R., & Westenberg, P. M. (2010). Social support from parents, friends, classmates, and teachers in children and adolescents aged 9 to 18 years: Who is perceived as most supportive?. *Social Development, 19*(2), 417–426.

Braun, V., & Clarke, V. (2012). Thematic analysis. In H. Cooper (Ed.), *Research methods in psychology* (pp. 57–71). Washington D.C.: American Psychological Association.

Brassai, L., Piko, B. F., & Steger, M. F. (2011). Meaning in life: Is it a protective factor for adolescents' psychological health? *International journal of behavioral medicine, 18*(1), 44–51.

Bronfenbrenner, U. (1979). *The ecology of human development.* Cambridge, MA: Harvard University Press.

Bronk, K. C. (2011). Portraits of purpose: The role of purpose in identity formation. *New Directions for Youth Development, 132,* 31–44.

Bronk, K. C. (2014). *Purpose in life: A critical component of optimal youth development.* Dordrecht: Springer.

Bundick, M., Andrews, M., Jones, A., Mariano, J. M., Bronk, K.C., & Damon, W. (2006). *Revised youth purpose survey* (Unpublished instrument). Stanford Center on Adolescence, Stanford CA.

Burrow, A. L., Agans, J. P., & Rainone, N. (2018). Exploring purpose as a resource for promoting youth program engagement. *Journal of Youth Development, 13*(4), 164–178.

Clemens, P., & Seidman, E. (2002). The ecology of middle grades school and possible selves: Theory, research and action. *Understanding Early Adolescent Self and Identity: Applications and Interventions, 133–164.*

Clydesdale, T. (2015). *The purposeful graduate: Why colleges must talk to students about vocation.* Chicago, IL: University of Chicago Press.

Damon, W., Menon, J., & Cotton Bronk, K. (2003). The development of purpose during adolescence. *Applied Developmental Science, 7*(3), 119–128.

Dawes, N. P., & Larson, R. (2011). How youth get engaged: Grounded-theory research on motivational development in organized youth programs. *Developmental Psychology, 47*(1), 259–269.

Deci, E. L., & Ryan, R. M. (2000). The "what" and "why" of goal pursuits: Human needs and the self-determination of behavior. *Psychological Inquiry, 11*(4), 227–268.

DuBois, D. L., & Silverthorn, N. (2005). Natural mentoring relationships and adolescent health: Evidence from a national study. *American Journal of Public Health, 95*(3), 518–524.

Eccles, J. S., & Midgley, C. (1989). Stage-environment fit: Developmentally appropriate classrooms for young adolescents. *Research on motivation in education, 3*(1), 139–186.

Eccles, J. S., Midgley, C., Wigfield, A., Buchanan, C. M., Reuman, D., Flanagan, C., et al. (1993). Development during adolescence: The impact of stage–environment fit on young adolescents' experience in school and in families. *American Psychologist, 48,* 90–101.

Futch Ehrlich, V. A., Deutsch, N. L., Fox, C. V., Johnson, H. E., & Varga, S. M. (2016). Leveraging relational assets for adolescent development: A qualitative investigation of youth–adult "connection" in positive youth development. *Qualitative Psychology, 3*(1), 59.

Gutowski, E., White, A. E., Liang, B., Diamonti, A. J., & Berado, D. (2018). How stress influences purpose development: The importance of social support. *Journal of Adolescent Research, 33*(5), 571–597.

Hamilton, M. A., Hamilton, S. F., DuBois, D. L., & Sellers, D. E. (2016). Functional roles of important nonfamily adults for youth. *Journal of Community Psychology, 44*(6), 799–806.

Hill, C. E., Knox, S., Thompson, B., Williams, E. N., Hess, S. A., & Ladany, N. (2005). Consensual qualitative research: An update. *Journal of Counseling Psychology, 52*(2), 196–205.

Hill, P. L., & Burrow, A. L. (2012). Viewing purpose through an Eriksonian lens. *Identity, 12*(1), 74–91.

Hill, P. L., Burrow, A. L., & Sumner, R. (2013). Addressing important questions in the field of adolescent purpose. *Child Development Perspectives, 7*(4), 232–236.

Hill, P. L., Sumner, R., & Burrow, A. L. (2014). Understanding the pathways to purpose: Examining personality and well-being correlates across adulthood. *The Journal of Positive Psychology, 9*(3), 227–234.

Hirsch, B. J., Deutsch, N. L., & DuBois, D. L. (2011). *After-school centers and youth development: Case studies of success and failure.* Cambridge: Cambridge University Press.

Hurd, N. M., Stoddard, S. A., Bauermeister, J. A., & Zimmerman, M. A. (2014). Natural mentors, mental health, and substance use: Exploring pathways via coping and purpose. *American Journal of Orthopsychiatry, 84*(2), 190.

Johnson, S. K., Tirrell, J. M., Schmid Callina, K., & Weiner, M. B. (2018). Configurations of young peoples' important life goals and their associations with thriving. *Research in Human Development, 15*(2), 139–166.

Kashdan, T. B., & McKnight, P. E. (2009). Origins of purpose in life: Refining our understanding of a life well lived. *Psihologijske Teme, 18*(2), 303–316.

Keels, M., Durkee, M., & Hope, E. (2017). The psychological and academic costs of school-based racial and ethnic microaggressions. *American Educational Research Journal, 54*(6), 1316–1344.

Koshy, S. I., & Mariano, J. M. (2011). Promoting youth purpose: A review of the literature. *New directions for youth development, 2011*(132), 13–29.

Liang, B., White, A., Mousseau, A. M. D., Hasse, A., Knight, L., Berado, D., et al. (2017). The four P's of purpose among College bound students: People, propensity, passion, prosocial benefits. *The Journal of Positive Psychology, 12*(3), 281–294.

Liang, B., Lund, T. J., Mousseau, A. M. D., & Spencer, R. (2016). The mediating role of engagement in mentoring relationships and self-esteem among affluent adolescent girls. *Psychology in the Schools, 53*(8), 848–860.

Lindell, A. K., & Campione-Barr, N. (2017). Continuity and change in the family system across the transition from adolescence to emerging adulthood. *Marriage & Family Review, 53*(4), 388–416.

Lund, T. J., Liang, B., Konowitz, L., White, A. E., & DeSilva Mousseau, A. (2019). Quality over quantity? Mentoring relationships and purpose development among college students. *Psychology in the Schools.*

Massey, E. K., Gebhardt, W. A., & Garnefski, N. (2008). Adolescent goal content and pursuit: A review of the literature from the past 16 years. *Developmental Review, 28*(4), 421–460.

Malin, H., Reilly, T. S., Quinn, B., & Moran, S. (2014). Adolescent purpose development: Exploring empathy, discovering roles, shifting priorities, and creating pathways. *Journal of Research on Adolescence, 24*(1), 186–199.

Malin, H., Ballard, P. J., & Damon, W. (2015). Civic purpose: An integrated construct for understanding civic development in adolescence. *Human Development, 58*(2), 103–130.

Malin, H., Liauw, I., & Damon, W. (2017). Purpose and character development in early adolescence. *Journal of Youth and Adolescence, 46*(6), 1200–1215.

Mariano, J. M., & Going, J. (2011). Youth purpose and positive youth development. In *Advances in child development and behavior* (Vol. 41, pp. 39–68). JAI.

Mariano, J. M., Going, J., Schrock, K., & Sweeting, K. (2011). Youth purpose and perceived social supports among ethnic minority middle school girls. *Journal of Youth Studies, 14*(8), 921–938.

Moran, S., Bundick, M. J., Malin, H., & Reilly, T. S. (2013). How supportive of their specific purposes do youth believe their family and friends are? *Journal of Adolescent Research, 28*(3), 348–377.

Murphey, D., Bandy, T., Schmitz, H., & Moore, K. (2013). *Caring adults: Important for positive child well-being.* Bethesda, MD: Child Trends.

National Academies of Sciences, Engineering, and Medicine. (2019). *The promise of adolescence: Realizing opportunity for all youth.* National Academies Press.

Pianta, R. C., Hamre, B. K., & Allen, J. P. (2012). Teacher-student relationships and engagement: Conceptualizing, measuring, and improving the capacity of classroom interactions. In S. L. Carstensen, A. L. Reschly, & C. Wylie (Eds.), *Handbook of research on student engagement* (pp. 365–386). Boston, MA: Springer.

Robinson, J., & Glanzer, P. (2017). Understanding student purpose types and student perceptions of the influences shaping them. *Journal of College and Character, 18*(2), 83–96.

Scales, P. C., Benson, P. L., & Roehlkepartain, E. C. (2011). Adolescent thriving: The role of sparks, relationships, and empowerment. *Journal of Youth and Adolescence, 40*(3), 263–277.

Spencer, R., Walsh, J., Liang, B., Mousseau, A. M. D., & Lund, T. J. (2018). Having it all? A qualitative examination of affluent adolescent girls' perceptions of stress and their quests for success. *Journal of Adolescent Research, 33*(1), 3–33.

Sumner, R., Burrow, A. L., & Hill, P. L. (2015). Identity and purpose as predictors of subjective well-being in emerging adulthood. *Emerging Adulthood, 3*(1), 46–54.

Sumner, R., Burrow, A. L., & Hill, P. L. (2018). The development of purpose in life among adolescents who experience marginalization: Potential opportunities and obstacles. *American Psychologist, 73*(6), 740.

Sellers, R. M., Copeland-Linder, N., Martin, P. P., & Lewis, R. L. H. (2006). Racial identity matters: The relationship between racial discrimination and psychological functioning in African American adolescents. *Journal of research on Adolescence, 16*(2), 187–216.

Steinberg, L. (2016). *Adolescence* (11th ed.). Columbia, MI: McGraw Hill.

Steinberg, L., & Morris, A. S. (2001). Adolescent development. *Annual Review of Psychology, 52*(1), 83–110.

Sterrett, E. M., Jones, D. J., McKee, L. G., & Kincaid, C. (2011). Supportive non-parental adults and adolescent psychosocial functioning: Using social support as a theoretical framework. *American Journal of Community Psychology, 48*(3–4), 284–295.

Theokas, C., & Lerner, R. M. (2006). Observed ecological assets in families, schools, and neighborhoods: Conceptualization, measurement, and relations with positive and negative developmental outcomes. *Applied Developmental Science, 10*(2), 61–74.

Tolan, P. H., & Deutsch, N. L. (2015). Mixed methods in developmental science. In W. F. Overton & P. C. Molenaar (Eds.), *Handbook of child psychology and developmental science, Vol. 1: Theory and method* (7th ed., pp. 713–757). Editor-in-chief: R. M. Lerner. Hoboken, NJ: Wiley.

Umana-Taylor, A. J., Quintana, S. M., Lee, R. M., Cross, W. E. Jr., Rivas-Drake, D., Schwartz, S. J., … Ethnic and Racial Identity in the 21st Century Study Group. (2014). Ethnic and racial identity during adolescence and into young adulthood: An integrated conceptualization. *Child Development, 85*, 21–39.

Varga, S. M., & Zaff, J. F. (2018). Webs of support: An integrative framework of relationships, social networks, and social support for positive youth development. *Adolescent Research Review, 3*(1), 1–11.

Williams, J. L., Tolan, P. H., Durkee, M. I., Francois, A. G., & Anderson, R. E. (2012). Integrating racial and ethnic identity research into developmental understanding of adolescents. *Child Development Perspectives, 6*(3), 304–311.

Wong, G., Derthick, A. O., David, E. J. R., Saw, A., & Okazaki, S. (2014). The what, the why, and the how: A review of racial microaggressions research in psychology. *Race and social problems, 6*(2), 181–200.

Yeager, D., & Bundick, M. (2009). The role of purposeful work goals in promoting meaning in life and in schoolwork during adolescence. *Journal of Adolescent Research, 24*(4), 423–452.

Yu, M. V. B., & Deutsch, N. L. (2019). Aligning social support to youth's developmental needs: The role of nonparental youth–adult relationships in early and late adolescence. *Applied Developmental Science*, 1–17.

Zimmer-Gembeck, M. J., Chipuer, H. M., Hanisch, M., Creed, P. A., & McGregor, L. (2006). Relationships at school and stage-environment fit as resources for adolescent engagement and achievement. *Journal of Adolescence, 29*(6), 911–933.

Chapter 8
Coming of Age on the Edge of Town: Perspectives in Growing up in a Rural Trailer Park

Katherine A. MacTavish

Abstract The study of the transition to adulthood has emerged as a hot topic research area as an increasing amount of scholarship considers pathways experienced by young people as they come of age. While much of this research has focused on urban and suburban populations, we have seen little attention paid of the experiences of rural youth. This analysis makes use of ethnographic data collected over the course of two decades in rural mobile home park. These data provide a unique opportunity to examine how that developmental context is experienced by young people as they transition to adulthood using a long range rather than point in time view of development.

Keyword Rural youth · Neighborhood effects · Marginality · Ethnography · Purpose development

8.1 Introduction

Upon receiving her second academy award for Best Performance by an Actress in a Leading Role, Hilary Swank declared, "I don't know what I did in this life to deserve all this. I'm just a girl from a trailer park who had a dream. I never thought this would happen." That Ms. Swank should bring up her trailer park childhood and having a dream seems particularly relevant for a volume focused on purpose and context. In the U.S. rural trailer parks or mobile home parks shelter approximately 5 million children and their families (Salamon & MacTavish, 2017). As a developmental context, this neighborhood form continues to be marginalized and all too often maligned by the toxic slur "trailer trash"; one of the last vestige of political incorrectness in our nation (Salamon & MacTavish, 2017). Ms. Swank's notion that having a dream is part of what carried her toward life success fits well with a growing body of research that connects *purpose*—that is, having a future-oriented or life aim goal—to a wealth of positive developmental outcomes (Bundick & Tirri, 2014; Damon, Menon, &

K. A. MacTavish (✉)
Oregon State University, Corvallis, USA
e-mail: kate.mactavish@oregonstate.edu

© Springer Nature Switzerland AG 2020   137
A. L. Burrow and P. Hill (eds.), *The Ecology of Purposeful Living Across the Lifespan*,
https://doi.org/10.1007/978-3-030-52078-6_8

Bronk, 2003; McKnight & Kashdan, 2009). Further, that research has suggested that purpose might develop and act in unique ways among people growing up in marginality (Sumner, Burrow, & Hill, 2018).

This chapter considers the experiences of a group of young people growing up, like Hilary Swank, in a trailer park. The chapter builds on an ethnographic project that examined rural trailer park life among families raising children (ages 8–9 years) and youth (ages 15–16 years old) (See Salamon & MacTavish, 2017). Drawing on longitudinal data collected a decade after the original field study, this analysis is focused on understanding how growing up on the edge of town shaped the developmental pathways of these same young people now in emerging (19–20 years old) and early adulthood (25–26 years old).

8.2   Place and Purpose

Trailer parks or mobile home parks as the families in our work refer to them, or manufactured home communities as the industry prefers function as our nation's leading source of unsubsidized, seemingly affordable housing at a time when the need for affordable housing has been termed a national crisis. Yet, trailer park residence presents families with a series of challenges. Exclusionary zoning regulations legally enforce geographic isolation and locate trailer parks on the edge of town far from the social resources of community and invariably adjacent to a community's least desirable and often toxic features—a waste water treatment facility, ditches or arroyos, train tracks, floodplains, and industrial operations (Ashwood, MacTavish, & Richardson, 2019). With a dense concentration of a community's younger, poorer and less well-educated residents, neighborhood life in a trailer park can be complicated by family experiences with divorce, residential mobility, economic hardships, and drug and alcohol use and abuse (Notter, MacTavish, & Shamah, 2008). And living in a trailer park brings with it the possibility of being socially denigrated merely based on address (Salamon & MacTavish, 2017). Yet, while these challenges are real (MacTavish, Eley, & Salamon, 2006, Salamon & MacTavish, 2006), for families of limited means, owning a singlewide trailer and siting that trailer on a rented lot in a trailer park also works to validate an optimism about achieving some version of the American Dream that would include broader life chances for their children (Salamon & MacTavish, 2017). Parents' financial sacrifices and hard work might in turn motivate precurser forms of purpose among children as they seek to honor their parents' (Moran, Bundick, Malin, & Reilly, 2012).

Rural location and unique features of small-town life bring additional potential developmental benefits for young people (Carr & Kafalas, 2009; Elder & Conger, 2000; Salamon, 2007). Community processes such as the collective investment in raising children seen as everyone's responsibility happen through small overlapping social world in which "everyone knows everyone" (Elder & Conger, 2000). Opportunities to engage in farm and ranch work as well as high visibility clubs, sports and other activities allow youth to make direct contributions to community life (Childress, 2000; Shamah, 2011; Shamah & MacTavish, 2018). Still, rural places vary in inclusive access to such resources (Carr & Kafalas, 2009; Duncan, 2014). A family with a "ne're do well" reputation (deserved or not) or an address on the "wrong side of the tracks" might find small town stigma and exclusion from resources to overcome (MacTavish & Salamon, 2006).

8.3 The Original Study

The original ethnographic study examined trailer park life among families raising children by looking across three distinct regions of the rural U.S.—the Midwest (white), Southwest (Hispanic), and the Mid-Atlantic (Black) (See Salamon & MacTavish, 2017). In each site, we recruited families with children who were 8–9 years of age, and families with youth who were 15–16 years of age. During a full year of field study in each site, we gathered interview and observational data. These data included education, work and family histories across generations along with data about parental and child/youth perceptions of neighborhood and community, future goals, and an accounting of how each respondent saw their lives as having been similar to or different from their parents.

To identify how children and youth were doing developmentally we referenced their parents' aspirations. Trailer park parents readily voiced dreams of assuring their child a way out of socially reproducing their working-poor class status. Statements like that of a mother of two who said, "*I did things backwards. I had kids, then got married and then chose a career. I hope my kids do things the other way around*" and that of a father of four who told us, "*I hope they can all find a job that will give them the income to support a family. I hope they finish school up to and including college. That they don't start a family until they're done [with school]*" revealed parents' hopes. In short, for study parents, success in life or *flourishing* was defined as: (1) a completed education (including some amount of college), (2) stability in career and in relationships, and (3) the avoidance of behaviors that endanger these achievements. Using these criteria, we identified three developmental pathways. We named these *Flourishing, Steady,* and *Floundering* to indicate how young people were positioned to move toward their parent's dreams.

Briefly, young people on a Flourishing pathway displayed academic and social success along with avoidance of problem behaviors, and thus appeared headed toward broader life chances. Young people on a Floundering pathway displayed academic failure, were socially marginalized, and persistently engaged in problem behaviors. These children and youth looked to be headed toward narrowed life chances. Young people on a Steady pathway, those in between, displayed developmental characteristics that led them toward reproducing their parents' class status.

Through a categorical analysis, we then found distinct developmental experiences in context associated with each pathway. Flourishing in middle childhood involved making an age appropriate transition from daily life that centered on the family home to daily life centered on neighborhood. Parents described flourishing children as being "*...out every minute the sun is up*". Deep engagement in the trailer park neighborhood among flourishing children was supported by parents' rules that allow sponsored access to the park. That kind of engagement led to a sense of mastery and ownership over the neighborhood context that was equated by children with knowing their "*...way around this whole trailer park*". In contrast, children on a Floundering pathway were disengaged from the neighborhood context, a pattern structured by parent's rules in response to fear of perceived neighborhood risks.

Flourishing in middle adolescence, in contrast, demanded another step of going away through complete disengagement from the trailer park neighborhood and deep embeddedness in middle-class worlds outside of the park. Flourishing youth, who had at one time been deeply embedded in their trailer neighborhoods as children, spoke about making critical choice in late childhood, to separate from the park. These choices often coincided with a realization of the stigma associated with park life. [more here about stigma] As one flourishing youth explained, "*I don't like living in a trailer park, but really I don't feel like I'm a part of it. I like [town] and that's where I belong.*" Parents of flourishing youth made major investments of time and resources to support engagement in the social world of town. Deep engagement in town offered access to resources like role models and mentors through participation in school, church and town activities. For floundering youth, the opposite was evidenced through withdrawal from the small town and isolation in the social world of the park. Floundering youth spoke about negative experiences with adults and peers in school and in community activities that left them hesitant interact in the small town outside their park.

8.4   The Follow-Up Study

About a decade ago, and squarely ten years after the original field studies, we launched a follow up study of the children (who were 9–10 years of age in our original study and who would at this point be 19–20 years of age) and the youth (who were 15–17 years of age and would at this point be 25–27 years of age). We hoped to examine whether our predictions for their development were accurate and to confirm whether the factors identified as important to producing *flourishing, steady, or floundering* pathways in middle childhood and adolescence persisted across developmental time. Most importantly, did the developmental benefits gained from access to the resourceful contexts of school, church, and small town sustain a positive trajectory allowing young people to further flourish as they made their way toward and into adulthood?

Social media sites like My Space and Facebook proved a means for locating at least a portion of the original samples. At that point, we made contact with seven of the original ten Illinois park youth and six of the original eight Illinois park children. Data collected through phone interviews, emails, and social media profile reviews with the Illinois group allowed us to consider a trailer-park effect with a longer-range view.

Our original analysis identified only one child among eight in the Illinois trailer park as on a flourishing pathway; six others were steady and the last floundering in their middle-childhood period. Among the ten Illinois park youth, two flourished, five were steady, and three floundered in middle-adolescence. This meant that at the age of eight or nine and fifteen or sixteen only three of the eighteen young people in the original Illinois sample appeared headed toward a life offering optimal choices and the chance at social mobility so hoped for by their parents.

Now as they reach their early to mid-twenties, using the same framework to consider developmental pathways, surprisingly we found the distribution changed. Looking first at the older cohort, four were now flourishing, four remained steady, and two continued to flounder. There is a clear shift to more positive trajectories than we originally anticipated for this group. Before we consider how young people stayed on the same positive trajectory, take the following longitudinal vignette of Will as an example of this positive shift.

8.5   Flourishing in Early Adulthood

The last time we spoke, in the spring of 1999, Will looked much like our other steady youth. He was by no means displaying the problematic behaviors that defined the floundering pathways of some park peers, but his grades had begun to slip during his sophomore year, so much so his mother contemplated pulling him out of football. Much of Will's leisure time was spent hanging out with park youth, mostly males, playing pickup ball and cruising the local BMX bike trails. Back then, Will dreamed of becoming a lawyer, yet he had little idea about what was required to make that happen. Will's mother, whose own education ended when she gave birth to Will shortly after her fifteenth birthday, spoke often of Will and his sister going to college, acknowledging it would take a scholarship to finance that goal. In short, despite having a dream, we did not anticipate Will would achieve that dream—he was classified as steady—headed toward reproducing the working-poor trailer park status of his mother.

Now ten years after that last contact, Will and I spoke by phone. I started by asking about the rest of high school. It was immediately evident from his response that he was much more interested in telling me about college. He stated immediately, "I graduated from high school and then went straight to _____ State University." Two years prior, he had completed a B.A. with a double major in history and political sciences having switched his major from journalism. He had since worked as a staff reporter for a small city paper. And come June, he would marry his long-term fiancé. At age of 25, Will had achieved exactly the kind of outcomes his parents and park parents more generally hoped for—he had completed the education he needed to land a stable job, he was involved in a meaningful relationship, and he was avoiding the life choices that might have derailed his dreams. Will then looked to be flourishing in early adulthood.

Like Will, all the Illinois youth who were flourishing in young adulthood had by definition achieved just what their parents outlined as successful development. All four obtained a college degree, were living on their own (not in a trailer park), had experienced successful relationships and were employed in a job that they define as a "step in a career path." In short, they displayed the markers we associate with a positive transition to adulthood (Settersten & Ray, 2011).

As we dug deeper over the next hour of the phone interview, it becomes evident how a combination of family, community, and government supports helped Will move beyond what we anticipated he would achieve. Will talked about his mother and step-father's efforts to stabilize family life through the purchase of a mobile home—their first foray into homeownership; about how his mother made it clear that "college was a requirement not an option." However, while he acknowledges his parents' efforts, he knows that these efforts worked only to place him on the edge of a pathway offering an opportunity toward social mobility. To make that leap to college, Will needed help navigating. He explained, "I was the first in my family to go to college. My parents didn't know anything about that. They didn't know about choosing a college, applying or how to fill out the FAFSA." Will told me of two other supports for his accessing higher education- a church mentor who knew the ins and outs of college (Will actually stayed with this mentor finishing out his senior year after his parents moved away from the area) and government assistance through a Pell-grant and subsidized student loans.

Finally, I asked Will how his life opportunities had compared to his parents and his peers. He told me he thought of his life as, "a lot different" from his parent and went on to explain that they had to deal with their own parents (Will's grandparents) substance abuse issues. Further, he added, "Growing up, my mom was young, her siblings were young when they became parents. Without kids—I don't know. Sometimes, I think I just don't realize the switch [to adulthood]." Comparing his progress toward adulthood with his peers, Will, who saw himself as an adult "in most ways", explained, "Well that depends. If I am thinking about kids from the church [middle class kids], they have had the same gradual transition [with options and opportunities]. For kids from the trailer park—most had kids. Then it was right away because that put them where they have more responsibility [and fewer choices]."

At that point, Will had constructed a social world far from the trailer park that was a three-hour distance by car. He told me he really has had no contact with peers from the park whom he saw himself as having little in common with. He said this is mainly from *"going away when others stayed"*.

This theme of *"going away when others stayed"* was shared by the other Flourishing young adults. The pattern of withdrawal from the park so necessary to a Flourishing pathway in adolescence seemed a necessary condition for flourishing in young adulthood as well. All four young adults located exited the trailer park–three headed-off to college in another town, and the other first joined the military and then attended college in another state. Shared in the stories of these four flourishing young adults was the experience of finding a sympathetic mentor who acted as a bridge to the middle-class world. One found a pastor, another young woman nannied for a middle- class family whom she says, "became more like my family than my real family," even helping to pay for college, and another had a helpful community college advisor. Affiliation with a college outreach program, targeting first generation students, supported two of these young adults as they navigated that new middle-class terrain. Access to financial support through government assisted student grants and loans—something they said their parents did not have—helped all four as well. Only one of the flourishing young adults maintained any connection with the park and in that case the connection was a tenuous tie to a sibling still living in he park.

8.6 Floundering in Early Adulthood

A clear pattern emerges for the Illinois floundering youth sample too. It is a pattern that includes continued isolation from the town, often spurred by perceptions of stigmatization and a corresponding embeddedness in the trailer park, or, in another marginal residential context such as the low rent apartments across the road from the trailer park, or a trailer park in another small town. With options constrained by a limited education and early parenthood, floundering young adults see little hope for altering the trajectory of their lives. In speaking about her work opportunities, one in this group, a high school dropout, explains, "It's been hard. Everything requires at least a high school education or more—college even. The opportunities are really limited. At twenty-seven, I don't see myself getting a college degree."

8.7 Flourishing and Floundering in Emerging Adulthood

A look at the longer-range outcomes of the younger Illinois cohort is also instructive. Using the framework already noted, we originally identified only one of the eight children on a flourishing pathway at 8 or 9 years of age, six on a steady pathway, and one on a floundering pathway seemingly headed toward narrowed life chances. Follow-up interviews with four of the younger group and Facebook contact with another two provided information on six of the eight in the original Illinois child sample. Looking at these young people now at 19–20 years of age, a shift in the distribution among our developmental pathways is apparent—but in a less positive way. Now, *none* appeared on a flourishing pathway with the original one flourishing child having slid onto a steady pathway as she entered adolescence. Six appeared positioned to reproduce their parents' working-poor class status, being steady that is, and another slipped to a floundering pathway.

These young people looked less well positioned to move toward the kind of future their parents envisioned as compared to the older cohort, the youth of the original study. Of the six original child sample, two did not finish high school, and another two finished in alternative programs that took them out of contact with mainstream peers. Only one young woman was living on her own (although a bit young for that to be the norm at this age), the others having bounced back home (often back into the same park) after failed attempts to move out. While most dabbled at coursework in a local community college, only one was enrolled full-time. One alone was working at a full-time job. The others had a marginal work status with part-time jobs largely in the fast food industry. One was looking at parenthood before his 20th birthday. As young people, they seemed to view their situations as interim or as one young woman put it, in a position of *"just waiting to be able to move forward."* They spoke of being developmentally derailed by family crisis including a parents' divorce or in one case sexual abuse by a stepfather. They shared optimism about the future but spoke of plans constrained by limited family resources with comments such as, "My family doesn't have a lot of money. Whatever I do, I will have to do on my own." Although they were not at this stage failures—in trouble with the law or dealing with drug or alcohol abuse—they were not achieving their or their parents' dreams either.

8.8   Reflection

Taking a longer-range view on young people's developmental experiences illuminates social and economic realities that shape the futures available to those growing up in the context of a rural trailer park. Success among the four flourishing young adults makes them in many ways like the *achievers* in Carr and Kafalas's (2011) small town in Iowa featured in their book "Hollowing out the Middle". As rural young adults, they made their way toward an urban future where they are now players in the middle-class arena. But of the remaining six steady and floundering, what Carr and Kafalas might term *stayers*, there is little expectation of their movement away from trailer-park life and their reproduction of their parents' working-poor class status or even downward mobility. Without access to middle class ladders, social mobility remained beyond reach for these youth. The patterns of social mobility we observe in our sample are not unlike those predicted for mobility among the full U.S. population. A recent report titled *Pursuing the American Dream* by the Pew Charitable Trust (2012) estimates that two-third of those raised in the bottom of the wealth ladder will remain on the bottom rungs as adults. For the other third, like our flourishing young people, social and economic mobility is a possibility although an estimate half of these will remain below the median in terms of income.

Given the current economic conditions, there is reason to be concerned about how the steady and floundering young adults will fare. In comparing her life to her parent's, one young woman who has floundered was quick to reply, "It's similar. My mom was pregnant at 17. They had to settle for things with a lack of education. They were responsible adults. They got married and had their own place. They have always lived on their own, always had a roof over head, always had food." Ironically, unlike her parents who had achieved trailer homeownership by age 20, she depended on public assistance [a HUD voucher] to help with rent on her trailer and food stamps to help provision the family. It is interesting to note that her parents now live with her, having experienced a health crisis and subsequent financial downfall that left them without housing.

Perhaps of even more concern are those in the younger cohort who were "just waiting to be able to move forward." To their credit, they had outpaced their parents in terms of educational attainment with high school completion the norm. Most had also avoided early parenthood, a pattern so evident among their parents. Yet they graduated high school at the height of the economic recession, when finding any job was challenging. As steady and floundering young adults they seemed left behind in their trailer-park neighborhood marooned from the opportunity to reach for their dreams.

It might seem that these stories cast a trailer-park neighborhood in a largely negative light. Yet we can see in Will's life history and that of others, attaining the dream of social mobility is a multi-generational project in which mobile-homeownership does play a critically important role in the family histories. The significant turning points in parents' lives that move them away from drug or alcohol abuse and toward more stable family life through the purchase of a trailer, for example, helped position their children for the next steps. Residential stability offered rural working poor and poor children the chance to form lasting relationships with small-town middle-class mentors like a teacher, a coach or a pastor so critical to a flourishing pathway. These small-town mentors, as I have illustrated, functioned as important ladders to social mobility. From this perspective, with each generation making incremental progress, it is not only the fast track achievers who are successful. And I question whether we honor the incremental intergenerational progress needed for mobility.

We can hear that echoed in Will's words as he reflects on what growing up in a trailer park has meant to him. He says, "Part of it, coming from where I did—coming from parents who were on social welfare...for us owning a mobile home was ...my parents had a lot of pride in that ownership. They saw it as a stepping stone to more success. Living there, I think I am predisposed to not assuming things about someone because of where they live. I had things assumed about me because of where I lived."

And in the words of another flourishing young adult: "It did [matter] only in that my family situation was less than ideal. Everything led me here... I mean if my life had turned out different, maybe then I would be more down on my parents. But I think it all made me stronger, a more compassionate person. I guess it gave me perspective. My husband is from a wealthy family where they think having to sell the boat is a tragedy when you need to reduce. My life gave me perspective, instead of always wanting more, I know that no matter what, this is the biggest and best home I have ever lived in."

8.9   Implications and Future Directions

While the work offered in this chapter did not directly focus on purpose, the findings suggest several implications and future directions for purpose research. First, the experiences of white, rural youth within our study shed light on a population still understudied in the purpose literature (Shamah & MacTavish, 2018). Sumner, Burrow and Hill (2018) describe how processes of liminality that stem from marginalization might work to attenuate youths' future thinking. They link this to the experiences of undocumented immigrant youth in the U.S. where purpose development is impeded when youth, faced with so many unknowns, find it difficult to imagine themselves in a future (Gonzalez, Suarez-Orosco, & Dedios-Sanguinetti, 2013). Our finding suggest parallel processes might be happening among low income, white young people coming of age in a rural economy that increasingly demands a college education. Actual and perceived barriers (e.g. money) seemed to discourage the pursuit of dreams. Further, an almost monolithic focus on higher education (that largely demands rural youth *go away* from their home town) versus trade school, for example, deters exploration of more personally meaningful pathways (Corbett, 2007). Additional research centering the experiences of rural, white youth seems needed if we are going to find ways to ensure these young people are not left behind in an economy that offers little means of imagining positive and predictable futures for themselves.

Second, the work offered here adds to questions around the "beyond-the-self" criteria in many definitions of purpose (e.g. Damon 2009). Youth in our study, much like the *Dreamers* described by Moran et al. (2012), adopted life aims motivated by a desire to achieve social mobility. For the small group of flourishing youth, that intention functioned as a "beacon" that motived engagement in behaviors that would support attaining that life aim and avoiding behaviors that might compromise it. While we did not ask specifically about the meaning behind life aims nor did outh articulate any meanings that would map onto beyond-the-self criteria. Perhaps, in the context of a rural trailer park, where managing stigma and overcoming financial constraints demands significant attention, little room is left for exploring loftier beyond-the-self aspects of purpose. That perspective aligns well with Glazier's (2009) review of Damon's work that states: "For most Americans, getting a job of some kind to support a family seems a sufficiently demanding purpose." Conversely, the words of flourishing youth make clear that they recognize how achieving social mobility will honor the efforts of their parents to stabilize family life and ensure access to broader life chances. That kind of focus on honoring family seems to embody a sort of beyond-the-self intention not well recognized in the current purpose literature. Again, additional research exploring possible intergenerational aspects of purpose might help us broaden how we think about beyond-the-self criteria.

Finally, our research adds to thinking about the role of social supports in purpose development. For flourishing youth in the trailer park, parents' encouragements to finish school, make good choices in romantic partners and to avoid mistake they themselves had made worked to set intentions in youth. Parents' investment of time, attention, and financial resources help to support flourishing youths' early effort to psychologically and socially separate from the park and connect them to the right groups that might support their future aims. Support from middle-class mentors proved critical as youth launched toward higher education. These kinds of supports are recognized in the purpose literature (e.g. Moran et al., 2012). Yet these same scholars name that the influence of purpose and social supports is complex. Does having purpose encourage youth to make strategic use of social supports or do those social supports make purpose possible? Our findings suggest both are perhaps true. Further, our findings suggest something else about social support. In going away, flourishing youth left behind social support systems that had been foundational to their success. Yet they continued to proceed toward their life aim and in fact continued to construct additional support networks. This pattern suggests that perhaps it is not only the supports themselves but the transferable skills acquired through accessing social supports that is important to purpose. As suggested by Moran et al. (2012), more research, including in-depth qualitative examination like that of Shamah (2011) might help clarify the complex processes between social supports and purpose.

References

Ashwood, L., MacTavish, K., & Richardson, D. (2019). The legal enforcement of spatial and environmental injustices in rural America. In M. Scott, N. Gallent, & M. Gkartzios (Eds.), *Routledge companion to rural planning*. London: Routledge.

Bundick, M., & Tirri, K. (2014). Student perceptions of teacher support and competencies for fostering youth purpose and positive youth development: Perspectives from two countries. *Applied Developmental Science, 18,* 148–162.

Carr, P., & Kafalas, M. (2009). *Hollowing out the middle: The rural brain drain and what it means for America*. Boston, MA: Beacon.

Carr, P., & Kefalas, M. (2011). Straight from the Heartland: Coming of age in Ellis, Iowa. In M. Waters, P. Carr, M. Kefalas, & J. Holdaway (Eds.), *Coming of age in America: The transitions to adulthood in the twenty-first century*. Berkeley, CA: University of California Press.

Childress, H. (2000). *Landscapes of betrayal, landscapes of joy: Curtisville in the lives of teenagers*. Albany, NY: State University of New York Press.

Corbett, M. (2007). *Learning to leave: The ironies of schooling in a coastal community*. Black Point, Nova Scotia: Fernwood Publishing Co.

Damon, W. (2009). *The path to purpose: How young people find their calling in life*. New York: NY: Free Press.

Damon, W., Menon, J., & Bronk, K. C. (2003). The development of purpose during adolescence. *Applied Developmental Science, 7,* 119–128.

Duncan, C. M. (2014). Worlds apart: Poverty and politics in rural America.

Elder, G., & Conger, R. (2000). *Children of the land: Adversity and success in rural America*. Chicago, IL: University of Chicago Press.

Glazier, N. (2009). *Purposeful youth: Is it asking too much? Education next*. Retrieved from https://www.educationnext.org/purposeful-youth/.

Gonzalez, R., Suarez-Orosco, C., & Dedios-Sanguinetti, M. (2013). No place to belong: Contextual concepts of mental health among undocumented immigrant youth in the United States. *American Behavioral Scientist, 57,* 1174–1199.

MacTavish, K., Eley, M., & Salamon, S. (2006). Housing vulnerability among rural mobile home park residents. *Georgetown Journal of Poverty Law and Policy, 13,* 95–117.

MacTavish, K., & Salamon, S. (2006). Pathways of youth development in a rural trailer park. *Family Relations, 55,* 163–174.

McKnight, P., & Kashdan, T. (2009). Purpose in life as a system that creates and sustains health and well-being: An integrative, testable theory. *Review of General Psychology, 13,* 242–251.

Moran, S., Bundick, M., Malin, H., & Reilly, T. (2012). How supportive of their specific purpose do youth believe their family and friends are? *Journal of Adolescent Research, 28*(3), 348–377.

Notter, M., MacTavish, K., & Shamah, D. (2008). Pathways toward resilience in a rural trailer park. *Family Relations, 57,* 613–624.

Salamon, S. (2007). *Newcomers to old towns: Suburbanization in the heartland.* Chicago, IL: University of Chicago Press.

Salamon, S., & MacTavish, K. (2006). Quasi-homelessness among rural trailer park families. In P. Cloke & P. Melbourne (Eds.), *International perspectives on rural homelessness.* London, UK: Routledge Press.

Salamon, S., & MacTavish, K. (2017). *Singlewide: Chasing the American dream in a rural trailer park.* Ithaca, NY: Cornell University Press.

Settersten, R., & Ray, B. (2011). *Not quite adults: Why 20-somethings are choosing a slower path to adulthood and why it's good for everyone.* New York: Bantam Books.

Shamah, D. (2011). Supporting a strong sense of purpose: Lessons from a rural community. *New Directions for Youth Development, 2011*: 45-58. https://doi.org/10.1002/yd.427.

Shamah, D., & MacTavish, K. (2018). Purpose and perceptions of family social location. *Youth and Society, 50,* 26–48. https://doi.org/10.1177/0044118X15583655.

Sumner, R., Burrow, A., & Hill, P. L. (2018). The development of purpose in life among adolescents who experience marginalization: Potential opportunities and obstacles. *American Psychologist, 73,* 740–752.

The Pew Charitable Trust. (2012). *Pursuing the American dream: Economic mobility across generations.* Accessed online: https://www.pewtrusts.org/~/media/legacy/uploadedfiles/wwwpewtrustsorg/reports/economic_mobility/pursuingamericandreampdf.pdf.

Chapter 9
The Shape of a Life: Gender and Its Influence on Purpose Development

Rachel Sumner

Abstract This chapter focuses on gender as an example of how social identity might contour the purpose development process, including purpose exploration and commitment, and the specific content of people's chosen purpose in life. Enacting gender roles over time can lead to the development of attitudes, skills, and behaviors that are aligned with societal expectations about one's gender, all of which may contribute to individuals' exploration of and commitment to purpose contents that are aligned with gender expectations as well. After outlining potential connections between gender and purpose exploration, commitment, and content, future directions for research are described, including: articulating costs associated with developing purpose in a patriarchal context, integrating intersectionality into research on purpose development, and moving beyond the gender binary to more accurately reflect people's lived experiences developing and maintaining a sense of purpose in life.

Keywords Gender · Purpose in life · Purpose development

> "Maybe we realize: it would have been possible to live one's life in another way. We can mourn because we didn't even realize that we gave something up. The shape of a life can feel like a past tense; something we sense only after it has been acquired." (Ahmed, 2017, p. 47)

How does one's sense of purpose in life take shape? What role does gender play in shaping the experience of cultivating and maintaining a sense of purpose? Much of the existing research on purpose in life fails to acknowledge the ways in which the experience of purpose development might be shaped by gender. Defined as a "central, self-organizing life aim that organizes and stimulates goals, manages behaviors, and provides a sense of meaning" (McKnight & Kashdan, 2009, p. 242), sense of purpose in life can be studied in many ways. Some scholars have focused primarily on the process of developing a sense of purpose in life, with others examining more closely the content of individuals' sense of purpose, and other work investigating outcomes

R. Sumner (✉)
Cornell University, Ithaca, NY, USA

© Springer Nature Switzerland AG 2020
A. L. Burrow and P. Hill (eds.), *The Ecology of Purposeful Living Across the Lifespan*,
https://doi.org/10.1007/978-3-030-52078-6_9

that are associated with having a sense of purpose in life. These three elements—purpose development, purpose content, and outcomes of having a sense of purpose in life—separately or in combination, have served as foundational concepts in the bulk of existing research on purpose in life.

An abundance of this existing research links the development of purpose in life to personal identity (e.g., Burrow, & Hill, 2011; Burrow, O'Dell, & Hill, 2010; Hill & Burrow, 2012), and some work explores connections between sense of purpose and social identities, or the identity groups that people are part of. Examples include studies on disability (Newman, Kimball, Vaccaro, Moore, & Troiano, 2019), ethnicity (Martinez & Dukes, 1997), gender (Pinquart, 2002; Xi, Lee, Carter, & Delgado, 2018), and socioeconomic status (Bowman, 2010; Pinquart, 2002). Given that all aspects of purpose development are experienced by individuals who have social identities and occur in contexts that have attached specific expectations to those social identities, there are many exciting possibilities for researchers interested in contributing to a more nuanced understanding of how social identities shape individuals' experience of developing a sense of purpose in life.

This chapter will focus on gender as an example of how social identity might contour the purpose development process, including exploration and commitment, and the specific content of people's chosen purpose in life. Having been described as "one of the most pervasive and enduring aspects of personal and social identity" (Bussey, 2011, p. 607), gender influences development through individual experiences and the social norms that shape these experiences, making it an interesting example of how social identity might affect purpose development and purpose content. Perhaps most individuals feel a sense of unlimited potential when it comes to their sense of purpose in life; maybe anything seems possible. It may be equally likely that most individuals feel their potential options for a sense of purpose are contoured or constrained by roles and expectations tied to their gender; as Sara Ahmed wrote, "it would've been possible to live another way." The fact that there is so much ambiguity about how people perceive their sense of purpose and their gender together reflects the vast amount of potential that exists for future research on this topic. Though some of the mechanisms and relationships described throughout this chapter might function similarly for other social identities' influence on purpose development, it should be noted that the relevant histories, power dynamics, and political realities of other social identities might affect their connection to purpose development differently.

When it comes to gender, these relevant histories, power dynamics, and political realities have contributed to the adoption and persistence of the gender binary in most of the United States (the cultural context that will be explored in this chapter). The gender binary is the idea that there are two genders and that someone is either a girl or a boy, and, as they age, a woman or a man. Given its prevalence, it is no surprise that the gender binary has seeped into the ways scholars conduct and describe their at earlier points in my time as a researcher, I myself have distributed surveys offering only two options ("woman" and "man") for participants to indicate their gender identity, and, even once I realized that this was a harmful perpetuation of the gender binary, I still excluded from statistical analyses participants who had identified as something other than "woman" or "man" because there were not enough of them to make statistically meaningful comparisons. I am not proud of this, and reflecting on it causes me to think about a quote widely attributed to Maya Angelou: "Do the best you can until you know better. Then when you know better, do better." I know better now, and I am trying to do better, though much of the existing research I cite throughout this chapter has treated gender like a binary. In an effort to accurately reflect the research that was done and not recklessly generalize (e.g., I cannot assume that an empirical finding based on the responses of people who identify as women would apply equally to anyone who does not identify as a man, such as people who identify as non-binary or agender), I will use the terminology used by the authors I am citing.

For example, social role theory is a framework that will be helpful in this exploration of gender's potential relationship to purpose development and purpose content. Social role theory posits that gender roles derived from the division of labor between the sexes include *descriptive* norms that describe how women and men are (Eagly, 2009; Eagly & Karau, 2002; Prentice & Carranza, 2002). Examples of such norms include that women are nurturing (because many are involved in childrearing) and men are providers (because of the expectation that they will work outside the household). Gender roles also include *prescriptive* norms that prescribe how women and men *should* behave, such as women *should be* nurturing and men *should be* providers. Enacting these gender roles over time can lead to the development of attitudes, skills, and behaviors that are aligned with societal expectations about one's gender (Eagly, 1997; Eagly & Wood, 1991; Wood & Eagly, 2002), all of which may contribute to individuals' exploration of and commitment to purpose contents that are aligned with gender expectations as well.

9.1   Gender and Purpose Development

9.1.1   Purpose Exploration and Gender

The process of developing a sense of purpose in life presents a number of potential opportunities for gender's influence. Typically beginning in adolescence, the purpose development process can continue through emerging adulthood and into midlife (Bronk, Hill, Lapsley, Talib, & Finch, 2009; Reker, Peacock, & Wong, 1987). Individuals developing a sense of purpose may engage in active periods of exploration, or considering various options that exist, followed by commitment, or choosing a purpose and working towards it (Blattner, Liang, Lund, & Spencer, 2013; Burrow, et al., 2010; Sumner, Burrow, & Hill, 2015). Three potential forms of purpose exploration that have been described by researchers include proactive exploration, or actively seeking out opportunities to engage with potential purposes in life, reactive exploration, consideration of one's purpose that is spurred by a transformative life event, and exploration via social learning, which involves learning about purpose from individuals who seem to have a clear sense of purpose in life (Hill, Sumner, & Burrow, 2014).

The development of one's sense of purpose in life is an inherently social process that often occurs in tandem with the development of personal identity (Burrow & Hill, 2011; Burrow et al., 2010; Hill & Burrow, 2012). Adolescents rely on the people around them—family, peers, teachers, mentors—to provide opportunities and support for their developing life aims (Bundick & Tirri, 2014; Liang et al., 2017; Malin, Ballard, & Damon, 2015; Moran et al., 2012). Even among adolescents experiencing various stressors that could present an obstacle to the development of this psychological asset, receiving social support from friends, teachers, parents, and/or employers was helpful (though not essential) to those who had cultivated a sense of purpose (Gutowski et al., 2018). The development of oneself as a gendered person is also inherently social, involving interactions between individuals and their parents, peers, culture, and media (Bussey, 2011; Eagly, 1997; Stockard, 1999). Although people do exercise agency in choosing and shaping their own environments and interactions (Bussey, 2011), these experiences and interactions are situated within societies that present social norms about how women and men are and should be (e.g., Eagly, 1997, 2009; Prentice & Carranza, 2002).

Given that purpose exploration takes place in a societal context replete with identity-related norms and expectations (Bronfenbrenner, 1977), it is easy to imagine how those norms and expectations applied to individuals of a particular gender could shape both the range and type of options that they explore. The sad reality is that people can experience severe consequences for pursuing long-term aims within communities that are not seen as being "for them," even if membership in that community is personally meaningful and could otherwise yield a sense of purpose in life. Imagine someone who identifies as a gamer and feels passionately about exploring a life of professional gaming, suspecting that this might culminate in a sense of purpose for them; within the online gaming community, where women are "harassed, threatened, and driven out," punished for "claiming voice, power, and the right to participate" (Solnit, 2014, p. 31), it seems that purpose exploration would be easier and more enjoyable for boys and men. Gender does not preclude anyone from exploring a sense of purpose in life connected to gaming and the online gaming community, but it is easy to imagine that one's experience of exploration in such a highly gendered context would be shaped by one's gender.

Expectations related to gender that exist in society also manifest in the home. There is evidence that adolescents are sensitive to the expectations of the adults who support their ongoing purpose development (Gutowski, White, Liang, Diamonti, & Berado, 2018), and these expectations could conceivably shape the contents of purposes that young people are encouraged to explore (or avoid). For example, a boy whose long-term aim is to help others may not thoroughly explore nursing as a potential way to enact his purpose in life if his family members say denigrating things about men who work as nurses, decline to provide him transportation to relevant opportunities that would enable him to learn more about nursing, and withhold emotional support related to his curiosity about nursing. In this hypothetical example, a child's exploration of his options related to purpose in life are being shaped by the expectations that others are applying to him because of his gender.

9.1.2   Purpose Commitment and Gender

As described at the beginning of this section, purpose exploration can culminate in the commitment to a purpose in life, and the sense of purpose fostered by this commitment has been linked to a number of positive outcomes related to psychological and physical health (e.g., Burrow, Sumner, & Ong, 2014; Hill, Jackson, Roberts, Lapsley, & Brandenberger, 2011; Hill & Turiano, 2014). Despite the obvious ways that identity-related norms and expectations might alter one's experience of purpose exploration, it remains unclear whether and how these societal pressures manifest in gender differences for overall sense of purpose in life.

Patterns in purpose-related gender differences vary across studies looking at sense of purpose. For example, Pinquart's (2002) meta-analysis revealed gender differences in sense of purpose *only* among the older subsample (70 years old or older), with males having slightly higher levels of purpose in life. This finding may be due to age differences, cohort effects, or a combination thereof; as gender expectations change over time, so too might their potential impacts on individuals' experience of purpose exploration and commitment. Burrow, Stanley, Sumner, and Hill (2014) found a correlation between gender and sense of purpose in a sample of adults, with male participants tending to have higher scores on a measure of purpose in life. Other research using a sample of adults found significant gender differences in reported sense of purpose in life, though in this study the female participants had significantly higher levels of purpose (Xi et al., 2018). A similar pattern, with women demonstrating greater sense of purpose in life, emerged in a different sample of midlife and older adults (Bundick, Remington, Morton, & Colby, 2019; assessing purposes that are oriented beyond oneself) and a sample of college students (Bowman, 2010). There are also studies that have found no significant relationship between gender and sense of purpose in life (e.g., Burrow, O'Dell, & Hill, 2010; Burrow & Rainone, 2017; Ko, Hooker, Geldhof, & McAdams, 2016), so it remains difficult to ascertain whether purpose commitment is generally characterized by gender differences or, as with many other things, gender similarity (Hyde, 2005). Even if persistent gender differences in scores of overall sense of purpose did emerge, the evolving nature of gender norms requires that researchers remain vigilant to potential changes in outcomes that might be affected by the prevalence and content of such norms; as suggested above, it could be the case that cohort and/or age effects are contouring the ways in which people of all genders are able to explore options and commit to a personally meaningful sense of purpose in life.

9.2   Gender and Purpose Content

There are myriad possibilities for purpose content, or which specific aim one commits to in order to derive a sense of purpose in life. Some contents can be grouped together based on their thematic similarity; striving for racial justice, trying to improve the environment, and helping others are different specific contents, but could all be described as having a prosocial orientation. Scholars have recognized four broad purpose orientations: prosocial, creative, financial, and personal recognition (Hill, Burrow, Brandenberger, Lapsley & Quaranto, 2010). The prosocial orientation is "defined by one's propensity to help others and influence the societal structure," financial orientation is "defined by goals of financial well-being and administrative success," creative orientation is "defined by artistic goals and a propensity for originality," and the personal recognition orientation is "defined by one's desire for recognition and respect from colleagues" (Hill, Burrow, Brandenberger, Lapsley, & Quaranto, 2010a, p. 174). There are obviously purposes that do not fall clearly into one of these existing overarching purpose orientations, but these four broad categories will be used to structure the following discussion of potential links between gender and purpose content, in order to connect to the previous research. For three of the four broad purpose orientations that have been studied in previous research, there are clear hypotheses about potential purpose-related gender norms informed by the existing literature, each of which is described below.

Stereotypes and social expectations associate women with communal, prosocial behaviors (Eagly & Karau, 2002; Eagly & Wood, 1991; Evans & Diekman, 2009), and this perceived link exists even among those as young as elementary school students (Heyman & Legare, 2004). Across numerous cultures, women do place greater value on prosociality than men do (e.g., Schwartz & Rubel, 2005; Xi et al., 2018) and they rate community involvement as a more important aspiration than men do (Kasser & Ryan, 1993). Internalizing this communal gender role is linked to the endorsement of goals and careers that involve caregiving and being social (Evans & Diekman, 2009; Roberts & Robins, 2000). Xi et al. (2018) found that women were more likely to endorse behaviors and attitudes consistent with altruism, and this difference explained much of the gap between their self-reported levels of sense of purpose in life and the relatively lower levels of sense of purpose reported by men. Additionally, a study of civic-oriented purposes found an association between gender and purposes focused on community service (Malin et al., 2015). With women being seen as more communal and prosocial in their behavior and their placing more importance on values or aspirations in this domain, a logical hypothesis is that people in the United States would have a descriptive gender norm linking women with prosocial purpose orientations.

Social behavior and expectations for men revolve more around agentic attributes, such as self-sufficiency, ambition, and acting as a leader (Eagly & Karau, 2002). Men tend to rate values related to power significantly higher than women do (Schwartz & Rubel, 2005), and they see themselves as being more agentic (Evans & Diekman, 2009). When asked to read about three powerful roles (such as politician or CEO), undergraduate men rated the positions more positively than women did, and importantly, as more possible for themselves (Lips, 2000). Men also see financial success as being important and more likely for themselves (Kasser & Ryan, 1993; Roberts & Robins, 2000), and when asked to define purpose in life, adolescent boys were more likely than their girl peers to include financial and/or occupational elements in their definitions (Hill, Burrow, O'Dell, & Thornton, 2010). Gendered expectations of men link them to power and financial success, leading to the hypothesis that people in the United States would perceive men as likely to pursue purposes related to personal recognition and financial orientation.

The purpose orientation related to creative pursuits is less conducive to formulating a clear hypothesis. Previous research on gender and creativity has been mixed, with studies finding that its relationship to gender depends on the kind of creativity task being assessed (Stoltzfus, Nibbelink, Vredenburg, & Hyrum, 2011) or the domain in which one is being creative (e.g., visual-artistic or science-analytic) (Kaufman, 2006). One study investigating gendered perceptions of creativity asked participants to rate poems for which the author's name was traditionally gendered as typically being a woman's name or a man's name. Perceived author gender did not significantly affect participants' ratings of the poem's creativity, suggesting that people do not hold strong views about one gender being more creative than the other (Kaufman, Baer, Agars, & Loomis, 2010). Thus, it is more difficult to make a clear prediction regarding gendered perceptions of the creative purpose orientation in the United States.

The findings described above convey a certain level of clarity about gender differences in self-reported goal endorsement and perceived gender differences in communal and agentic traits. Moving into more speculative territory, I think these findings suggest that descriptive norms related to purpose content (i.e., "women do pursue prosocial purposes...") exist. If so, then social role theory posits that they are accompanied by parallel prescriptive norms (i.e., "women *should* pursue prosocial purposes...") (Eagly, 2009). There are social incentives for behaving in ways that are consistent with the social norms and expectations of one's gender (Bussey, 2011; Eagly & Karau, 2002), so, if the hypothesized descriptive norms related to purpose content exist, girls and women might anticipate and/or encounter fewer social barriers if they pursue a prosocial purpose, while boys and men might find it more socially acceptable to work towards a purpose that is oriented towards personal recognition or financial success. Though there is evidence that gender is related to whether the content of one's purpose is directed towards oneself or others, with females overrepresented among those whose purpose is other-oriented (Bronk & Finch, 2010), existing research on purpose content has failed to acknowledge the ways in which gender norms might impinge on individuals' perceived or actual freedom to pursue *any* purpose.

9.3   Three Future Directions in the Study of Gender Identity and Purpose in Life

How much *do* people feel free to pursue any purpose, regardless of gendered expectations? This is one of many research questions spurred by the simultaneous consideration of gender identity and purpose in life. Below, I will highlight three future directions for research on the relationship between gender identity and purpose in life (both its development and overall sense): articulating costs associated with developing purpose in a patriarchal context, integrating intersectionality into research on purpose development, and moving beyond the gender binary to more accurately reflect people's lived experiences developing and maintaining a sense of purpose in life. I am highlighting these not because they are the most important or the most urgent (though I believe they are important and urgent), but because I think these directions would help scholars more thoroughly connect the experience of purpose in life to the cultural, historical, and individual contexts in which it is developed and pursued.

9.3.1   Pursuing Purpose in a Patriarchal Context

The prevalence of stereotypes and gender norms linking communal values and behaviors to women while agentic values and behaviors are linked to men is one manifestation of the patriarchy in contemporary American society. This system centers the experience of men and facilitates their access to power and, as is true of any hierarchical system with entrenched and systematic inequities, it "has profound ramifications that influence and limit how we think about ourselves and others, how and with whom we interact, and the opportunities and choices we have about how to lead our lives. Although in some instances there are positive effects, there are costs and harmful consequences for all of us, though in different ways" (Goodman, 2001, p. 103). Some of these positive effects and costs can be expected to emerge in the purpose development process if, as I have postulated, there are descriptive and prescriptive gender norms related to purpose contents. The positive effects and costs will differ, however, depending on one's gender and whether the content of one's purpose in life is consistent with gendered expectations.

For those pursuing a purpose content consistent with what is expected of their gender, people who identify as men might experience benefits stemming from purposes aimed at financial success and/or personal recognition. In a study looking at the connection between having a sense of purpose in life and both income and net worth, Hill, Turiano, Mroczek, and Burrow (2016) found that gender did not moderate the positive relationship between purpose and financial outcomes. That study considered overall sense of purpose in life as the predictor, however, and it seems likely that a study investigating income and net worth across different purpose contents would yield differences between those who aim for financial success and those who aim to help others. The benefits accruing to people who identify as women and pursue prosocial purposes are less likely to be financial and more likely to be psychological: indeed, Xi et al. (2018) found that women's greater endorsement of altruistic behaviors and attitudes fostered their having a stronger sense of purpose in life, and being committed to a purpose is associated with a host of benefits, including higher levels of positive affect, life satisfaction, self-esteem, and happiness (Kiang & Fuligni, 2010; Paradise & Kernis, 2002; Sumner et al., 2015).

The existence of hierarchical gender expectations might interfere with individuals' ability to identify and pursue a personally meaningful sense of purpose in life. For example, recent research found that, among undergraduate men, endorsing a masculine norm of power was negatively related to their psychological well-being (a measure that includes a subscale capturing sense of purpose in life) (Kaya, Iwamoto, Brady, Clinton, & Grivel, 2019). If the decision to pursue a life aim of financial success or personal recognition is driven by a belief that men should be powerful, then that purpose may not ultimately be personally meaningful and therefore not associated with the host of benefits typically experienced by people with a sense of purpose in life.

Because the norms associated with gender roles can act as a social mechanism that shapes behavior, the existence of gender-related norms attached to different purpose contents could also have serious implications for those whose desired purpose conflicts with what is expected of them. One recent piece of evidence that speaks to this possibility is a study of undergraduate men in the United States which found that greater gender role conflict was linked to lower scores on measures of psychological well-being, including autonomy, environmental mastery, personal growth, positive relationships, self-acceptance, and purpose in life (Cole et al., 2019). Indeed, those authors suggest that "one possibility is that gender role conflict makes more difficult to work toward self-determined goals when these goals are inconsistent with traditional masculine norms" (Cole et al., 2019, p. 9). Individuals who violate expectations experiencing social consequences for doing so, such as female leaders who violate the expectation that women are more communal than agentic and are therefore seen as less likable and less effective as leaders (Eagly & Karau, 2002; Heilman & Okimoto, 2007). It is therefore plausible that those experiencing tension between a purpose in life that feels authentic to them and the purpose that might be expected of them based on their gender may disengage from the purpose development process altogether, leading to lower levels of commitment to a sense of purpose and, presumably, less access to the host of beneficial outcomes associated with purpose commitment.

9.3.2 Intersectionality and Purpose in Life

It stands to reason that variation between individuals who share a social identity can lead to differences when it comes to cultivating and enacting one's sense of purpose. For example, within a group of people who identify as women there could be differences in the strength of one's belief in the gendered nature of purpose, one's endorsement of traditional gender roles, and one's commitment to the gender binary, all of which could be expected to contour the purpose development process. People who share a social identity might also have different experiences developing their sense of purpose in life because they do not have *all* of the same social identities in common. Individuals hold multiple social identities, each of which is connected to a broader societal system of power and, in combination, these identities and systems of power shape their experiences in life (e.g., Crenshaw, 1991). For example, researchers have suggested that "Girls, in particular, must sometimes go against their ethnic traditions and family expectations to be involved in civic activities" (Malin et al., 2015, p. 121), highlighting that gender might interact with ethnicity to shape purpose exploration, commitment, and content.

When asked to describe themselves, people often provide answers that reflect their numerous social identities (e.g., race, gender, socioeconomic status) (Rogers, this volume; Way & Rogers, 2015), and acknowledging the intersectional nature of identities in future work on gender and purpose development could yield findings that more closely reflects individuals' lived experiences. How do social identities, in combination, shape which purpose contents feel possible and which are actually attainable? For example, some people cultivate a sense of purpose in life related to having and caring for a family; is a purpose in life oriented around family equally accessible to everyone, regardless of gender and other social identities? Thirteen percent of workers in the United States have access to paid parental leave (U.S. Department of Labor, 2014), so the intersection between socioeconomic status and gender likely informs decisions about who pursues a purpose in life that entails being a parent and having a job. For those whose sense of purpose in life includes being a parent to adopted children, gender status and gender identity may combine to inform whether and how to pursue that purpose: in forty-four states transgender applicants seeking to adopt or foster children are "vulnerable to extra scrutiny or denial simply for being transgender" (Lambda Legal, n.d.). There are huge racial discrepancies in pregnancy-related deaths, with African-American, Alaska Native, and Native American women dying at a rate approximately three times higher than white women (Rabin, 2019), so the intersection of race and gender may inform whether and how someone pursues a sense of purpose that involves birthing children.

Previous research suggests other specific combinations of social identities that, when considered simultaneously, can also elucidate important features underlying the development and pursuit of one's sense of purpose in life. For example, age, gender, and highest level of education seem to interact in ways that contour the purpose development process. Adolescence and emerging adulthood are developmental periods that are well-suited to exploring one's options for a purpose in life (Arnett, 2000; Bronk et al., 2009), so it may be that if gender differences exist among people in these age groups, they would be more likely to manifest in experiences of purpose exploration rather than commitment or content. Even within emerging adults, there may be different patterns that emerge between those who are in college and those who are not: college students' responses tend to be more similar to each other's than responses collected from adult samples (Peterson, 2001) and gender differences in values among college student samples tend to be smaller than those in community samples (Schwartz & Rubel, 2005). Women college students, in particular, tend to be more similar to men (both in college and out) than women who are not in college. Whether this is due to self-selection bias (women with more "masculine" values choosing to go to college) or a process of homogenization that occurs during college remains unclear, but it suggests that scholars interested in understanding connections between gender and purpose development in emerging adulthood should be mindful of the role that education status can play in shaping these outcomes. Gender differences in purpose commitment or content may be most likely to emerge among adult samples because individuals in this age range have likely had more time to work towards a particular purpose, specializing in one thing over others, which might cause small differences that exist earlier in life to become larger over time. In particular, the financial and personal recognition purpose orientations may be difficult to actualize in high school or college, so any potential gender differences in endorsement of these purpose orientations could be hard to detect before adulthood.

9.3.3 Moving Beyond the Gender Binary

Once we start considering the patriarchy's role in shaping purpose development, we will have to start questioning some of the assumptions that underlie and uphold this system. "The insistence that there is a naturally biologically based world of sex differences is at the heart of patriarchal thinking," (hooks, 2003, p. 83), as is the insistence that there are only two genders: women and men. There are compelling reasons for the psychological literature to move beyond the rigid binary conception of gender, with existing work in neuroscience, behavioral neuroendocrinology, and psychology offering legitimate challenges to the gender binary and raising necessary questions about its role in future research (outlined beautifully by Hyde, Bigler, Joel, Tate, & van Anders, 2019). If scholars are interested in creating an accurate and comprehensive research literature on purpose development and outcomes linked to having a sense of purpose in life, then we cannot include in our studies *only* people who identify as either a girl/woman or a boy/man and we must ask research questions about gender that do not limit the experience of it to only one or the other.

   I am concerned that the potential connections between gender identity and purpose development I have described throughout this chapter may be taken as a manifestation of gender fatalism which, as described by Sara Ahmed, "rests on ideas about nature as well as time; what 'will be' is decided by 'what is'" (2017, p. 25). Adherents to the gender binary might read this chapter and find themselves wondering about how being a woman or being a man contours one's experience of purpose development. I am not claiming that people of any gender are destined to pursue a specific type of purpose because of their gender identity. I am hoping that readers find themselves wondering about gender in a broader sense, encapsulating the ways in which the experience of gender in the United States—being socialized in a patriarchal culture that reinforces a gender binary and has clear norms about who is (and who should be) agentic or communal—might be affecting the ways that individuals explore their options for a purpose, whether they commit to a sense of purpose in life, and what purpose content they choose to pursue. As people cultivate and maintain their sense of purpose in life, what are the implications of doing so in a context where people of their gender are not often portrayed as powerful and rational? What are the implications of developing purpose in a context where they rarely interact with people of their gender doing caregiving work? What are the implications for their purpose development to grow up in a context where they see very few people of their gender represented at all?

In addition to catalyzing new research questions, a commitment to moving beyond the gender binary might spur the reconsideration of questions that have already been explored. There are demonstrated links between religious or spiritual practice to sense of purpose in life (e.g., Rosenkrantz, Rostosky, Riggle, & Cook, 2016), but Hopwood (2019) notes "that there is a paucity of data to fully understand the direct impact of religion and spirituality on gender-diverse populations of any specific age group" (p. 131). While religious and spiritual involvement in other populations has been associated with a deeper sense of purpose in life (Rosenkrantz et al., 2016), Hopwood (2019) describes unique challenges that may complicate the relationship between religion/spiritualty and purpose in life for gender-diverse individuals, including the risk of being rejected from a place where one had previously felt a sense of belonging and feeling distress upon experiencing discrimination stemming from specific religious messages or communities that reject transgender and non-binary people.

9.4   Conclusion

There are many opportunities to pose novel research questions and revisit former questions with a more inclusive lens, and there is an abundance of existing work on which to build a more comprehensive picture of purpose development. It is clear that having a sense of purpose in life can be beneficial to one's physical and psychological well-being (e.g., Burrow et al., 2014b; Hill et al., 2011; Hill & Turiano, 2014) and that researchers are increasingly interested in understanding how social identities might affect individuals' experience of the purpose development process (e.g., Cole et al., 2019; Newman et al., 2019; Sumner, Burrow, & Hill, 2018). This chapter has outlined some potential connections between one social identity—gender—and purpose exploration, commitment, and content, in addition to some specific considerations for future research on the topic. Existing research on gender provides clear frameworks for investigating how this social identity may be shaping the development of this psychological asset and, as "one of the most pervasive and enduring aspects of personal and social identity" (Bussey, 2011, p. 607), gender and its influence could easily become more pervasive in research on purpose exploration, commitment, and content. As we continue to conduct research, let's not mourn because we gave up a comprehensive understanding of how social identities shape the experience of purpose development; it is possible to live in another way.

References

Ahmed, S. (2017). *Living a feminist life*. Durham, NC: Duke University Press.

Arnett, J. J. (2000). Emerging adulthood. A theory of development from the late teens through the twenties. *American Psychologist, 55,* 469–480.

Beal, S. J., & Crockett, L. J. (2010). Adolescents' occupational and educational aspirations and expectations: Links to high school activities and adult educational attainment. *Developmental Psychology, 46,* 258–265.

Blattner, M. C., Liang, B., Lund, T., & Spencer, R. (2013). Searching for a sense of purpose: The role of parents and effects on self-esteem among female adolescents. *Journal of Adolescence, 36,* 839–848.

Bowman, N. A. (2010). The development of psychological well-being among first-year college students. *Journal of College Student Development, 51,* 180–200.

Bronfenbrenner, U. (1977). Toward an experimental ecology of human development. *American Psychologist, 32,* 513–531.

Bronk, K. C. (2008). Humility among adolescent purpose exemplars. *Journal of Character Education, 6,* 35–51.

Bronk, K. C. (2011). The role of purpose in life in healthy identity formation: A grounded model. *New Directions for Youth Development, 132,* 31–44.

Bronk, K. C., & Finch, W. H. (2010). Adolescent characteristics by type of long-term aim in life. *Applied Developmental Science, 14,* 35–44.

Bronk, K. C., Hill, P. L., Lapsley, D. K., Talib, N., & Finch, H. (2009). Purpose, hope, and life satisfaction in three age groups. *Journal of Positive Psychology, 4,* 500–510.

Bundick, M. J., Remington, K., Morton, E., & Colby, A. (2019). The contours of purpose beyond the self in midlife and later life. *Applied Developmental Science.* https://doi.org/10.1080/10888691.2018.1531718.

Bundick, M. J., & Tirri, K. (2014). Student perceptions of teacher support and competencies for fostering youth purpose and positive youth development: Perspectives from two countries. *Applied Developmental Science, 18,* 148–162.

Burrow, A. L., & Hill, P. L. (2011). Purpose as a form of identity capital for positive youth adjustment. *Developmental Psychology, 47,* 1196–1206.

Burrow, A. L., O'Dell, A. C., & Hill, P. L. (2010). Profiles of a developmental asset: Youth purpose as a context for hope and well-being. *Journal of Youth and Adolescence, 39,* 1265–1273.

Burrow, A. L., & Rainone, N. (2017). How many likes did I get?: Purpose moderates links between positive social media feedback and self-esteem. *Journal of Experimental Social Psychology, 69,* 232–236.

Burrow, A. L., Stanley, M., Sumner, R., & Hill, P. L. (2014a). Purpose in life as a resource for increasing comfort with ethnic diversity. *Personality and Social Psychology Bulletin, 40,* 1507–1516.

Burrow, A. L., Sumner, R., & Ong, A. D. (2014b). Perceived change in life satisfaction and daily negative affect: The moderating role of purpose in life. *Journal of Happiness Studies, 15,* 579–592.

Bussey, K. (2011). Gender identity development. In S. J. Schwartz, K. Luyckx, & V. L. Vignoles (Eds.), *Handbook of identity theory and research* (pp. 603–628). New York: Springer.

Cole, B. P., Baglieri, M., Ploharz, S., Brennan, M., Ternes, M., Patterson, T., et al. (2019). What's right with men? Gender role socialization and men's positive functioning. *American Journal of Men's Health, 13*(1), 1557988318806074. https://doi.org/10.1177/1557988318806074.

Crenshaw, K. (1991). Mapping the margins: Intersectionality, identity politics, and violence against women of color. *Stanford Law Review,* 1241–1299.

Eagly, A. H. (1997). Sex differences in social behavior: comparing social role theory and evolutionary psychology. *American Psychologist, 52,* 1380–1383.

Eagly, A. H. (2009). The his and hers of prosocial behavior: an examination of the social psychology of gender. *American Psychologist, 64*(8), 644.

Eagly, A. H., & Karau, S. J. (2002). Role congruity theory of prejudice toward female leaders. *Psychological Review, 109,* 573–598.

Eagly, A. H., & Wood, W. (1991). Explaining sex differences in social behavior: A meta- analytic perspective. *Personality and Social Psychology Bulletin, 17,* 306–315.

Evans, C. D., & Diekman, A. B. (2009). On motivated role selection: Gender beliefs, distant goals, and career interest. *Psychology of Women Quarterly, 33,* 235–249.

Goodman, D. J. (2001). The costs of oppression to people from privileged groups. *Promoting diversity and social justice: Educating people from privileged groups* (pp. 103–125). Thousand Oaks: Sage.

Gutowski, E., White, A. E., Liang, B., Diamonti, A. J., & Berado, D. (2018). How stress influences purpose development: The importance of social support. *Journal of Adolescent Research, 33,* 571–597.

Heilman, M. E., & Okimoto, T. G. (2007). Why are women penalized for success at male tasks? The implied communality deficit. *Journal of Applied Psychology, 92,* 81–92.

Heyman, G. D., & Legare, C. H. (2004). Children's beliefs about gender differences in the academic and social domains. *Sex Roles, 50,* 227–239.

Hill, P. L. & Burrow, A. L. (2012): Viewing purpose through an Eriksonian lens. *Identity: An International Journal of Theory and Research, 12,* 74–91.

Hill, P. L., Burrow, A. L., Brandenberger, J. W., Lapsley, D. K., & Quaranto, J. C. (2010). Collegiate purpose orientations and well-being in early and middle adulthood. *Journal of Applied Developmental Psychology, 31*(2), 173–179.

Hill, P. L., Jackson, J. J., Roberts, B. W., Lapsley, D. K., & Brandenberger, J. W. (2011). Change you can believe In: Changes in goal setting during emerging and young adulthood predict later adult well-being. *Social Psychological and Personality Science, 2,* 123–131.

Hill, P. L., Sumner, R., & Burrow, A. L. (2014). Understanding the pathways to purpose: Examining personality and well-being correlates across adulthood. *The Journal of Positive Psychology, 9,* 227–234.

Hill, P. L., & Turiano, N. A. (2014). Purpose in life as a predictor of mortality across adulthood. *Psychological Science, 25,* 1482–1486.

Hill, P. L., Turiano, N. A., Mroczek, D. K., & Burrow, A. L. (2016). The value of a purposeful life: Sense of purpose predicts greater income and net worth. *Journal of Research in Personality, 65,* 38–42.

Hooks, B. (2003). *Communion: The female search for love.* Perennial.

Hopwood, R. A. (2019). Religion, Spirituality, and Health Behaviors: Intersections with Gender Diversity and Aging. In *Transgender and Gender Nonconforming Health and Aging* (pp. 131–150). Cham: Springer.

Hyde, J. S. (2005). The gender similarities hypothesis. *American Psychologist, 60,* 581–592.

Hyde, J. S., Bigler, R. S., Joel, D., Tate, C. C., & van Anders, S. M. (2019). The future of sex and gender in psychology: Five challenges to the gender binary. *American Psychologist, 74,* 171–193.

Kasser, T., & Ryan, R. M. (1993). A dark side of the American dream: Correlates of financial success as a central life aspiration. *Journal of Personality and Social Psychology, 65,* 410–422.

Kaufman, J. C. (2006). Self-reported differences in creativity by ethnicity and gender. *Applied Cognitive Psychology, 20,* 1065–1082.

Kaufman, J. C., Baer, J., Agars, M. D., & Loomis, D. (2010). Creativity stereotypes and the consensual assessment technique. *Creativity Research Journal, 22,* 200–205.

Kaya, A., Iwamoto, D. K., Brady, J., Clinton, L., & Grivel, M. (2019). The role of masculine norms and gender role conflict on prospective well-being among men. *Psychology of Men and Masculinities, 20,* 142–147.

Kiang, L., & Fuligni, A. J. (2010). Meaning in life as a mediator of ethnic identity and adjustment among adolescents from Latin, Asian, and European American backgrounds. *Journal of Youth and Adolescence, 39,* 1253–1264.

Ko, H. J., Hooker, K., Geldhof, G. J., & McAdams, D. P. (2016). Longitudinal purpose in life trajectories: Examining predictors in late midlife. *Psychology and Aging, 31,* 693–698.

Lambda Legal (n.d.). *FAQ About Transgender Parenting*. https://www.lambdalegal.org/know-your-rights/article/trans-parenting-faq.

Liang, B., White, A., Mousseau, A. M. D., Hasse, A., Knight, L., Berado, D., et al. (2017). The four P's of purpose among college bound students: People, propensity, passion, prosocial benefits. *The Journal of Positive Psychology, 12,* 281–294.

Lips, H. M. (2000). College students' visions of power and possibility as moderated by gender. *Psychology of Women Quarterly, 24,* 39–43.

Malin, H., Ballard, P. J., & Damon, W. (2015). Civic purpose: An integrated construct for understanding civic development in adolescence. *Human Development, 58,* 103–130.

Martinez, R. O., & Dukes, R. L. (1997). The effects of ethnic identity, ethnicity, and gender on adolescent well-being. *Journal of Youth and Adolescence, 26,* 503–516.

McKnight, P. E., & Kashdan, T. B. (2009). Purpose in life as a system that creates and sustains health and well-being: An integrative, testable theory. *Review of General Psychology, 13,* 242–251.

Moran, S., Bundick, M. J., Malin, H., & Reilly, T. S. (2012). How supportive of their specific purposes do youth believe their family and friends are? *Journal of Adolescent Research, 28,* 348–377.

Newman, B. M., Kimball, E. W., Vaccaro, A., Moore, A., & Troiano, P. F. (2019). Diverse pathways to purpose for college students with disabilities. *Career Development and Transition for Exceptional Individuals, 42,* 111–121.

Paradise, A. W., & Kernis, M. H. (2002). Self-esteem and psychological well-being: Implications of fragile self-esteem. *Journal of Social and Clinical Psychology, 21,* 345–361.

Peterson, R. A. (2001). On the use of college students in social science research: Insights from a second-order meta-analysis. *Journal of Consumer Research, 28,* 450–461.

Pinquart, M. (2002). Creating and maintaining purpose in life in old age: A meta-analysis. *Ageing International, 27,* 90–114.

Prentice, D. A., & Carranza, E. (2002). What women and men should be, shouldn't be, are allowed to be, and don't have to be: The contents of prescriptive gender stereotypes. *Psychology of Women Quarterly, 26,* 269–281.

Rabin, R. C. (2019, May 7). Huge Racial Disparities Found in Deaths Linked to Pregnancy, *The New York Times*. Retrieved from https://www.nytimes.com/2019/05/07/health/pregnancy-deaths-.html.

Reker, G. T., Peacock, E. J., & Wong, P. T. (1987). Meaning and purpose in life and well-being: A life-span perspective. *Journal of Gerontology, 42,* 44–49.

Roberts, B. W., & Robins, R. W. (2000). Broad dispositions, broad aspirations: The intersection of personality traits and major life goals. *Personality and Social Psychology Bulletin, 26,* 1284–1296.

Rosenkrantz, D. E., Rostosky, S. S., Riggle, E. D., & Cook, J. R. (2016). The positive aspects of intersecting religious/spiritual and LGBTQ identities. *Spirituality in Clinical Practice, 3,* 127–138.

Schwartz, S. H., & Rubel, T. (2005). Sex differences in value priorities: Cross-cultural and multimethod studies. *Journal of Personality and Social Psychology, 89,* 1010–1028.

Solnit, R. (2014). *Men explain things to me*. Haymarket Books.

Stockard, J. (1999). Gender socialization. In J. S. Chafetz (Ed.), *Handbook of the sociology of gender* (pp. 215–227). New York: Kluwer Academic/Plenum Publishers.

Stoltzfus, G., Nibbelink, B. L., Vredenburg, D., & Hyrum, E. (2011). Gender, gender role, and creativity. *Social Behavior and Personality, 39,* 425–432.

Sumner, R., Burrow, A. L., & Hill, P. L. (2015). Identity and purpose as predictors of subjective well-being in emerging adulthood. *Emerging Adulthood, 3,* 46–54.

Sumner, R., Burrow, A. L., & Hill, P. L. (2018). The development of purpose in life among adolescents who experience marginalization: Potential opportunities and obstacles. *American Psychologist, 73,* 740–752.

U.S. Department of Labor, Bureau of Labor Statistics (2014). *Leave benefits: Access, civilian-workers, national compensation survey, March 2014*. Retrieved from https://www.bls.gov/ncs/ebs/benefits/2014/ownership/civilian/table32a.htm.

Way, N., & Rogers, O. (2015). They say black men won't make it, but I know I'm gonna make it. In K. C. McLean & M. Syed (Eds.), *The Oxford handbook of identity development*. USA: Oxford University Press.

Wood, W., & Eagly, A. H. (2002). A cross-cultural analysis of the behavior of women and men: Implications for the origins of sex differences. *Psychological Bulletin, 128,* 699–727.

Xi, J., Lee, M. T., Carter, J. R., & Delgado, D. (2018). Gender differences in purpose in life: The mediation effect of altruism. *Journal of Humanistic Psychology*. https://doi.org/10.1177/002216 7818777658.

Chapter 10
"I Just Can't Be Nothin": The Role of Resistance in the Development of Identity and Purpose

Leoandra Onnie Rogers

Abstract Identity is a core developmental task for adolescents as they seek to answer the questions "who am I?" and "who will I become?" (Erikson, 1968). In this way, identity is germane to purpose; it is a compass that guides and directs how individuals engage with the world. For individuals whose identities are marginalized by oppressive stereotypes, a healthy identity and positive sense of purpose requires resistance to society's negative expectations. This chapter draws from in-depth interview data with adolescent Black boys about their racial and gender identities to show three resistance strategies that young people employ to develop a positive sense of identity and purpose in a society defined by inequality and oppression. Acknowledging societal oppression and the role of resistance makes visible the potential of identity and purpose to be transformative—developmental resources that serve to transform and liberate the self and others.

Keywords Identity development · Resistance · Purpose · Black boys · Racial identity

10.1 Introduction

Q: What are some of the good things about being Black, things you like about it?

"I'm just glad to be Black you know, even though there's like a lot of stereotypes...Like, Black men really don't like to grow up, either they're like drug dealers or gang bangers, or end up dead or something like that, or end up in jail. No, since I'm Black I feel like I gotta, you know, achieve somethin' other than that, you know? I've got goals to do.

Q: Do you like that? That you have the—

Yeah! It keeps me focused. ... Like they say Black men probably won't make it, but I know I'm going to make it and even if I don't make it I'll still try to do something. I just can't – it's not me, I just can't be nothin'; I've got to do something."

—Devin, 14 years old, Black boy

L. O. Rogers (✉)
Northwestern University, Evanston, IL, USA
e-mail: onnie.rogers@northwestern.edu

© Springer Nature Switzerland AG 2020   165
A. L. Burrow and P. Hill (eds.), *The Ecology of Purposeful Living Across the Lifespan*,
https://doi.org/10.1007/978-3-030-52078-6_10

As a developmental psychologist and identity scholar, my research explores how young people come to understand who they are and who they want to become—the development of identity. Devin, the adolescent Black boy quoted above, was a participant in one of my research studies. In this interview excerpt, he discussed what he liked about being Black and why this was an important part of his identity. "I'm just glad to be Black," Devin explained, "even though there's like a lot of stereotypes." Racial identity scholars refer to this as racial identity centrality and evaluation—the importance and positive feelings about one's racial group (e.g., Sellers et al., 1998). Although there is much to analyze from the angle of racial identity development, I highlight here that Devin's response intersects *identity* and *purpose* as mutually constituted and reinforcing constructs. First, it is noticeable that Devin responds to a question about what he likes about being Black with an explicit and spontaneous reference to future orientation, goals and motivation—who he wants and does not want to be. Second, Devin expresses a fear of being/becoming "nothing"—of not being or doing anything of value or significance to society (drugs, gangs, in jail, dead). This threat comes in the form of stereotypes. It is not the task-specific threat, such as fear of not performing well on an exam (Steele & Aronson, 1995), but the more ominous "threat in the air" (Steele, 1997), that he, by virtue of his being Black *and* male in America, lacks the capacity to become anything of value or to contribute to society. Finally, in response to this fear, Devin expresses a deep yearning and assertion *to be*: "I just can't be nothin'; I've got to do something." In this way, the core question that defines identity, "Who am I?" is inextricable from the question of purpose: "What and how will I contribute?"

The human being's desire to "be", to have a sense of self and feel a sense of purpose in the world is universal to the human experience, and is itself not novel. Philosophers, theologians, and scholars across disciplines have written for centuries about the human yearning for a life with purpose and meaning (Erikson, 1959; Frankl, 1963; Maslow, 1962; Steger, Frazier, Oishi, & Kaler, 2006). Indeed, Erikson (1968) wrote that "identity is necessary as the anchoring of man's transient existence in the here and now" (p. 42). Yet, young people like Devin grow up in a society defined by structural oppression, and dehumanizing stereotypes perpetuated by prevailing ideologies of white supremacy and patriarchy. These young people are forced to contend with being told, both implicitly and explicitly, that they possess nothing of value, or have anything to offer, because of their identities. The current chapter centers how the sociocultural context undermines the identities of particular persons as it relates to the development of purpose. Acknowledging oppression as a fundamental disruption of one's humanity (Freire, 1970/2000), reveals that the path to affirming one's identity and establishing a sense that purpose is not without obstacles (e.g., Sumner, Burrow, & Hill, 2018). This approach flows from a developmental framework that 'reimagines' social and emotional development as a process of resistance (Rogers & Way, 2018). In a culture where the hegemonic ideologies of white supremacy, patriarchy, and capitalism persist, individuals must learn to question, resist and reject societal "norms" that are harmful to the self (Gilligan, 2011; Rogers & Way, 2018; Turiel, 2003).

In this chapter, I use the resistance framework and research with Black adolescent boys to consider what the development of purpose means, what it sounds like, and what it requires of those growing up in contexts of dehumanization. First, in alignment with previous perspectives, I outline my approach to identity development and purpose as interlocking constructs (e.g., Hill & Burrow, 2012). Next, I discuss the salience of the sociocultural context, specifically the social hierarchy and dehumanization that are the backdrop for these developmental processes (Rogers & Way, 2018). Finally, I present data illustrating three resistance strategies that Black boys use to navigate oppression as their identities develop and affirm their purpose in a broken society.

10.2 Defining Identity and Purpose

I adopt Erikson's psychosocial identity theory (1968) to conceptualize the development of identity and purpose, which intentionally locates the development of the self as nested within, and inextricable from, the social and cultural context. Erikson's writings on identity also made evident that identity and purpose were overlapping and interlocking processes, which is the assumption I take in this chapter (e.g., Hill & Burrow, 2012; Hill, Burrow, & Sumner, 2013).

Erikson (1968) introduced identity as a developmental and psychological construct that was a necessary and universal aspect of healthy development of individuals and societies. He defined *identity* as an invigorating sense of sameness and continuity that individuals develop through exploration, integration of past experiences and roles, and ultimately clarity about and commitment to one's own sense personhood (Erikson, 1968). Identity has been described by others as "an anchor in sea of possibilities" (Schwartz, 2005, p. 294), owing to its directional and motivational force in an individual's life course.

Purpose can be defined as a "self-organizing life aim that organizes and stimulates goals, manages behaviors, and provides a sense of meaning" (McKnight & Kashdan, 2009, p. 242). Like identity, purpose is like an internal compass that guides behaviors and shapes one's social and emotional interpretations and reactions to daily tasks and choices as well as future aspirations (e.g., Kiang, 2012; Hill et al., 2013), and is one of the ways of individuals contribute to the world beyond the self (e.g., Damon, Menon, & Bronk, 2003). In this way, identity and purpose seem to be mutually reinforcing developmental processes that together underlie positive well-being, life satistifaction, learning and success (e.g., Kiang & Fuligni, 2010; Hill et al., 2013; Sumner et al., 2018). This is not to say that identity and purpose are synonymous or interchangeable terms, but rather that the two inform each other and share a joint goal of moving one through the life course with meaning (e.g., Hill & Burrow, 2012). In this chapter, I consider where and how purpose surfaces in the construction of identity.

Identity is a process that unfolds over time as part of the whole of human development. In Erikson's psychosocial theory, *identity versus role confusion* is the 5th stage in the 8-stage lifespan model. Each stage is marked by a developmentally relevant 'crisis', beginning with *trust versus mistrust* during infancy and concluding with *integrity versus despair* in old age. Each crisis pivots on a conflict between the self ("psycho") and the other ("social"). The resolution of each crisis denotes a potential turning point, a fork in the pathway where development will proceed one direction or another. During the adolescent years, 13–18 years old, individuals enter the "identity crisis" as they work to integrate past experiences and social roles that will guide life choices for career, relationships, and ultimately generativity and contribution to society writ large. In this way identity is foundation for the development of purpose.

Erikson proposed that this 'identity crisis' was universal; a normative part of development, a fact of growing up in any culture, time, and place. There were two possible outcomes of this crisis: *identity,* a sense of clarity and wholeness, or *role confusion*—a term referring to identity uncertainty and incoherence (Erikson, 1968). Those who successfully navigated the crisis emerged with a strong sense of self and were prepared to move on to healthy, positive relationships, investing in others and giving back to society; being generative and ending life with a sense of purpose and fulfillment. However, those who stagnate in *role confusion* face emotional and social stunting; failing to develop meaningful intimate relationships, and subsequently are inward focused, detached from others, and unfilled and unable to contribute to the world later in life.

The crisis of identity, like all of the crises in Erikson's model, hinges on the social context: the norms, expectations, opportunities afforded to one by the culture in which they reside. For identity, the primary crisis is between *who am I and who do I want to be?* Versus *who does society (parents, peers, culture) say that I am and should be?* As such, it is necessary to understand the sociocultural context in which identity development unfolds.

10.3   Centering the Sociocultural Context of Dehumanization

The ecological context of human development has been conceptualized as multi-layered, moving from the most proximal contexts that influence a child, such as family and peers, to the more distal ones, like laws, polices, and cultural ideologies (Bronfenbrenner, 1994; Spencer, 2008). Each level of the developmental context is, however, mutually reinforcing and situated within the other. This chapter focuses on the cultural ideologies that reside in the macro-level of the ecological system (Way, Gilligan, Ali, & Noguera, 2018; Way & Rogers, 2017).

The United States has longstanding ideologies that affect youth development (Rogers & Way, 2018; Spencer, 2008; Way et al., 2018). From the beginning, America has been marred by historical racism, and narratives of dehumanization have played a pivotal role in the creation and maintenance of systemic oppression. Dehumanization is both a structural (cultural/economic) and psychological process whereby groups of people are ranked in terms of their humanness. In a racist, white supremist society, White people are at the top of the hierarchy of humanness—with White, straight, economically-stable men at the very top. All "others" are ranked below on the basis of race, sexuality, social class, gender and the so on. Historically, Black people in the United States were considered property, not human beings, a subjection that justified and sanctioned slavery (Alexander, 2012; Omi & Winant, 1994). Subsequently, persons racially designated as "Black", a legal determination of 1/32nd "Negro blood", were counted primarily as property, not as humans. Even with the abolition of slavery, Black persons were legally deemed second-class citizens and not afforded the same basic civil rights, liberties and practices, as persons designated racially as "White." Notably, these racial designations were, and continue to be, socially constructed—calculated to maintain a system of power and inequality that privileges whiteness (Omi & Winant, 1994; Sidanius & Pratto, 1999). It is this foundation of racial dehumanization that continues to undergird the system of race and racism today (Alexander, 2012; Omi & Winant, 1994).

In a recent set of social psychology experiments, researchers have found that "blatant dehumanization"—an explicit belief that some groups of humans are indeed 'less human' than others—persists across countries. Kteily and colleagues used a newly developed and rather simple measure to assess such "blatant dehumanization" (Kteily, Bruneau, Waytz, & Cotterill, 2015). Across a number of studies, Kteily and colleagues showed thousands of participants an image that depicted an image progression showing the evolution of an ape to a (hu)man; at the far left was an ape on all fours, and at the far right an upright man with human features. Below the image progression was a simple sliding bar with percentages ranging from 0 to 100; "0%" indicating not human at all (e.g., ape) and "100% indicating fully human. Participants in the studies were shown the name of a social group, for example, Europeans, or Muslims, or Blacks, and then asked to slide the bar along the bottom of the image to indicate the "human-ness" of the group, from 0 to 100% human (or evolved). Much to their surprise, even such a crude measure showed nauseating effects: groups that are stigmatized in society (in the United States and across the world) are rated as "less human." Americans, on average, rated Black people as 75% human, and significantly less human than other racial and ethnic-dominant groups (e.g., Whites, Europeans) (Kteily et al., 2015).

When Erikson first wrote about identity, he also recognized that social hierarchy and marginalization were relevant to factors and processes. "[E]conomic, ethnic, and religious marginality," Erikson wrote, "provide poor bases for positive identities" (p. 196). Certainly, marginality refers to the tangible social inequality that is perpetuated through structural systems and policies, such residential segregation, housing discrimination, employment, and education (Alexander, 2012). But society's "typologies" and stereotypes—or dehumanizing beliefs—about groups are also a relevant pathway for undermining identity development. These are not benign ideas but "negative [cultural ideologies] rooted in a hierarchy of humanness in which some humans (i.e., men, White people, and rich people) are considered 'more human' than others" (Rogers & Way, 2018, p. 311).

The context of dehumanization is relevant to identity because it means that the 'conflict' or 'crisis' that individuals must navigate for identity formation is tied to the dehumanizing stereotypes and beliefs held by society. Stereotypes, in this way, matter not simply as attitudes that individuals hold but as broader "master narratives" that uphold the hierarchy of humanness; they are the messages, widely-shared and accepted within a culture, that justify dehumanization (Hammack & Toolis, 2015; McLean & Syed, 2015; Rogers & Way, 2018). Stereotypes can be 'accurate' or 'inaccurate', they can be 'positive' or 'negative', but regardless of their content, all stereotypes contribute to the "shared storylines" that live in our collective consciousness and shape our views of others—and ourselves (Nasir, Snyder, Shah, & Ross, 2012).

For example, Black males are stereotyped as violent and aggressive, as problems that need to be "fixed" (Noguera, 2009; Ferguson, 2000; Rogers & Brooms, 2019). If society expects Black males to be rappers, criminals, thugs and athletes, what is required for them to construct a different sense of identity or aspire to a different purpose? This is the "crisis" or "conflict" that defines identity formation, according to Erikson (1968). Generally, the examples used to describe the conflict of self and society in identity development focus on interpersonal preferences or career aspirations; for example, an adolescent aspires to be an artist but their parents want them to be a doctor. Or, examples are given for conflicts related to religious or political affiliation: an adolescent raised in a devout Catholic family grows into their own beliefs in agnosticism. In Erikson's terms, such tensions are focal to the identity crisis that individuals must resolve. However, there are more fundamental issues at hand in a society that dehumanizes particular groups on the basis of their identities—particularly Black people. Indeed, W. E. B. DuBois, in writing about the Black experience in 1903, asked: "How does it feel to be a problem?"

Although negotiating parental expectations about one's career or religious choice are relevant conflicts, to face a socially imposed "conflict" over one's humanity is qualitatively distinct. Sexuality minority youth, for example, whose parents do not affirm their identity, encounter a crisis that is not simply about who they are dating but about their fundamental sense of belonging and value and rights as a full human being (Hammack & Toolis, 2015). The prevailing racist ideologies and stereotypes that position Black people as "less human" and thus less worthy of care and respect (Epstien, Blake, & Gonzalez, 2017; Kteily & Bruneau, 2017), change the nature and meaning of the conflict. From this vantage point, the question of identity, and of purpose, becomes: *How does one achieve the human task of a healthy sense of identity and understanding of their purpose in a society that views you as deficient, dangerous, and less than human?* The answer to this question requires the framework of resistance—critical acknowledgment that transformation and liberation is inseparable from normative human development (Rogers & Way, 2018; Way & Rogers, 2017).

10.4 The Role of Resistance

To address the fact that marginalization was a "poor basis" for identity development, Erikson proposed the concept of "negative identity"—an identity outcome that results from all of society's negative expectations. In response to marginalization, Erikson (1968) wrote, a young person may form "a negative identity ... putting his energy into becoming exactly what the careless and fearful community expects to be–and make a total job it" (p. 196). Erikson's explanation of 'negative' identity outcomes among marginalized groups acknowledged the responsibility of oppression, but also marks the personhood of marginalized peoples as *only* negative and defined by oppression. Consequently, it is difficult to imagine, from Erikson's starting point, that there is an alternative pathway to positive identity for minoritized individuals, let alone what such a path would look like. However, becoming exactly what the racist (white, dominant) society wants is not the only identity option or outcome. That is, beyond the experience of "being" a problem, individuals respond to and resist this position. Although we often discuss the ways in which youth are influenced by and socialized into cultural norms and expectations, less often does our study of young people center them as active agents responding to and challenging the social structures as part of their own development (e.g., Anyon, 1984; Liben, 2017).

Rogers and Way (2018; Way & Rogers, 2017) proposed *resistance as a developmental process*, which rests on two assumptions: (a) the dominant culture perpetuates oppression via a set of ideologies that reinforce a hierarchy of humanity; (b) young people have the capacity and innate desire to resist such oppression (Anyon, 1984; Fine, Tuck & Yang, 2013; Gilligan, 2011). A major benefit of the resistance framework is that it centers deconstructing inequality and liberation as essential to healthy development. Thus, healthy identity cannot be defined only by positive individual-level well-being or scholastic success; rather a healthy identity encompasses an identity that embeds resistance to the inequality that structures dehumanization (Rogers, 2018; Rogers & Way, 2018; Turiel, Chung, & Carr, 2016). Likewise, a healthy sense of purpose, in a culture of inequality, would encompass a resistance that transforms the self and liberates others. For example, a young person may find purpose in aspiring to become a doctor not so much because of the prestige of the profession, or even the economic mobility it might provide, but perhaps because of her desire to address racial disparities in health outcomes.

This perspective on purpose brings into a view what I will term "transformative purpose"—a definition and an approach to studying purpose that embeds the navigation and ultimately transformation of inequality as core to purpose. That is, transformative purpose is not separate from but hinges on equity and justice. I draw this terminology from the emergent social and emotional learning (SEL) framework put forth by Jagers and colleagues, "transformative SEL" (Jagers, Rivas-Drake, & Williams, 2019). The "transformative" notion calls for traditional SEL frameworks to critically interrogate inequality in the very definition and measurement of SEL programming and research, and to assess the effectiveness of SEL by its impact on inequality. The shift to transformative SEL recognizes that conceptualizing and assessing social and emotional skills and strategies without naming the racist and oppressive realties that young people face is not only insufficient and ineffective but also counterproductive for promoting equitable outcomes (Jagers et al., 2019). Therefore, transformative SEL centers the outcome of equity at the outset. A similar rationale could be applied to the study of purpose. In a context of oppression, the development of purpose is deemed "healthy" and "good" not only if it benefits the individual within the existing structures but when it transforms oppressive structures. Understanding the forms of resistance that youth engage as they develop their identities can shed light on how young people come to construct their identities and sense of purpose in transformative ways.

10.5   Strategies of Resistance to Oppression: Finding Identity and Purpose

The aim of this empirical example is to reveal the role of resistance as integral to the development of identity and purpose that is transformative and liberating. The data presented here come from a longitudinal mixed-method study focused on the identity development of Black adolescent boys attending an all-boys high school, and the interview data were analyzed to describe patterns of racial and gender identity and resistance to racial and gender stereotypes (see Rogers, 2018; Rogers & Way, 2016). This chapter places these identity narratives in a framework of purpose, revealing that resistance offers a meaningful lens for understanding the development of purpose in contexts of social marginality and oppression.

I use interviewing as a methodological approach to center phenomenology. By listening to young people describe their identities, we hear how purpose is interwoven into their identity process and that resistance is key to its development. I first present what Black boys know about how they are perceived by others—their view of themselves from the eyes of others. Then, against this sociocultural context, I present the three resistance strategies that Black boys used to make sense of their identities with a sense of purpose in the world.

In the eyes of others. When asked what others think about Black boys, there was consensus that Black males are seen as *unsuccessful, bad and violent*. Others people saw them as "killers", "beaters", "stealers", and "cheaters"; "the gangster in the hood who sells crack." For example, Brandon (9th grade) said others think "Blacks can't succeed in nothing, they're always stealing, killing, all this violence." Franklin (10th grade) explained that "most people don't think African-Americans are smart; not talented, not well-behaved." Omar (10th grade) simply said: "Oh man, they think we are just niggers." Asked to expand on this, he explained: "Like uh, they think we're all ignorant. You know, disrespectful and wild." The message from society is clear and negative: to be Black and male is to be a problem.

Black boys recognized that the stereotypes came with behavioral expectations. "Especially a Black male," Devin explained (10th grade), "you're supposed to be this tough guy, don't mess with me and stuff like that." The expectation for toughness was paired with athletic prowess and strength, as definitional of Black boys. Kirk (9th grade), gave the following example:

> Like, when we walk into the track meet they expect us to be like the real fast ones. Like we, we might not have even seen them, they think we gonna run fast and be sprinter, just 'cause, I guess 'cause we [are] Black.

Cameron (9th grade) made explicit the link between identity and purpose, and the ways stereotypes shape this connection: "You know, most people will say Black men are for sports and going to basketball and football and trying to get to the pros." Black boys, by virtue of their identity, have a particular purpose in society—to be an athlete, to be tough, to be bad and violent. And Black boys, in the normative work of identity development, are attuned to who they are 'supposed to be' in the eyes of society. Such expectations must be considered as we seek to understand their path to defining a sense of purpose. Below I discuss three strategies employed by Black boys to navigate these stereotypes.

Accommodation. The strategy of accommodation resembles Erikson's notion of 'negative identity' where young people seem to secure their identities by "becoming exactly what the careless and fearful community expects" them to become (Erikson, 1968, p. 196). For example, Omar, a 9th-grader, explained that what he likes about be Black is that "like a lot of people are scared of us; that's great." It is "great" to be seen as scary Black male, he explained, because it is "funny to see that fear in people." Rather than question or challenge this negative perception, he seems accept it, even if he does not actually fit the box.

Defining oneself in accordance with the stereotypes is not simply about identity in the present, it is about where one is headed—and how he will invest in others. Like Devin, quoted above, Omar also suggests that being Black is important and positive, and gives him direction:

> Because it's good for me to be Black because now I have a chance at setting a goal for Black people. Well like now the percentage of Black people graduating is real low, so if I could just get that one percent to be me it will make it a little bit better. When I graduate I can do something to help more Black people to get involved. Then as it keeps going and going a lot of other people get involved and then everybody can be one whole again.

Omar links his racial identity to his desire "to help more Black people" in a positive manner, suggesting a purpose beyond himself (e.g., Damon et al., 2003), and acknowledging indirectly the historical oppression in which his academic aspirations are rooted (e.g., Oyserman, Grant, & Ager, 1995; Sumner et al., 2018). Still, within this thread of resistance and optimism who Omar sees that he *can* be different than the stereotypes, we also hear how society's dehumanization imposes itself on how Black boys imagined their future:

> Q: When you think about your future, what do you hope for?

> A: Man, to be alive, yeah because this is wild, I'll be like man I hope I don't get shot. Because I already know, yeah. I'm the hood guy; a lot of people know me and that's kind of good and

kind of bad at the same time. So I just make sure I always be right, so I know okay, I know they ain't goin' to try to kill you when I'm sleeping so I'm all good.

Q: And when you think about your future, what do you worry about?

A: Man, I think I'll worry about me being bad; I don't know. I'll be kind of tempted sometimes, like 'man, you need that money dog'; I'm trying to be good now ... .I ain't trying to be locked up {laughs}. I can't do that, no, no, no. I'm too little to go to jail.

The threat to his livelihood, first of all, disrupts the assumption that a future feels secure and possible for all youth. Omar articulates this precarity, and as he describes what his future might hold, he focuses who he does *not* want to be yet fears he will become: "bad." His guiding light is to "be" good, which suggests an internalizing of the narrative that he is not inherently good and must actively work *not to become* the bad person he his "tempted" to be. The question for the study of identity and of purpose is how the sociocultural context formed this path of development—and how we create alternative pathways that affirm their personhood.

Exceptionalism. Black boys in this research study also used exceptionalism as a strategy to negotiate the stereotypes. In this way, their identities and sense of purpose was defined by being separate, different, and better than "other Black people" or the "regular Black male."

Deon, a 9th-grader, described himself: I'm [a] tall, Black, handsome young man. ... I love God. I'm a positive man."

When asked what being a "positive man" means to him, he explained:

Um, not like the other men on the street that would, um, go and sell drugs, get high. And do the all the ordinary stuff like uh, like another Black man would: leave out on his wife or kids when she about to have a kid or somethin'. I don't care if I have twenty kids, I'm gonna be there for every last one of 'em. Because I wouldn't want to end up like my father. I wouldn't want to see my kids cry every night tryin' to see where their father at or nothin' like that.

Deon draws a clear contrast between his ideal self as a "positive man" and feared self as a Black male stereotype (a drug user and absent father), revealing how identity is tied to that which he wishes to avoid. Deon defines his identity, and correspondingly his sense of purpose, by *not* becoming what society expects (Way, Santos, Niwa & Kim-Gervey, 2008). But, this subjective definition also suggests that he believes the stereotypes accurately described the "ordinary" Black man, but simply do not apply him personally.

Jaire (10th grade) described himself similarly, suggesting that his value is rooted first in proving that his *not* like the (stereo)typical Black male:

I would say that I'm a very intelligent, articulate young man ... And someone who is genuinely a well-behaved person, a well-dressed or groomed person...

Jaire's general self-description stood in direct contrast to how he says *other people* view Black people: "just lazy and acting out and don't care about their educations." Asked to explain what he likes most about himself, Jaire makes this comparison and his exceptionalism explicit:

I love the fact that different people think of me to be um a more complex individual and a more intelligent individual. Because there's no 14-year-old – let's be real, young African American male 14-year-old, you know, that can use different words in different situations and say different things and give his opinion about Barack Obama or the state the economy is in, the Iraq war, and different situations or the lesbian movement or whatever.

Positioning himself in a conversation of power (i.e., politics), Jaire describes himself as intelligent, which is a sign of his resistance to and rejection of the "negative identity" that society has created for him as a Black boy. But, much like Deon, he at the same time adheres to the belief that Black males, as a social group, are not intelligent, well-behaved, or valued citizens. The resistance strategy of exceptionalism is a double-edged sword: it both allowed boys to resist stereotypes by separating themselves from *other* Black people; but such a resistance also disconnects them from relationships with others and does not address the system of inequality (Rogers, 2018). It is not liberating because it reinforces the very stereotypes they wish to avoid.

The narrative of exceptionalism, while positive in some respects and offering Black boys a counter narrative and pathway for who they are and can become, simultaneously works to undermine the goal of collective liberation. That is, when boys responded to the stereotypes by viewing themselves as exceptions to the stereotypes, they implicitly (and some explicitly) perpetuated stereotypes as "true" rather than socially constructed. Robinson and Ward (1991) refer to this as "resistance for survival"—it is a short-term strategy that may promote individual progress, but does not facilitate the liberation or success of the collective whole.

Resistance for liberation. The final strategy, resistance for liberation, is one that involves seeing and naming the stereotypes and injustice and rejecting it—for oneself and for others. There is a recognition that one's own liberation is tied to the liberation of others—to the dismantling of the system, in cultivating and demanding a more caring and humane culture (Robinson & Ward, 1991; Rogers, 2018; Ward, 2018). Marcus (9th grade), explained "like guys aren't supposed to be feminine or guys aren't supposed to be sensitive or stuff, or show their feelings, or cry." But from his view, "Of course you gonna cry 'cause that's like human nature, you supposed to cry, that's why um, you have tear ducts in your body." He rejects the tough male stereotype, explaining:

Cause um, I guess society thinks that if um, men or boys act feminine that they're gay or they just assume that they gay or things like that. And I think that's a bad stereotype because you know, some … Guys need to express their feelings too.

Marcus explained how society's stereotypes a problematic for but went on to articulate why resistance to such stereotypes is key to liberation and a sense of wholeness and transformation. Telling others they cannot express their feelings or conflating emotionality with homosexuality, Marcus said: "just makes you look less of a human. I don't think that's a good stereotype because that's like telling kids not to care about anything that happens." As Erikson (1968) wrote about negative identity, it is a "careless" culture that undermines identity. Marcus recognizes that the carelessness is in the community and not in Black boys themselves. The humanity of Black boys thus requires resistance and gives purpose to their resistance.

Of course, the constraints of stereotypes extend beyond emotionality of boys. Devin (9th grade) also illustrates this resistance in the context of his racial identity:

> Q: So what do you think it means to be Black?
>
> A: Well, like what I think it means and what other people like society want it mean is not the same. Like [the class discussion] got me thinking about statistics and stuff like that. That's what everybody want it to be; they don't want being Black to mean being intelligent and stuff like that. They want it to be being ignorant, ghetto and whatnot. That's what I think. Well that's what *they* want it to mean; that's not what it means to me. I think it means to be like having pride in yourself you know, having to prove something, like what I said previously, that's what I think it means.
>
> Q: Why do you think society wants it to mean something negative?
>
> A: Because they don't want to you know they don't want to be wrong you know. They want to be right. They're actually saying like, they want to keep us in our place and stuff like that. They don't want us to be equal to them.

Devin is aware that there is a larger system at work, a system that perpetuates inequality, and in response, Devin defines being Black as resistant to this system: "It means to me that I've got something to prove to the people, you know, to be successful and also to prove it to myself that I can be successful." The purpose in such resistance is not simply to 'prove the stereotype wrong' but to affirm his identity.

Such affirmation is key to liberation and gives meaning to the resistance. After describing the society's view of Black people as ignorant, drug dealers and gang bangers, Devin explains that he doesn't believe stereotypes are true at all:

> No, because *I am Black* and I've been around Black people all the time. I mean, I thought that for a moment you know all you see on the news, you know? But, like all my friends don't gang-bang, none of my friends do.

Defining Blackness based on his lived experience rather than society's narrative, Devin acknowledges that he found himself believing the stereotypes "for a moment" but then grounding his knowledge about Black people in the reality of his own life ("my friends don't gang-bang") rather than what the media tells him he knows that they aren't true. Ahmad gave a similar response when I asked him how he would describe Black people:

> I'd say [Black people are] hard workin', for what I see around in my family. Like, my mamma, my daddy they not rich or whatever but they work hard to take care of me and my brothers and sisters all that stuff. ... And like I said stereotypes that White[s] have toward us that Black[s] are ignorant, you know, gang-banger, thugs, whatever, so um I say Black people are underestimated 'cause not all Black people are like that.

Rather than lazy and unsuccessful, Ahmad knows what he sees—"hard working" Black people who are "underestimated." Cameron (9th grade) similarly explained that the good thing about being Black to him is "Knowing that Black people are good." Like Devin, Ahmad and Cameron both know a simple yet essential truth—Black people are not what society says they are—they are "good" and "hardworking"; they are human.

Acknowledging the hierarchies of inequality, and listening to how adolescent Black boys negotiate them, reveals that strategies of resistance, and that there is a sense of purpose in resisting stereotypes, in righting a system that threatens one's humanity. Growing up in a system and a culture where dehumanization and inequality are normative realities, not only requires that one learn and accommodate to the existing norms and values but also, for their own humanity and the humanity of others, to question, resist, and reject those cultural ideals that are indeed harmful to the self—and others (Rogers & Way, 2018; Way et al., 2018).

Freire (1970/2000) called for such critical interrogation and repudiation of oppression as the work of becoming more fully human—it is, according to Freire, the human's "ontological vocation"—or purpose. We can, then, think of the development of identity and purpose as the work young people are engaged in—and that we must nurture and support. And, in doing so, we also nurture our own ontological vocation of becoming more fully human. The importance of "socializing agents" (Schachter & Ventura, 2008) in the identity development of young people is well documented. Parents, other adults, peers, siblings, the media are all socializing sources that will influence how a young person develops identity, but we mostly focus on the unidirectional impact of such processes—that is, how socializing agents impact the young person. A transactional view of identity, however, acknowledges that self and society are "jointly constructed … with implications not only for the individual … [but also] for relationships, communities, societies, and cultures" (Rogers, 2018, p. 286). In this way, socializing agents may themselves find a sense of purpose in nurturing within young people the capacity to resist and transform inequality.

In my own research at The Boys School, an all-Black, all-male high school, I also interviewed teachers and administrators about how they came to teach in this particular school serving this particular student population (see Rogers, 2018; Rogers & Brooms, 2019). One of the focal findings from these data is that educators felt a clear sense of purpose not only in teaching but in being a role model and fostering within Black boys a sense of purpose to resist and reject negative stereotypes. For example, one teacher, Ms. B., explained why it was important to her, as a Black woman, to teach at this school and do this work:

> I just feel it's important to provide something back to the community, basically help Black people. If you're a Black person that has been successful, I think it's really important, especially now, to do something that directly affects the Black community.

Much like the Black boys in my study, teachers suggest that their identities ("if you're a Black person …") are tied to purpose, and that in supporting Black boys, this teacher nurtures her own sense of purpose. Another teacher, Mr. S., explained that the reason he teaches young Black boys was to "change the images in their minds" and help "them to understand that they're not an island to themselves; they're interconnected." For Mr. S., the impact of this message was not about individuals but societies:

> There is an interconnected nature between each of these young men and that if each and every one of them individually achieves they will be better, not only be better young men for their families, they'll be better citizens and thus improve our nation. I mean it goes community, society, and nation and it's just a logical progression.

In both of these examples we hear the transactional impact of transformative purpose. This perspective offers another lens on the *how* and *why* of socializing agents; it also brings into view questions about how such socialization can contribute to disrupting inequality and cultivating liberation within others—and within the self.

Where inequality and oppression are the norm, resistance becomes a vital tool for the development of healthy identities and societies. Freire (1970) argued that dehumanizing another was not only harmful to the other but also to the self; "the oppressor … is himself dehumanized because he dehumanizes others …" (Freire, 2000). On the other side, then, nurturing the humanity of others may indeed be self-humanizing and offer a pathway to fulfilling one's ontological purpose.

10.6   Conclusion

The development of identity and purpose—solidifying who one is and one's role and contribution in society—are not exempt from the oppressive sociocultural context that actively undermines the humanity of marginalized peoples. For this reason, although resistance to oppression is itself universal (Freire, 2000), it is often most evident among the most socially marginalized, for their path of development is littered with stereotypes (Rogers & Way, 2018). In other words, it was through listening to the identity narratives of Black adolescent boys that we could see how the definition and interpretation of purpose in a diverse society requires a deep reckoning with the structural inequalities and injustices that plague society, as well as individuals' resistance to it. In a similar fashion, it was through listening to the voices of women, marginalized and excluded from the dominant discourses of psychology, that Dr. Carol Gilligan (1993) discovered that the "ethic of care", alongside moral rationalization, was a relevant and central dimension of human morality—for women *and* men. The role of resistance offers a new way to think about and measure what purpose means, how it forms, and why it matters. Keeping transformation at the center means, first and foremost, that we see and fully acknowledge that there are structural issues to transform, and secondly it appreciates the capacities of young people (and all of us) to do such transformational work. If our approach to normative development does not acknowledge inequality or the capacities to resist and transform it, we undersell the efficacy of science to positively change the lives of young people—and the world.

References

Alexander, M. (2012). *The new Jim Crow: Mass incarceration in the age of colorblindness.* New York, NY: New Press.

Anyon, J. (1984). Intersections of gender and class: Accommodation and resistance by working-class and affluent females to contradictory sex role ideologies. *Journal of Education, Boston, 166,* 25–48.

Bronfenbrenner, U. (1994). Ecological models of human development. *Readings on the Development of Children, 2,* 37–43.

Damon, W., Menon, J., & Cotton Bronk, K. (2003). The development of purpose during adolescence. *Applied Developmental Science, 7,* 119–128. https://doi.org/10.1207/S1532480XADS0703_2.

Epstein, R., Blake, J., & Gonzalez, T. (2017). *Girlhood interrupted: The erasure of Black girls' childhood..* https://doi.org/10.2139/ssrn.3000695.

Erikson, E. H. (1959). Identity and the Life Cycle. *Psychological Issues, 1,* 1–171.

Erikson, E. H. (1968). *Youth and crisis.* New York: WW Norton & Company.

Ferguson, A. A. (2000). *Bad boys: Public schools in the making of masculinities.* Ann Arbor, MI: University of Michigan Press.

Fine, M., Tuck, E., & Yang, K. W. (2013). An intimate memoir of resistance theory. In E. Tuck & K. W. Yang (Eds.), *Youth resistance research and theories of change.* New York, NY: Routledge.

Frankl, V. E. (1963). *Man's search for meaning.* New York, NY: Washington Square Press.

Freire, P. (1970/2000). *Pedagogy of the oppressed.* New York, NY: Continuum. http://www.historyisaweapon.com/defcon2/pedagogy/pedagogychapter1.html.

Gilligan, C. (1993). *In a different voice: Psychological theory and women's development.* Harvard University Press.

Gilligan, C. (2011). *Joining the resistance.* Cambridge, UK: Polity Press.

Hammack, P. L., & Toolis, E. E. (2015). Putting the social into personal identity: The master narrative as root metaphor for psychological and developmental science. *Human Development, 58,* 350–364. https://doi.org/10.1159/000446054.

Hill, P. L., & Burrow, A. L. (2012). Viewing purpose through an Eriksonian lens. *Identity, 12,* 74–91. https://doi.org/10.1080/15283488.2012.632394.

Hill, P. L., Burrow, A. L., & Sumner, R. (2013). Addressing important questions in the field of adolescent purpose. *Child Development Perspectives, 7,* 232–236. https://doi.org/10.1111/cdep.12048.

Jagers, R. J., Rivas-Drake, D., & Williams, B. (2019). Transformative social and emotional learning (SEL): Toward SEL in service of educational equity and excellence. *Educational Psychologist, 54,* 162–184. https://doi.org/10.1080/00461520.2019.1623032.

Kiang, L. (2012). Deriving Daily Purpose Through Daily Events and Role Fulfillment Among Asian American Youth. *Journal of Research on Adolescence, 22,* 185–198. https://doi.org/10.1111/j.1532-7795.2011.00767.x.

Kiang, L., & Fuligni, A. J. (2010). Meaning in life as a mediator of ethnic identity and adjustment among adolescents from Latin, Asian, and European American backgrounds. *Journal of Youth and Adolescence, 39,* 1253–1264. https://doi.org/10.1007/s10964-009-9475-z.

Kteily, N. S., & Bruneau, E. (2017). Darker demons of our nature: The need to (re) focus attention on blatant forms of dehumanization. *Current Directions in Psychological Science, 26,* 487–494. https://doi.org/10.1177/0963721417708230.

Kteily, N., Bruneau, E., Waytz, A., & Cotterill, S. (2015). The ascent of man: Theoretical and empirical evidence for blatant dehumanization. *Journal of Personality and Social Psychology, 109,* 901–931. https://doi.org/10.1037/pspp0000048.

Liben, L. S. (2017). Gender development: A constructivist-ecological perspective. *New perspectives on human development* (pp. 143–144). https://doi.org/10.1017/cbo9781316282755.010.

Maslow, A. (1962). *Toward a psychology of being.* Princeton, NJ, US: D Van Nostrand. xi 214 pp., https://doi.org/10.1037/10793-000.

McKnight, P. E., & Kashdan, T. B. (2009). Purpose in life as a system that creates and sustains health and well-being: An integrative, testable theory. *Review of General Psychology, 13,* 242–251. https://doi.org/10.1037/a0017152.

McLean, K. C., & Syed, M. (2015). Personal, master, and alternative narratives: An integrative framework for understanding identity development in context. *Human Development, 58,* 318–349. https://doi.org/10.1159/000445817.

Nasir, N. S., Snyder, C. R., Shah, N., & Ross, K. M. (2012). Racial storylines and implications for learning. *Human Development, 55,* 285–301. https://doi.org/10.1159/000345318.

Noguera, P. A. (2009). *The trouble with black boys: … And other reflections on race, equity, and the future of public education.* John Wiley & Sons.

Omi, M., & Winant, H. (1994). *Racial formation in the US: From the 1960s to the 1990s.* New York, NY: Routledge.

Oyserman, D., Gant, L., & Ager, J. (1995). A socially contextualized model of African American identity: Possible selves and school persistence. *Journal of Personality and Social Psychology, 69,* 1216–1232. https://doi.org/10.1037/0022-3514.69.6.1216.

Robinson, T., & Ward, J. V. (1991). "A belief in self far greater than anyone's disbelief": Cultivating resistance among African American female adolescents. *Women and Therapy, 11,* 87–103. https://doi.org/10.1300/J015V11N03_06.

Rogers, L. O. (2018). The "Black Box": Identity development and the crisis of connection among Black adolescent boys. In N. Way, A. Ali, C. Gilligan, & P. A. Noguera (Eds.), *The crisis of connection: It's roots, consequences, and solutions* (pp. 129–150). New York, NY: New York University Press.

Rogers, L. O., & Brooms, D. (2019). Ideology and identity among White male teachers in an all-Black male high school. *American Educational Research Journal.* https://doi.org/10.3102/000 2831219853224.

Rogers, L. O., & Way, N. (2016). "I have goals to prove all those people wrong and not fit into any one of those boxes" paths of resistance to stereotypes among black adolescent males. *Journal of Adolescent Research, 31,* 263–298. https://doi.org/10.1177/0743558415600071.

Rogers, L. O., & Way, N. (2018). Reimagining social and emotional development: Accommodation and resistance to dominant ideologies in the identities and friendships of boys of color. *Human Development, 61,* 311–331. https://doi.org/10.1159/000493378.

Schachter, E. P., & Ventura, J. J. (2008). Identity agents: Parents as active and reflective participants in their children's identity formation. *Journal of Research on Adolescence, 18,* 449–476. https://doi.org/10.1111/j.1532-7795.2008.00567.x.

Schwartz, S. J. (2005). A new identity for identity research: Recommendations for expanding and refocusing the identity literature. *Journal of Adolescent Research, 20,* 293–308. https://doi.org/10.1177/0743558405274890.

Sellers, R. M., Smith, M. A., Shelton, J. N., Rowley, S. A., & Chavous, T. M. (1998). Multidimensional model of racial identity: A reconceptualization of African American racial identity. *Personality and social psychology review, 2,* 18–39. https://doi.org/10.1207/s15327957pspr02 01_2.

Sidanius, J., & Pratto, F. (1999). *Social dominance: An intergroup theory of social hierarchy and oppression.* Cambridge, UK: Cambridge University Press.

Spencer, M. B. (2008). Phenomenology and ecological systems theory: Development of diverse groups. In W. Damon & R. M. Lerner (Eds.), *Child and adolescent development: An advanced course* (pp. 696–735). New York: Wiley Publishers. https://doi.org/10.1002/9780470147658.chp sy0115.

Sumner, R., Burrow, A. L., & Hill, P. (2018). The development of purpose in life among adolescents who experience marginalization: Potential opportunities and obstacles. *American Psychologist, 73,* 740–752. https://doi.org/10.1037/amp0000249.

Steele, C. M. (1997). A threat in the air: How stereotypes shape intellectual identity and performance. *American Psychologist, 52,* 613–629. https://doi.org/10.1037/0003-066X.52.6.613.

Steele, C. M., & Aronson, J. (1995). Stereotype threat and the intellectual test performance of African Americans. *Journal of Personality and Social Psychology, 69,* 797–811. https://doi.org/10.1037/0022-3514.69.5.797.

Steger, M. F., Frazier, P., Oishi, S., & Kaler, M. (2006). The meaning in life questionnaire: Assessing the presence of and search for meaning in life. *Journal of Counseling Psychology, 53,* 80–93. https://doi.org/10.1037/0022-0167.53.1.80.

Turiel, E. (2003). Resistance and subversion in everyday life. *Journal of Moral Education, 32,* 115–130. https://doi.org/10.1080/0305724032000072906.

Turiel, E., Chung, E., & Carr, J. A. (2016). Struggles for equal rights and social justice as unrepresented and represented in psychological research. In *Advances in Child Development and Behavior, 50,* 1–29. JAI. https://doi.org/10.1016/bs.acdb.2015.11.004.

Ward, J. V. (2018). Staying woke: Raising Black girls to resist disconnection. In N. Way, A. Ali, C. Gilligan, and P. A. Noguera (Eds.) (Ch. 3). *The crisis of connection: Its roots, consequences, and solutions.* New York, NY: New York University Press.

Way, N., Ali, A., Gilligan, C., & Noguera, P. (Eds.). (2018). *The crisis of connection: Roots, consequences, and solutions.* New York, NY: NYU Press.

Way, N., & Rogers, L. O. (2017). Resistance to dehumanization during childhood and adolescence: A developmental and contextual process. In N. Budwig, E. Turiel, & P. D. Zelazo (Eds.), *New perspectives on human development* (p. 229–257). Cambridge University Press. https://doi.org/10.1017/CBO9781316282755.014.

Way, N., Santos, C., Niwa, E. Y., & Kim-Gervey, C. (2008). To be or not to be: An exploration of ethnic identity development in context. *New Directions for Child and Adolescent Development, 2008*(120), 61–79. https://doi.org/10.1002/cd.216.

Chapter 11
When Passion Serves a Purpose: Race, Social Networks, and Countering Occupational Discrimination

Adia Harvey Wingfield

Abstract Sociological research provides extensive analysis of the racial disparities present in contemporary workplaces. However, there is less attention to the
strategies and tools black workers use to offset potential challenges. This paper
examines how early motivation for pursuing careers provides a sense of purpose
that becomes integral for black professionals in the health care industry. Sense of
purpose compels black professionals to develop strategies that buffer against racial
workplace discrimination, particularly in high-status occupations.

Keywords Race · Occupational discrimination · Purpose · Social networks

Most of the research on race and work documents that black workers face extensive disadvantages ranging from hiring discrimination (Bertrand & Mullainathan,
2004; Pager, 2007) to differential treatment in the workplace (Roscigno, 2007) to
blocked avenues for promotion and advancement (Bell & Nkomo, 2003). Yet we
know less about the social psychological factors that serve as a buffer for black
workers in environments where they are underrepresented. This is particularly true
for black professionals, who frequently work in predominantly white settings that
can be hostile, unwelcoming, or replete with racial biases (Ray, 2019).

   In this chapter, I consider how a sense of purpose plays an important role in
shaping the ways black professionals proactively attempt to offset potential workplace discrimination. For black workers who anticipate that they will face racial bias,
developing a sense of purpose provides additional motivation for coping with racial
challenges they may encounter. It foments a sense of commitment and dedication
to professional careers that becomes necessary and useful in predominantly white
environments that can be uncomfortable spaces.

A. H. Wingfield (✉)
Washington University in St. Louis, St. Louis, MO, USA
e-mail: ahwingfield@wustl.edu

© Springer Nature Switzerland AG 2020   183
A. L. Burrow and P. Hill (eds.), *The Ecology of Purposeful Living Across the Lifespan*,
https://doi.org/10.1007/978-3-030-52078-6_11

11.1 Background

Research has consistently shown that challenges abound for black professional workers. In an early study of the black middle class, Feagin and Sikes (1995) showed that despite the class advantages that accompanied employment in professional occupations, black workers still encountered marginalization, stereotypes from colleagues, supervisors, and customers, and presumptions of incompetence and low skill. For black women, these issues are complicated by intersections of race and gender, leaving them absent crucial mentoring relationships, social networks, and subject to unique forms of harassment (Bell & Nkomo, 2003; Yanick & Feagin, 1998). These workers are less likely to receive tips and advice about navigating professional environments (Royster, 2003), but more likely to face discriminatory processes in the form of blocked avenues to promotion and increased risks of termination (Roscigno, 2007). These occupational challenges create pronounced emotional and personal consequences for black workers, including but not limited to racialized emotion management, increased anger, frustration, and stress (Cose, 1993; Evans, 2014).

We know, in short, that the contemporary contours of racial discrimination in the workplace present significant obstacles for black workers. But we know less about how they cope with these challenges, and still less about how they take proactive strategies to cope with environments widely known to be difficult spaces in which to thrive and advance. Thus, this chapter raises several questions in an attempt to consider how black professional workers prepare for the racial issues they encounter in predominantly white spaces, and presents the concept of purpose as a major factor that enables them to persist past daunting occupational hurdles.

To show how purpose matters in black professional workers' lives, this chapter poses several key questions. How do black health care workers come to believe that this is the career for them? What creates the idea that doing health care work is their purpose, the work which they are meant to do? What factors make health care an appealing profession as opposed to other areas of employment? And what role does race play in shaping these determinations?

11.2 What Exactly Is Purpose?

Sociologists have yet to establish a cogent theory of purpose, but there are some insights from various researchers and theorists. While they do not focus explicitly on purpose, sociologists have long wrestled with the question of why social groups engage in certain behaviors. Rational choice theorists such as George Homans and James Coleman argue that human behavior is driven primarily by self-interest, and that people are motivated to accrue certain forms of capital (human, social, and/or economic) in order to advance. The pioneering sociologist W.E.B. DuBois contended that racial differences mattered in shaping behaviors, suggesting that whites acted to maintain the "psychological wage of whiteness" which indicated that no matter how socially, economically, and culturally disadvantaged they were, they could still view themselves as better than their black counterparts. Thus, sociological theorists have been able to offer a basic framework for why groups enact various behaviors, whether driven by a desire to maintain racial privilege, economic advantages, or other factors.

This paper builds on these existing theories, and envisions purpose as a motivator that explains what would otherwise be innocuous, mundane behaviors. In this chapter, I focus less on what shapes everyday behavior, and more on what makes black workers imbue their actions, behaviors, and choices with additional meaning. Purpose then becomes a form of resiliency and drive, the guiding force that compels black workers to maintain a course of action even in the face of significant racialized obstacles. For black workers in predominantly white settings, purpose thus becomes a strategy for undermining and challenging workplace racial discrimination.

11.3   Research Design and Methodology

The results of this study are based on intensive interviews with 60 black workers in the health care industry. The data from which these results are drawn is a study of how economic and cultural changes are impacting black professionals. Health care thus produced a topical site in which to study these changes due to the growing commodification and privatization of this industry coupled with its growing calls for increased diversity.

Of the black respondents in this study, 26 were doctors, 23 were nurses, and 11 were technicians. The focus on three separate occupational categories allowed for comparisons across the occupational spectrum, and allowed me to highlight areas where there were both similarities and differences between workers in different employment categories. Respondents hailed from a variety of categories in health care work, including fields as varied as obstetrics/gynecology, anesthesiology, and internal medicine.

I located respondents through a variety of methods. Initially I began with a snowball sample where I began with respondents I knew or who acquaintances knew in these professions, and asked if they would be willing to refer me to potential respondents. Though snowball sampling runs the risk of replicating data to the extent that respondents share similar social networks, it is also a particularly useful methodological strategy for targeting difficult-to-reach populations. Given the underrepresentation of black men in nursing (2%) and black women in medicine (3%), this methodological approach allowed me to access populations that otherwise might have been quite challenging to locate.

Interviews took place from 2014–2017 and were typically conducted in my office, the respondent's office, or a neutral location such as a local coffee shop. In most cases, interviews were audio recorded and later professionally transcribed. In the few cases where respondents did not agree to be interviewed, I took detailed notes during the interview instead. Data were coded according to themes that emerged deductively. All respondents' names and identifying details have been changed to protect their privacy.

11.4 Findings

The remainder of this chapter answers two questions: what shapes black health care workers' sense of purpose? And how does this sense of purpose act as a buffer against potential or perceived racial discrimination? I find that many black health care workers inculcate a sense of purpose that cements into a firm commitment to find employment in this industry. That purpose helps them develop tools to offset contemporary racial discrimination, particularly the outsize importance organizations often place on social networks in hiring and advancement.

Hill, Sumner, and Burrow (2014) argue that individuals may follow several different pathways towards developing a sense of purpose. Proactive individuals actively seek out a sense of purpose, and are motivated to find something that becomes a primary goal. Others follow a more reactive path where they respond to changing life circumstances. Still a third path involves role models who provide insights into potential goals and ideals that constitute a sense of purpose. How an individual develops a sense of purpose can influence their openness to new experiences as well as the extent and level of their commitment to that purpose.

Respondents in this study conformed to two of the pathways identified in the extant literature. Generally, respondents shared an early interest in pursuing careers in health care, and this initial exposure formed the foundation of their purpose. However, this early exposure generally took the form of a response to changing life circumstances, in the form of responding to illnesses; or interactions with a mentor who helped spark respondents' interest in and commitment to a career providing health care. While the findings do not indicate whether following these paths leads to differences in level of commitment or openness to new ideas, they do suggest that both the reactive and role modeling routes can take on heightened significance for blacks employed in predominantly white workplaces.

11.4.1 Establishing the Sense of Purpose: Early Interest in Health Care

For many black doctors, nurses, nurse practitioners, and physician assistants (PAs), this is a decision made early on in life. Many of the health care professionals I interviewed reported a very early sense that they were destined for work in this field. Thinking back to her teenage years, Emma, a nurse, remembered the moment she realized not just that nursing was her calling, but that she specifically wanted to work with babies: "I knew once I got in high school that [nursing] was what I wanted to do. I was actually watching a television show on TV about nurses that took care of special care infants in the NICU and I was like, 'That's me. That's what I want to do.' And ever since then, I stuck with it and the more I learned about it, especially when I got into college in the nursing program, I was like, 'Yeah, this is definitely what I'm supposed to be doing.'" This chance exposure to a television program established Emma's lifetime interest in nursing and the career trajectory that followed. Later on, when she gained more exposure to health care work, it reinforced her sense that nursing was work that fulfilled a sense of purpose.

Julia, a pediatrician, shared a similar story. Her very early interest in both children and science made pediatrics a perfect match: "I've always had an affinity towards children in general, just growing up. I like to tell the story about how I was 11 years old when my sister was born. So I watched her grow up and that I think really just sparked an interest in children. And I was thinking about careers as I got older. I was thinking about teaching maybe, but science always intrigued me, so I felt like being a pediatrician would be the best of both worlds. To have that science background and then be able to work with kids on a daily basis. A lot of people say they want to be pediatricians, but I did know fairly early on and I kind of stuck with it. Even through medical school". Julia describes never really wavering from this career choice despite settling on it at a precociously early stage.

For doctors, nurses, and midlevel providers, early exposure mattered. This early interest typically derived from one of two factors. These health care workers either had early exposure to someone in the medical industry who made a strong impression on them, or they dealt early on with someone who had serious health care issues. In some cases, respondents themselves coped with health issues. These experiences in formative years laid the foundation that motivated these workers to pursue health care work, sometimes against daunting odds.

11.4.2   Role Modeling: Early Exposure to Health Careers

Langston offered an interesting story about a doctor he encountered in his formative years and the impact that doctor had on him. When I spoke with Langston, he was no longer practicing medicine but, after an illustrious career, launched a nonprofit designed to expose people of color to medicine. We spoke in his sunny office surrounded by his awards, photos with local politicians, and rows of books. When I asked him how he first got interested in medicine, he told me:

"Well, I've wanted to be a doctor virtually all my life. Really from about
age 5. Because I had a role model, Dr. Grant. My father [who provided
ambulance service], whenever he would go to take someone down to
see Dr. Grant, which was frequent in the black community because rather
than going in separate segregated waiting rooms for the three white doctors
in town, the blacks, if they could afford it, would prefer to be taken down

to see Dr. Grant. Dr. Grant impressed me. He was important. He had
powers that no one else had. He would always seem mysterious. There was
something powerful and magical and very important and mysterious about
him. I wanted to be like him".

Langston grew up in the deep south during the era of legal segregation. As a black physician, Dr. Grant stood out as an important contrast to the narrow occupational fields in which blacks were typically concentrated. As Langston describes, this lent him an air of mystery and importance. In a time when very few blacks held powerful, high status positions, Dr. Grant stood out as someone unusual and inspiring.

Marisol, a nurse practitioner, tells a similar story about a family background in health care: "I figured that I might go into nursing, just because I knew... my family has a big background in healthcare... or medicine, to be exact. My mother's a physician, my uncle's a physician, my grandfather was a physician, my grandmother was a midwife. And specifically, my grandfather was a OBGYN. My uncle was a OBGYN. My mom started off an OBGYN but she went into pathology. So I always had that interest, that background of women's health".

Notably, despite the family history of working in medicine, Marisol opted to become a nurse practitioner. When I asked her why, she stated that despite the long family history, she had never had interest in being a doctor and that medical school "wasn't in her plan". In her case, her family's lengthy involvement in the health care industry sparked a general interest in this work and in women's health in particular, but did not crystallize into a desire to pursue medicine as a doctor.

Theresa, another nurse practitioner, described a close family member who exposed her to the field as well:

"My aunt is a nurse. My favorite aunt is a nurse and she's always told me stories about things that have gone on at her job and things of the sort. So that's what got me interested in nursing. She would tell me about a lot of exciting things that would go on at work in terms of caring for people, people and their symptoms when they would come in. She also did labor and delivery. The one story that I actually think of is a particular story she was just telling me about a labor and delivery patient who was in a whole lot of pain, and acting out a bit. And she was telling me how she helped calm her down and how they ended up having a healthy happy baby. She did quite a bit. And just how she bonded with her coworkers and she bonded with a lot of the patients, like all of those things are what really stuck out in my head".

For Theresa, the most attractive aspect of her early exposure to nursing was the opportunity to care for people while building relationships with patients and coworkers. This is consistent with the construction of nursing as a field where caring, rather than technical proficiency, is critical. Clearly both are required for this work, but nursing has long been portrayed as an occupation where (mostly women) workers care for patients rather than diagnosing and treating them.

For many doctors and nurses, an early role model was essential to shaping an interest in the health care field. As Marisol's and Edgar's examples show, this person did not necessarily have to be someone who worked in the same profession they would later pursue. However, the initial exposure to the power, social relationships, and intrigue of health care proved an early lure to the field.

11.4.3 Reactive Processes to Developing Purpose: Dealing with Illness

Other respondents were drawn to health care work because they had direct experience with someone suffering from illness. In many cases they watched family members coping with a chronic, persistent medical condition. In some instances, they faced illnesses themselves. Overall, seeing the ways in which family members coped with health problems–and more importantly, navigated the health care system—sparked an interest in pursuing careers in this field.

Melinda, a phlebotomist, offers an example of this when she considers what led her to this profession: "Because there was a lot of my family members that were basically getting sick, they needed care for… I started out working with mentally disabled, and then I went from working with mentally disabled and went to school for medical assistant and went from medical assistant to phlebotomist". Melinda found herself in the position of caring for many of her ill family members. For her, moving into doing this work in a paid capacity became a natural progression.

Alexandria, a geneticist, shared a similar story of how she first became attracted to medicine: "I've always been fascinated with medicine, and I think a lot of that stemmed from the fact that I saw my grandmother go through so many different health conditions, so many different barriers while I was a child growing up. So it was just something that always piqued my curiosity". Note that while Alexandra was not responsible for providing direct care, observing the barriers her grandmother faced in getting care left a mark. Alexandra's trajectory suggests that seeing the medical racism some black patients encounter can serve as an impetus for pursuing work in the health care industry.

For Darius, a physician's assistant, it was his mother's health care problems that attracted him to the work. He told me, "I've always wanted to do health care. My mom was always sick. This exposed me to the need in the field at a young age. And I grew up in a really small town. Where I'm from there's not a lot of advanced practice providers, so I saw how hard it was for her". Note that for Darius, the context of living in a relatively rural area that was medically underserved exacerbated the challenges his mother encountered. Overall, however, seeing the way that his mother often fought for care and struggled with her health in that environment opened his eyes to the potential of a career in health care.

Finally, Aaliyah is a neonatologist whose interest in medicine grew out of her own struggles with chronic conditions. She acknowledges that her own serious health problems gave her extensive exposure to the medical system. "I got interested in being a doctor because of my own medical condition. So I have severe asthma. That's how I got interested in medicine, and then I always liked working with children. That's how I got interested in pediatrics. Once I was interested in pediatrics I liked high acuity work. I liked the diagnostic process, so I was really drawn to neonatology. I like not specializing in one organ system and I like intensive care, so neonatology seemed perfect for me". Aaliyah clearly tracks the connection between how her own illness sparked her initial focus on health care, and then her own interests shaped the specific trajectories she took once in the field. While struggling with asthma offered an early introduction to the health care system, her own personal affinity for children, diagnostic work, and intensive care combined to make neonatology a good fit for her.

Being driven to health care work as a result of observing an ill family member is not necessarily unique to black professionals in this field. I spoke with Rhonda, a white woman working as a charge nurse on a labor and delivery floor, who shared a pretty similar story: "I got hurt a lot as a kid playing sports. And I saw all my father's injuries. So we were at the hospital a lot. And even as young as five years old, I was fascinated by what they do. I've wanted this career since then. I like the family friendliness, the work-life balance". Rhonda's story, on its face, parallels what I heard from many black health care workers. The distinction, however, lies in the scope. Given that blacks en masse have worse health outcomes than their white peers, blacks are more likely to cope with health challenges and issues that could potentially expose them to careers in this line of work. These adverse health outcomes could, ironically, have the potential to put them on a career path to work in this industry.

For black professionals in health care, early exposure to the field mattered. Thus, while many respondents described the significance of role models in the health care industry, many others were drawn to this work as a result of first or second hand exposure to the way family members (or they themselves) coped with persistent health issues. Whether respondents got this exposure on the patient side or practitioner side, being aware of how health care could make a difference was enough to spark an interest in the field that put them on their current career paths.

An important component of this early commitment to health care is that it meant many black workers were unprepared or unwilling to consider any other career choices. As a result, they were adamant that being a doctor or nurse was the only line of work they could or would do. This level of focus meant that many black doctors excelled in high school and college because they knew they would need top grades to navigate postsecondary school and find work. Additionally, and perhaps more importantly, it provided a purpose and an internal motivation to seek solutions when faced with situations that could give rise to occupational discrimination.

11.5 Obstacles to Purpose: Covert Discrimination in Health Care

Respondents noted that beginning at the postgraduate level, outcomes were driven much more by social connections and networks than they were by objective measures. Peer groups, social ties, and relationships could determine everything from study groups to fellowship opportunities to employment. For blacks in nursing and medical programs, however, this presented a complication. The emphasis on social networks meant that it was very easy for black students to be left out and excluded from opportunities that were available to their white peers.

Edgar, a surgeon affiliated with a university hospital, also discussed how heavily medicine relies on networks. Like Ella, he believed the reliance on networks could lead to discriminatory outcomes for black candidates when it comes to hiring:

> "Hiring is no different than in corporate America. Although there
> are certain constraints that are put on you, most people, when they
> put a job out there, they already know who they're hiring. So they'll
> go through a rudimentary process to say, 'Oh yes, we opened this up,
> we put the job description in the journal, however, the job's already
> filled.' We actually just talked about that last night with regard to trying
> to create some diversity here. How do we make sure that process is done
> fairly? And that's a hard thing to do because each department
> has its own hiring and chairmen have their own thoughts of who they
> want to hire. Pretty much the person is selected first and then second the
> job is listed. It's just via friendships. People recommend them. But yeah,
> [black doctors] a lot of times are left out of the loop on that because
> we're not networked in that same circle".

Edgar is very candid in noting that friendships and personal recommendations make the difference. This leaves highly qualified workers who do not have the right connections at a disadvantage. And it does not escape him that black doctors are more likely to be among those that lack those social ties.

Adewale, an anesthesiologist in his thirties, shared similar observations about the way that networking matters in the medical profession: "It's an old boys club. It's the situation where you're an equally qualified candidate, and because Joe Smith's father and mother and brother and uncle all went to the same institution, and know every surgeon and every physician and every nurse in the department, you're not going to be necessarily the top of the list or the remembered name at the end of the day compared to Joe Smith who everyone knows already". I heard other doctors use the "old boys club" metaphor to characterize medicine. Given the racial consequences of this heavy reliance on social networks, it is perhaps important to note that this old boys club is open much more to white boys than black ones.

Lest we assume this mostly affects doctors, Marisol, a nurse practitioner, suggests that social networks are equally important for finding jobs in nursing: "I find that women of color [in nursing programs] are typically pushed to more public health departments, community clinics, health departments. Whereas the more, I guess you could say white, Caucasian… but statistically, the more affluent students are given assignments of private practices, OBGYN offices, the plush offices. So that then when they graduate, they have this experience and the network that they can draw on. Whereas the students of color don't necessarily have those same connections. So it becomes harder to get into that marketplace".

There is extensive empirical support for black health care workers' perceptions that relying on social networks leads to subtle forms of racial discrimination. Despite the fact that it has been outlawed for nearly half a century, racial discrimination still plays a role in hiring. Yet it rarely takes on the sort of overt, obvious forms present in previous generations. Job ads will not read "whites only need apply," and employers will not state that they discriminate based on race—quite the opposite! But employers can (and do) espouse discriminatory beliefs and attitudes about prospective black workers, as long as they do not openly attribute these to race outright. Instead, they use assumptions about culture, work ethic, and even names as a proxy for race (Bertrand & Mullainathan, 2004; Kirschenman & Neckerman, 1991; Rivera, 2014; Roscigno, 2007). Racial discrimination persists, even if it is not called by that name.

When it comes to hiring, employers routinely stereotype blacks as lazy, unmotivated, and undesirable workers. This applies to both black men and women, though there are some ways that gender intersects with race to shape the particulars of the stereotypes used. Employers associate a "single mother element" with black women regardless of their parental status, and attach these stereotypes to their assumptions about black women's credibility and reliability (Kennelly, 1999). Hiring managers believe black men lack "soft skills" like personability, approachability, and work ethic that would make them desirable workers (Moss & Tilly, 1996). When matched with otherwise identical resumes, employers even prefer white men *with criminal records* to black men with no history of involvement in the criminal justice system (Pager, 2007). Hiring discrimination thus presents a serious obstacle for blacks accessing certain jobs.

As these health care workers observed, even when hiring happens through informal connections, black workers are typically disadvantaged. The saying that "it's not what you know, it's who you know" certainly describes a common pattern of capitalizing on connections and friendships in order to secure work. But even these social ties are racially structured in ways that can exclude blacks and minimize access to jobs. Whites routinely reserve tips, leads, and information about jobs for other whites in their social networks (Royster, 2003). Even in high-status, elite professional service jobs like finance, consulting, and law, recruiters show a bias towards applicants with social and cultural hobbies that are more likely to be the province of upper class whites–e.g., polo, squash, or lacrosse rather than boxing, pool, or bowling (Rivera, 2014). Social networks, then, can be a key mechanism of hiring discrimination. Furthermore, even though she overstated the specific numbers in nursing, Marisol is correct that discriminatory processes can have material consequences, as professional blacks still face wage inequality relative to whites even when controlling for education, work experience, and region (Wilson & Rodgers III, 2016).

11.6 Managing Networks, Managing Discrimination

For many blacks across a variety of fields, these conclusions are not surprising. Employment discrimination has been a fact of black life for centuries. But because black doctors' and nurses' commitment to health care created a sense of purpose and determination to achieve their occupational dreams, they did what blacks have always done: attempted to work the system. They saw very early on that to achieve their longstanding goals of becoming doctors or nurses, they could not simply rely on hard work alone. Instead, they coupled this with intentional efforts to construct social networks that would pay off for them and hopefully reduce possibilities of casual, covert discrimination.

Bella offers an example of this. She is a 34 year old internal medicine doctor who comes from humble beginnings. Bella immigrated to the US from Sierra Leone as an infant but is now an American citizen. A first generation college student, she attended an elite, highly selective research university for her undergraduate degree. It was here that she began actively using her connections to guide her path into medicine.

Bella was very open about deliberately using her connections to advance. "I was fortunate that by the time I started to apply, I had a lot of friends who had already been through it. And my sister in law was also at the time in her fourth year of medical school. So I had a lot of people really there to support me. My friends who were proofreading my essays repeatedly… There's so much that I think that had I not had people who had been through it and mentored me through the application process, it would have been very difficult to know what areas of the application to really focus on. What is critical, where do you not want to make any mistakes. So I think that definitely helped me out in terms of getting into medical school. And then just even understanding what schools to apply to and what not to apply to".

She continued, "I would say with my networking, a lot of it was my alumni network that I reached out to and I had four really good friends who went through that process as well. And who also called on my behalf. Definitely having people recommend– it's almost like having legacy. Parents went to the school and you can say hey, my daughter is going here. Put in a good word for her". Bella's conscious decision to use her networks proved critical for gaining acceptance to the medical school of her choice. She took advantage of the connections an elite school offered, and surrounded herself with friends who were also on or had already navigated the track to medical school. These connections eased her application process considerably. Though Bella did not go through life with these sorts of ties, she was able to use her alumni network strategically to construct social networks that functioned like the legacy processes which can help children of alumni attend selective institutions. She believed that doing so created essential social capital that facilitated her acceptance into her first choice medical school.

Adewale, the anesthesiologist mentioned earlier, also actively used his networks to address a setback during the match system where graduating medical students land in their first jobs:

"This match system is supposed to be fair, however, the residency program
is going to pick who they think are the best applicants. So the question that
you asked me was can I point to a specific point in which my network helped
me to get where I needed to go. So in my process of going from medical school to residency, I did not match. So that next period becomes what's called a scramble, which means of all those programs, some may have one or two spots left over. Now all of those applicants who got an interview but did not get a spot, or maybe didn't get an interview, are all writing and faxing and emailing trying to get those one or two spots left over. And it's times like those when some of my mentors and professors I knew were able to speak to a program director and say 'Hey, I know this guy, didn't make an interview selection. Maybe there were too many, maybe you skipped over him. Take a look again. I can vouch for this guy.' Or 'I've seen him work. He's a hard worker, he had a couple of grades drop off or he had to take time off or maybe she got pregnant or family issues got in the way.' So then there becomes that verbal element, that personal element that is missed, or supposedly missed during that interview process. And I can say for sure that in my particular case, that that happened for me more than once. And I appreciated it. I did not think it was a handout because I knew that I was qualified as evidenced by my current position, but it didn't hurt".

Social networks were essential for Adewale to move into the medical field. By attending a top caliber medical program, he was able to rely on those links and his relationships with professors and advisors in ways that permitted his career to advance.

Ricky, a surgeon, realized during medical school that white students had very different networks than he did. Once he realized this, however, he immediately made conscientious efforts to insert himself into them:

"I was really struggling and was concerned about if I was going to
make it through the program, honestly. Then I had this conversation
with this kid one day while we were walking to class. He said something
to me about their study group. Study group?! I didn't even know these
dudes had a study group! So I asked him if I could sit in with them. Come
to find out, not only are these guys all studying together, but they
would ask the professor about stuff that was going to be on the exam.
I didn't even know that was allowed! That was how I passed my
neurology class—studying with those guys, working with the group.
And please believe, once I saw how they had it set up, and how they
were relying on each other, I made friends with my white class mates
and my Asian classmates and my South Asian classmates as well as
my black classmates and Latino classmates".

For those who are familiar with the way postgraduate programs in many fields work, it may seem self-evident that Ricky could have linked up with fellow students to form study groups and benefit from their collective knowledge. But he also characterizes this as a very informal process that was not widely shared or known among the few black students in his medical school program. Indeed, he only learned through happenstance that this particular group existed at all, and he had no idea that asking the professor specific questions about the exams was permitted. Thus, while other students also found the course difficult, Ricky was unaware that they addressed this by working together and in concert with the professor to pass an especially difficult class. Once he learned that this was the case, he made certain to restructure his social networks accordingly.

Social networks matter for nurses too. Emma, the nurse in a neonatal intensive care unit (NICU) acknowledges that her connections helped her secure her current position: "I actually ended up in the medical surgical unit first. It was more so an easier place to get into because it's not specialized so you don't need any special training and they're more open to new grads. But I kind of knew a few people that transferred from the medical surgical unit to women's health and they kind of helped me get my foot in the door in that area. But I knew that's what I wanted to do". Emma's early aspirations involved nursing in the NICU, although this is a harder field to enter as a recent nursing school graduate. As she notes, however, she was able to use her connections to people in that area in order to ease her transition into this more specialized field.

Although occupational discrimination in health care can take this covert, ostensibly nonracial form of relying on social networks, this process undoubtedly has racial implications. Blacks notice as early as medical and nursing school that connections matter more than their educational performance or technical skills. What is significant here, however, is the finding that when faced with this pattern of colorblind discrimination, black doctors and nurses take steps to address it by actively forming ties with white peers who can provide the connections and referrals that lead to their advancement.

Other studies have shown that social relations are a key component of how individuals maintain purposeful pursuits (Ryff, 1989). This research builds on those findings by showing that black workers in professional occupations intentionally form and leverage these networks in an effort to create a bulwark against potential and suspected racial discrimination. These workers develop a purpose early on in life, but the establishment and maintenance of these social relationships help them to challenge the casual, implicit racial assumptions built into the credentialing and hiring processes in health care work.

11.7 Summary

For black workers in the health care industry, purpose is an important, if understudied, component of their ability to withstand and respond to occupational obstacles. These workers' pathways into this field are often set in early years, where they are exposed to role models or the importance of quality care. This develops into an unshakable commitment to health care work. That commitment comes in very handy for black workers who frequently confront occupational discrimination in the workplace, and pushes them to construct and leverage social networks very strategically as a way of integrating themselves into professional settings.

Social ties are integral to advancing in the modern workplace, and health care occupations are no exception. Respondents were quite aware of this fact. As a result, black professionals simply have to be intentional and decisive when constructing and using their social networks. Carefully developing and using these connections is not an option, but a critical decision that helps to avoid the ways social networks can maintain exclusionary processes and result in covert racial discrimination. A sense of purpose about their role in the medical field helps to achieve this.

Future sociological research could consider expanding the concept of purpose more fully. The findings here indicate that a sense of purpose, formed through personal circumstances and role models, helps inculcate black professionals with the motivation to enact strategies to offset racial workplace challenges. Thus, future studies could examine other ways that purpose helps underrepresented workers in other social institutions develop tools they need to succeed. Garcia-Lopez's (2008) study of Chicana attorneys suggests that their commitment to communities of color helps motivate them to establish their own firms when the racial and gender discrimination they encounter in predominantly white practices becomes unbearable. It may be that for other workers of color, purpose is a common thread that shapes occupational decisions more than we know.

References

Bell, E., & Nkomo, S. (2003). *Our separate ways*. Cambridge, MA: Harvard Business Press.

Bertrand, M., & Mullainathan, S. (2004). Are Emily and Greg more employable than Lakisha and Jamal? A field experiment on labor market discrimination. *American Economic Review, 94*(4), 991–1013.

Cose, E. (1993). *Rage of a privileged class*. New York: Harper Perennial.

Evans, L. (2014). *Cabin pressure*. Lanham, MD: Rowman and Littlefield.

Feagin, J., & Sikes, M. (1995). *Living with racism*. Boston: Beacon Press.

Garcia-Lopez, G. (2008). Nunca Te Toman En Cuenta [They Never Take You Into Account]: The Challenges of Inclusion and Strategies for Success of Chicana Attorneys. *Gender & Society 22*(5): 590–612.

Hill, P. L., Sumner, R., & Burrow, A. (2014). Understanding the pathways to purpose: Examining personality and well-being correlates across adulthood. *Journal of Positive Psychology, 9*(3), 227–234.

Kennelly, I. (1999). That single mother element. *Gender and Society, 13*(2), 168–192.

Kirschenman, J., & Neckerman, K. (1991). 'We'd love to hire them, but …': The meaning of race for employers. *The Urban Underclass., 203*, 203–232.

Moss, P., & Tilly, C. (1996). 'Soft' skills and race: An investigation of black men's employment problems. *Work and Occupations, 23*(3), 252–276.

Pager, D. (2007). *Marked*. Chicago: University of Chicago Press.

Ray, V. (2019). A theory of racialized organizations. *American Sociological Review, 84*(1), 26–53.

Rivera, L. (2014). *Pedigree*. Princeton, NJ: Princeton University Press.

Roscigno, V. (2007). *The face of discrimination*. Lanham, MD: Rowman and Littlefield.

Royster, D. (2003). *Race and the invisible hand*. Berkeley, CA: University of California Press.

Ryff, C. D. (1989). Happiness is everything, or is it? Explorations on the meaning of psychological well-being. *The Journal of Personality and Social Psychology, 57*(6), 1069–1081.

Yanick, J. S., & Feagin, J. (1998). *Double burden*. New York: Routledge.

Wilson, V., & Rodgers III, W. M. (2016). Black-white wage gaps expand with rising wage inequality. *Economic policy institute* (pp. 1–65).

Chapter 12
How Practicing Our Purpose Aim Contributes to a Cultural Common Good, and Vice Versa

Seana Moran

Abstract Life purpose is fundamentally ecological: individual life purpose aims interacting with cultural resources generate momentum in individual lives and in cultures. A dynamic life momentum loop model highlights how a purpose practice starts with a purpose aim (mental representation of a specific prosocial effect), filtered by personal meaning (significance or importance), that influences perception of situational resources (a subset of a culture's shared meanings, artifacts, practices and "behavioral defaults" stored in the "common good") to initiate opportunities to enact the envisioned prosocial effect, and afterward evaluate perceived feedback for effectiveness. Cultures also develop and, with increasing multicultural contact, individuals can influence and be influenced by multiple common goods. Repetitions of this purpose practice loop generate individual life momentum and shared cultural momentum.

Keywords Youth · Purpose · Culture · Meaning-making · Ecological · Developmental

12.1 How Practicing Our Purpose Aims Contributes to a Cultural Common Good

A life purpose aim is a reason *to* live by envisioning something beyond oneself here-and-now to live *for* (Frankl, 1959). This chapter elaborates an ecologically dynamic life momentum model to understand how purpose aim, when practiced, is a dynamic psychological force for our own lives to proceed as well as for us to influence each other's lives and potentially contribute to the common good of our shared culture.

Purpose practice is an ecological process of finding useful resources and opportunities in everyday situations to make envisioned prosocial effects. The life momentum

S. Moran (✉)
ImagiNations, Arlington, MA, USA
e-mail: SMoranImagiNations@gmail.com

model posits that our *purpose aim* is (a) a *criterion* for perceiving everyday experiences as potential opportunities and for perceiving feedback to evaluate effectiveness, and (b) a *template* for enacting our aimed-for prosocial effect. Our aim starts our *purpose practice* to filter perceptions of everyday situations as suitable venues to create prosocial effects, stimulate intention to act, follow our aim's template for enactment, and evaluate how well we did. Purpose aim helps us determine when and how to proceed with our purpose practice in order to increase our odds of benefiting others and our culture.

The life momentum model makes explicit, from an individual's perspective, the dynamics of an individual's purpose aim "looping" through personal meaning, intention, action, and effect (a) to *feedforward* and make a situational prosocial effect and perhaps a lasting contribution to the common good and (b) to *feedback* and regulate the aim's own clarity and strength. The model also notes from a cultural perspective (a) how what is valued in the common good influences the options individuals have for their purpose aim and (c) how individuals from different cultural backgrounds interacting in situations may diversify or transform the common good or create multiple parallel common goods, which can expand the resources individuals have for their own purposes.

This chapter launches a dynamic conceptualization within the purpose research community and, by extension, the purpose education community...with a caveat. I draw on existing studies and theories as support for specific assertions I make about the dynamics of purpose aim and practice. But most of these prior sources provide only *indirect* support for the following reasons: They usually are based on correlational analyses of data collected at one time point so they cannot directly address dynamics over time. Most are based on purpose measures that do not require respondents to state a specific purpose aim as an anchor for the respondents' other responses (e.g., Ryff, 1989; Steger, Frazier, Oishi, & Kaler, 2006), so they cannot provide direct insight on how a focal aim functions to launch a specific prosocial effect. Furthermore, although many sources don't state a theory of purpose function, those that use a framework often rely on models of hierarchical components (such as meaning being "a part of" purpose or vice versa; e.g., Costin & Vignoles, 2019; Martela & Steger, 2016) or dimensions ("a purpose" = meaning + intention + engagement; Damon, 2008), so they do not address how the constructs themselves can change or can transform each other over time.

Still, I must start somewhere or we will get nowhere—that is how innovation works (Moran, 2016a). I bring in sources beyond purpose research, psychology and education to include disciplines like physics and biology that may have metaphors or models that could be useful. I include studies, theories and commentaries that address any part of the life momentum model, including sources that link to psychological constructs beyond purpose aim itself that may play dynamic roles in purpose practice. For example, emotions relate both to meaning-making and to feedback because they signal *felt* personal significance, and they indicate the state of our relationship to the environment. Similarly, intention relates to future orientation, future time perspective, and agency because the designs we make for our lives depend in part on whether we are forward-looking, how far forward we imagine, and whether we believe we are capable to move forward. My hope is that reinterpreted prior work dynamically may help our collective thinking to move forward.

Overview of the chapter. The life momentum model is a new way of understanding life purpose and it has yet to be directly tested. So I consider this chapter a series of propositions: First, purpose practice is a dynamic ecological force because it creates a reciprocal, symbiotic relationship between individuals and life situations that co-produce cultural ecosystems. Second, not everyone has a purpose aim, but practicing purpose has been touted as beneficial to self, others, and communities. Third, a purpose aim guides and evaluates individuals in aligning their actual effects in situations with their mental representation of a meaningful, specific prosocial effect. Fourth, these prosocial effects can ripple beyond the situation and into the common good, which means a purpose aim builds not only momentum in individuals' own lives but also in their culture. Fifth, individuals from different cultures in interaction means multiple cultural common goods and a wider variety of purpose aims are in play, which presents additional opportunities and challenges for making prosocial effects.

12.2 Dynamics: Purpose as a Psychological Force

Dynamics address how linked entities interact as forces on each other over time. In psychology, dynamic approaches use data collected at multiple time points to discover *when* and *how* specified psychological constructs (i.e., perception and meaning) emerge, change, transform, and stabilize each other: What threshold does a construct need to surpass for a new status to arise? How does one construct's function change another construct's function over time?

Dynamic methods could be helpful to address impasses of correlational methods in life purpose research. Although dynamic theories were prevalent in developmental psychology with Lewin and Vygotsky in the 1930s (see Lewin, 1951; Moran & John-Steiner, 2003, for reviews), recently as new tools have become available, theorists and methodologists have returned to dynamics (Van Geert, 1998), including for purpose-related constructs like identity (Lichtwarck-Aschoff, Van Geert, Bosma, & Kunnen, 2008). However, a coherent, ecological-dynamic model of life purpose aim and practice has been lacking in the life purpose literature, and I am not aware of any empirical papers that directly examine the dynamics of purpose practice.

Yet, several life purpose researchers have hinted at a need for dynamic models in their calls for time-dependent measures, interactions, and feedback. For example, Burrow, Hill, Ratner, and Sumner's (2018) and Hill, Burrow, and Sumner's (2013) characterization of purpose as "where am I going?" requires directed pursuit toward a specific aim over time (temporal motion). Their use of "agency" requires consideration of *self*-control of one's own actions rather than simply responding to contextual stimuli (interaction and feedback), and their use of "contexts" requires considering how individuals contribute as well as consume resources (interaction and transformation). McKnight and Kashdan's (2009) review of purpose and related concepts includes many reciprocal relations, such as between purpose and meaning (feedback).

Modeling purpose practice through feedforward and feedback loops. See Fig. 12.1 for a diagram of the life momentum model, which got its name from the direction, speed and commitment to a specific prosocial aim that is maintained by a person repeatedly using the processes in the model to make—and learn from making—contributions to others. Two repositories of contributions (the rectangles) anchor the model. The first is the purpose aim, which is a mental representation of an ideal prosocial effect a person wants to make in their lifetime, usually built over time into a repository of imagined and remembered personal prosocial effects. The representation is not of a specific act (i.e., doing surgeries), but rather of the helpful effect the

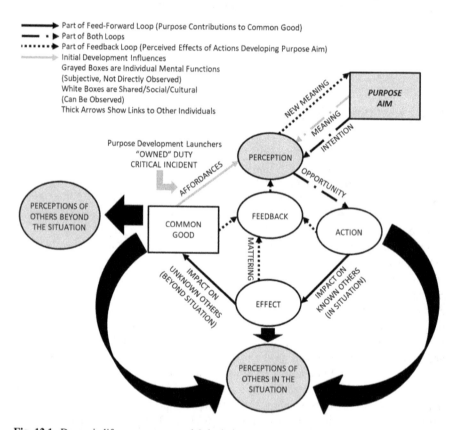

Fig. 12.1 Dynamic life momentum model depicting purpose practice generated by purpose aim. Model focuses on one person's purpose aim to influence perception (upper right), which starts the purpose practice within a situation. But an individual does not practice purpose in isolation because other people are part of the situation. So links to the perceptions of other individuals within (bottom) and beyond (left) the situation are also shown. Individual purpose practices are linked through perception of each other's contributions (thick arrows)

person wants to have on others (e.g., eradicating cleft palates in children, or reducing deaths by heart defects). The second is the common good, which is a repository of aggregated contributions in a culture that grows through social contagion of prosocial effects beyond the situation that originated the effect. Most specific prosocial effects don't make it into the common good because they mimic the already existing "defaults" or are not shared widely enough beyond their originating situation.

Purpose aim and common good are linked in two reciprocal feedforward loops and one feedback loop comprising transformative processes (the ovals and arrows). Purpose aim feeds forward to regulate the common good through effects that are socially shared, become widely used, and are saved cross-generationally. The common good feeds forward to regulate individuals' purpose aims through offering resources that could be used to make prosocial effects.

Feedback is a pathway in which one repository regulates itself through the influence of transformations that eventually return to the same repository. The purpose aim's mental representation is maintained or updated from feedback from the actor's own feelings and insights. But the most important feedback comes from others within the situation who are affected by the actor's efforts, and possibly from people beyond the situation who learned about the actor's prosocial effect through social learning. This feedback forms new meanings to clarify the purpose aim's template for finding further opportunities to practice.

The feedback loop is dependent in part on the feedforward loop: feedback can't occur if there is not at least an attempt to enact a purpose aim to create an effect that feeds forward a potential contribution toward the common good. Given this life momentum model, what are the ecological implications of purpose aim and purpose practice?

12.3 Ecology: Moving from Contexts to Affordances

Ecology studies the dynamics of living organisms in a habitat. A habitat is a circumscribed setting that provides resources for organisms to fulfill their needs. The best-known ecological framework in psychology is Bronfenbrenner's (1979) systems model that "layers" environmental resources from nearest to farthest in influence on a focal person. These environmental layers unidirectionally influence the person and can bidirectionally influence each other. But Bronfenbrenner minimizes how the person also can influence these contexts through actions or meanings that could change how the contexts "work" for the person.

For this reason, Gibson's model of perceived affordances (Gibson & Pick, 2000) and Lewin's (1951) model of life spaces and psychological events are more appropriate frameworks for an ecologically dynamic view of purpose aim and practice. Gibson's affordances are contextual resources transformed in a person's perception to be important and useful for specific goals. Lewin's life space defines the subset of a culture's meanings and opportunities that is subjectively possible for a person, of which the person during their lifetime actually experiences a subset of these possibilities as psychological events. A psychological event means something happened that was made salient to the person's perceptions, beliefs, emotions and behavior.

Within a psychological event, a purpose aim brings together a person's anticipated future possibilities as a force to influence the person's current perception and action (Lewin, 1951). A purpose aim does not predict the future, it makes the subjective future salient in the current situation to increase the probability that the situation might afford an opportunity for the anticipated prosocial effect to occur.

I am aware of no life purpose studies that are based on Lewin's and Gibson's work, and most statistical studies do not include a specific purpose aim. However, case studies of purpose exemplars convey narratives of how precocious youth draw resources from their experiences in increasingly sophisticated ways to pursue their purpose aims (Bronk, 2012; Malin, Ballard, & Damon, 2015; see also Moran, 2020 for a theoretical view). Similarly, a few statistical studies could be interpreted as providing indirect support for individuals making the future psychologically present: (a) a study of how stronger sense of purpose and self-direction toward the future is related to lower impulsivity in the present (Burrow & Spreng, 2016), and (b) a study of how stronger future orientation—a deliberate focus on later possibilities that help planning and goal-setting behaviors—is associated with lower violent behavior in the present (Stoddard, Zimmerman, & Bauermeister, 2012). Both studies suggest that our subjective conceptions of our personal future can keep us from doing something rash in current situations that might affect our future life spaces.

Ecosystems comprise interactions from a subjective point-of-view. In an ecological view of life purpose practice, individuals comprise the organisms, and life situations comprise proximal habitats that manifest a subset of a larger cultural habitat. Individuals simultaneously are psychological persons (we have a unique perspective on the world) and social actors (others can perceive how we behave through their own unique perspectives). How we practice our purpose aim will be strongly influenced by our perceptions and experiences and not necessarily by what "objectively" happened. Subjectivity matters (e.g., it's not how fast the molecules are moving in an item, measured objectively as temperature, but rather that the item feels hot or cold *to me*). Ecologically, there are many phenomena in a situation. But a specific phenomenon only matter to me when it becomes usable to pursue my purpose aim—when an item, subjectively determined, becomes an "affordance" (Heft, 2013).

An individual's subjective perspective encompasses their personal past and present, anticipated future, and salient cognitive, emotional and social capacities. The situation as a habitat for the individual comprises what the individual perceives as affordances from: (a) the available social-cultural artifacts and tools; (b) the accumulated cognitive, emotional and social capacities of *other* individuals participating in the situation; and (c) the culturally shared "default" understandings, value, uses, and relationships of various resources accumulated and saved from past individuals' efforts. Since each participant in the situation also is an *I*, the situation could be construed as very different combinations of affordances because each person subjectively selects based on different purpose aims or needs.

Individuals produce the ecosystem. Ecologically, "having" a general sense of purpose has no force because it provides no template for the person to enact a prosocial effect, nor criteria by which the person can scan or search the situation for affordances and evaluate their own efforts. Without a purpose aim to find affordances tailored to an envisioned prosocial effect, a person generally will navigate the situation based on extrinsic incentives. With a purpose aim, the person can *self*-regulate perception so the situation's resources are not the sole stimuli influencing their behavior.

The ecological advantage of a purpose aim is that it makes perception of a situation more agentic and efficient. Purpose aim sifts and organizes perceptions faster. It generates "motivated perception" to view the world in terms of opportunities to enact prosocial effect: we see what can help us realize our desired outcome, sometimes even shifting our perceptions to help us persist despite challenges (see Burrow, Stanley, Sumner, & Hill, 2014, for extended discussion). So the person does not miss *this* specific opportunity before them.

With a purpose aim, the person does not generally *wish* for something to happen because they can more efficiently find ways to *make* something happen. As examples, to a professional canoe builder, a perceived wooden log becomes "my next project in sustainable carpentry," or to a climate activist, perceived heavy traffic signals "drivers who needs to be educated." A blighted empty lot may mean "dangerous location to be patrolled" to a police officer, "affordable housing development" to a builder, and "community garden" to a neighborhood leader.

12.4 Purpose Practice: Generating Prosocial Effects

Purpose practice is desirable but elusive. The life momentum model focuses on one person's purpose *aim* starting a feedforward loop of psychological and social processes that, combined, equals *practicing* purpose. Although not always focused on a specific aim, the notion of purpose in general has become a socially desirable developmental objective in the twenty-first century (Hill, Burrow, & Sumner, 2013) as studies report numerous psychological benefits to individuals who "have" at least a general sense of purpose, even if they don't report a specific purpose aim (reviewed in Bronk, 2014; McKnight & Kashdan, 2009).

Young people are trying to engage purpose in some way. Half of college freshmen believe, at least conceptually, that sense of purpose is important (Molasso, 2006). Three of four college upperclassmen are somewhat or greatly searching for a sense of purpose, and most college students discuss purpose-related topics and sometimes purpose aims with friends (Keyes, 2011). The few studies that address purpose aim also find positive trends. Over time, high school and college students tend to view purpose practice as interactions of goal-setting, prosociality and commitment (Bronk, 2014; Malin, Reilly, Quinn, & Moran, 2014; Moran, 2014). Yet, the pursuit of a specific purpose aim is difficult. Only 23% of high school graduates and 42% of college sophomores and juniors report engaging a specific purpose aim (Moran,

2009). Only about 15% to 33% adult Americans feel even a general sense of purpose or purpose aim in their work (reviewed in Keyes, 2011).

The mechanisms by which a purpose aim functions in a person's life are not well understood, and many existing research findings may not mean what researchers think they mean. Feeling a general sense of purpose is much less committed than practicing a specific purpose aim by finding situations to enact the aim's prosocial effect. Purpose definitional dimensions of meaning, intention, engagement and beyond-the-self impact (Moran, 2009) or of scope, strength, and awareness (McKnight & Kashdan, 2009) when operating separately are not likely to produce the coherence of a purpose practice that coordinates these dimensions to increase the chances of a prosocial effect. Psychological benefits to oneself associated with sense of purpose do not show the same long-term implications as a purpose aim to benefits others (Hill, Burrow, Brandenberger, Lapsley, & Quaranto, 2010).

Life purpose aim focuses on prosocial effect. Prosocial effect is the crux of an ecological model for purpose aim. Focusing on what people intend to do to maintain or build the common good, not consume from the common good, makes purpose practice *sustainable*. A world of only self-oriented life goals is not sustainable. If everyone consumes shared resources only for their own benefit without care to maintain or replace resources, that is the definition of a "tragedy of the commons" (Hardin, 1968), a fundamentally ecological event of the breakdown of the interdependent relationships among organisms in a habitat.

Prosocial effect means helping others who are present in the situation (e.g., direct effect of helping family, Kiang, 2012). Contribution means "to bestow together." Contributions are prosocial effects shared beyond the specific situation to become normalized as part of the common good (e.g., inviting students' mothers to become part of an English as Second Language course so the families and the broader neighborhood integrate better, Moran & Opazo, 2019; e.g., sharing cultural traditions, creating innovations, or changing societal structures, Folgueiras & Palou, 2018; Moran, 2010).

The assertion that purpose aim must benefit something beyond the individual is controversial. Several scholars side-step or reject the idea of "beyond-the-self" impact as too ambiguous, too fraught with moral overtones, or too subjective to measure well (e.g., Hill et al., 2013; Waddington, 2010). On closer scrutiny, this criticism is untenable if scholars also continue to promote youth purpose as a way to improve both individuals and society (Moran, 2019a). First, if prosocial effect is not the focus of a purpose aim, then societies could end up producing more Hitlers because, without prosocial effect, Hitler is considered "purposeful" (Bronk, 2014). Prosocial effect need not be on the grand scale of exemplars (Colby & Damon, 1992; Oliner & Oliner, 1988), and is more likely to be found in quotidian efforts within daily life (e.g., Coles, 1993; Loeb, 2010) that might ripple through mimicry, reciprocity, collaboration, and social diffusion. Second, if purpose is not distinguished from solely self-benefiting life goals, and youth are educated to "do whatever you want because you are the center of your world," then American extreme individualism can become a societal cancer not only in the US but abroad as more individuals become self-centered (e.g., Hedayati, Kuusisto, Gholami, & Tirri, 2017; see also Moran, 2019a).

A prosocial orientation for life purpose is supported by past studies. Sense of purpose is related to understanding that one's efforts affect others (Bronk & Finch, 2010; Kiang, 2012) and contributes to the community (Johnson et al., 2018; Stoddard & Pierce, 2015; see special issue, Moran, 2018b). Prosocial types of aims developed in college relate to a concern for the future in middle age whereas creative, financial and personal recognition life goals do not (Hill et al., 2010). In a study of how youth conceive of life purpose aims, the second largest group (33%) comprised "givers," most who defined purpose *in terms of* beyond-the-self impact and who were pursuing a prosocial aim. A majority felt strongly certain and confident that this was their true purpose and that they could realize it—exceeding the other groups oriented toward achievement, God, or support (Moran, 2014).

One of the few studies to attempt building a developmental trajectory for purpose aim and practice (albeit only with two data points two years apart) suggests the beyond-the-self dimension of purpose may be foundational (Malin et al., 2014). Consideration of others was the common theme of the youngest cohort of middle-schoolers who shared specific purpose aims. This consideration manifested as "empathic awareness," an emotional beyond-the-self orientation to help others less fortunate. At later age stages, youths learned to represent their prosocial purpose aims cognitively and linguistically. Older youth were 35% more likely to specify beyond-the-self reasons for their specific "one most important focus" (Moran, Bundick, Malin, & Reilly, 2013). Although more developmental research is needed, it is interesting that the prosocial dimension may be the launchpad for meaning and intention, not the other way around.

12.5 Purpose Aim: Aligning Envisioned and Actual Effects

Feedback helps us calibrate what we aim for with what influence we actually have on others. In addition to the purpose aim's mental representation functioning as a feedforward criterion *before acting* for assessing if there are affordances in a situation and generate intentions, there is the criterion function of purpose aim *after acting* against which actual effects are judged by those in the situation who benefited. Thus, the life momentum model also focuses on one person's purpose aim benefiting from a feedback loop of evaluations of the effects of the person's actions.

Purpose is neither a characteristic or direct cause of action (Moran, 2017). First, it is not enough to take action and perform well: the action must make something positive happen for others in the situation to generate feedback. We cannot accurately judge by ourselves whether our actions create a prosocial effect in the situation, much less whether it ripples to become a contribution to the common good. What counts as a prosocial effect stems from an ecosystemic evaluation aggregating how others perceive what we've done as beneficial to them. Perceptions of feedback are "made meaning of" to stay "on target" in relation to the purpose aim's criterion of effectiveness (Marken, 2009). Second, saying "purposeful action" misses how the purpose aim most directly influences *perception* (Marken, 2002). We need the input of others to maintain and clarify our purpose aim over time so it functions better as an affordance seeker.

This calibration function of a purpose aim is partially supported by recent findings that, translated into the terms of the life momentum model, suggest purpose aims are reinforced or clarified by meaning-making of one's role within the situation. For example, sense of purpose is related to expected perceptions to enjoy, be seen as helping others, and feel positive emotions in an upcoming service-learning situation (Moran & Garcia, 2019). These expectations hint at criteria that students use to determine if they will be making a difference. Another study provides an example of alignment: sense of purpose and increasing the salience of a purpose aim can make a situation look less effortful or more achievable than the person would perceive it to be otherwise (Burrow, Hill, & Sumner, 2016), so the person adjusts perception to stay aligned with the purpose aim. If a purpose aim does not stay calibrated, its influence on perception can become weaker or misdirected, and momentum can be "derailed" (Burrow, Hill, Ratner, & Fuller-Rowell, 2018), which is why practice in keeping the purpose aim top of mind is important to its effective functioning. Feedback makes the purpose aim salient throughout the purpose practice.

Acting in situations that may provide near-term social feedback on observable prosocial effects (e.g., community service; Malin et al., 2015; Moran, 2018a) is usually easier for calibrating purpose aim than acting in situations where the expected beneficiaries of one's efforts may not be present, such as occurs for purpose aims for systemic change (e.g., building tolerance, justice, or innovation in the culture; Malin, 2015; Quinn, 2014). Interacting with people directly provides immediate feedback, whereas social change and creative work take more time and produce more ambiguous feedback (Moran, 2010). So those who pursue change-oriented aims may require a particularly strong mental representation of their desired effect (Moran, 2010) and belief in the changeability of the world (Quinn, 2014). Even with a strong purpose aim, some change-oriented youth still may not see their own efforts as prosocial, especially with creative work for which clear feedback may only come if one's creation becomes a contribution to the common good and spreads widely (Moran, 2010; Moran, 2020).

Few life purpose studies have directly included feedback as a variable. One study found that educational "simulation" activities that provide early forms of feedback can develop or strengthen at least a sense of purpose: when students understand how people in the future will depend on what they are learning now, students glimpse how they matter and better regulate their actions even during boring tasks (Yeager & Bundick, 2009; Yeager et al., 2014).

A series of studies on service-learning provide similar insights. A six-country study of whether recent community service work increased students' sense of purpose (Moran, 2018a) found that the act of serving related to a positive change in sense of purpose, so the action itself had some feedback influence. But what mattered most for higher-than-average positive change in sense of purpose was students' noticing the beneficial effects of their work on others, especially if the work was initially unfamiliar to the students. Another study showed informative feedback on volunteering efforts, even for service tasks the youth did not enjoy, correlated with stronger prosocial contribution and purpose commitment (Shin et al., 2018). In yet another study, receiving feedback that service-learners' efforts were effective strengthened students' clarity of meaning and intention (Opazo et al., 2018): the experience of expending effort for the betterment of others helped these students realize which specific aspects of helping were most important to them, guiding them to clarify what to do next. Finally, a case study in Spain explored how the common good can provide feedback (Moran & Opazo, 2019). One service-learner teaching Spanish to immigrant children noticed an opportunity to teach mothers along with their children. After several weeks, the mothers shared stories with the service-learner about how much easier their daily tasks and neighborhood integration were because they could better speak the local language, and they invited her to their homes so she could see the results herself, which allowed her to see a change in the whole community that rippled from her teaching efforts.

Finally, a small exploratory study using a computer simulator provides clues for why prosocial aims can be difficult in dynamic environments when feedback is clearer for short-term, self-benefiting markers of success. The study examined how well two leaders' decisions drew on reasoning based on the purpose aim each espoused at the start of the simulation (Shippen & Moran, 2014). At the end of each round, leaders made a decision and justified it. Then the simulator provided feedback by calculating new values for markers of success based on the combined effects of both leaders' decisions. Each leader selected one of four aims that represented what they cared about most within the simulated scenario. Two aims were self-benefiting by building their own prestige, and two were prosocial focusing on their people's well-being or the sustainability of both organizations. Leaders who espoused self-oriented purpose aims resulted in graphs showing either stable alignment of decision reasons across all rounds of play, or one-round "blip" misalignment followed by a quick rebound. Their aims didn't need to be that strong because the simulator dynamics worked in their favor by rewarding the self-benefiting markers of success over the short-term. Leaders espousing prosocial aims resulted in turbulent graphs: they tried to reason at as prosocial a level as they could, given the panic they felt at short-term feedback that assaulted their prestige, and many ended the simulation with prosocial reasoning. But their graphs showed how much more effort and stamina may be needed to persistently decide based on prosocial reasoning and not become reactionary to noisy self-benefiting feedback in a dynamic environment.

During calibration, meaning may feel more salient than the purpose aim. Dynamically, meaning and purpose are not synonyms. Many prior life purpose models and measures use purpose and meaning interchangeably or they inconsistently subordinate one to the other (e.g., George & Park, 2016; Martela & Steger, 2016). One reason for this confusion may be because the timing and sequence of purpose aim and meaning-making are entangled. One is not categorically superordinate to the other, but rather dynamically each's influence on the other depends on which comes first. Over time, they are reciprocal; but at any given moment, one may be the influencer and the other the influenced. Developmentally, personal meaning predates a functioning purpose aim since youth usually build their aim by cohering experiences that they felt were personally significant (Malin et al., 2014; Martela & Steger, 2016; McKnight & Kashdan, 2009).

Once a purpose aim is committed to, the aim influences meaning to evaluate significance of situations through the specific lens of prosocial effect (Colby & Damon, 1992; McKnight & Kashdan, 2009). As the aim is increasingly enacted and strengthened, it becomes more self-reinforcing. Although it still can undergo tweaks of clarity as a criterion and a template, the mental representation of the prosocial effect stabilizes through its dual ability to perceive what is relevant and ignore what isn't. Purpose practice is subjective, especially because the meaning-making aspect of purpose practice is subjective (King & Hicks, 2009).

Meaning is more fluid and changeable than purpose aim because it is constantly trying to weave experience into coherence (Martela & Steger, 2016). Meaning (importance/significance) does a lot of the work of calibration because it is the conduit between purpose aim (mental representation/criterion for prosocial effect) and perception of the situation. Meaning is how alignment or misalignment of aim and effect is *felt*, and feelings often register in consciousness before cognitions. Upon receiving feedback, meaning's "what is important to me" directs the person's: (a) monitoring of the alignment of perceived and aimed-for effects: is my effort working as expected? (b) launching of further intentions, especially if a misalignment is found: what do I do next? and (c) clarifying of the purpose aim: how can I tweak my mental representation moving forward to be a better template and criterion?

Yet the purpose aim may need to be made salient to keep meaning-making in line with the purpose aim for two reasons: (a) situational stimuli are always bombarding us for attention and can be demanding (Moran & Gardner, 2018), and (b) meaning-making processes are used by many other psychological functions beyond purpose (see Moran, 2019a; Moran & John-Steiner, 2003).

Burrow et al.'s (2014) and Burrow and Hill's (2013) studies provide indirect support of the meaning-purpose connection through their intervention for participants to make their purpose aim salient by writing about it before entering a challenging situation. Even though these studies did not include actual purpose aims in their analyses, the act of focusing on a purpose aim increased its influence on the meaning-making of situations involving an ethnically diverse train car and a mountain climb. From a life momentum model perspective, it is possible that the purpose aim reduced other meaning-making influences on perception, such as general worldview or recent media or a map/diagram of the potential problems of these situations, so that the purpose aim could generate an intention to make a prosocial effect and could evaluate the situation in prosocial terms. In these studies, that prosocial effect equated with reducing negative mood.

From a subjective perspective, meaning addresses what is important to me, partially based on what I already understand through past experiences and partially based on how I feel, so that I can "make sense" of what's going on in a way that helps me get my bearings. Otherwise, the world appears incomprehensible because there are too many possible stimuli to attend to (see Moran, 2019a, for review). Purpose aim is one "pull" on meaning-making: its representation built from a lifetime of prosocial effects gives meaning a lens to help perception deliberately look for opportunities. A strong purpose aim can make meaning's job easier by quickly discarding stimuli that are extraneous or irrelevant to the purpose aim. With a strong purpose aim, meaning tends to be well integrated and "loyal" to the aim. A person is more likely to adapt the meaning of the situation to the purpose aim's criterion, if possible. But sometimes, feedback may stimulate new meaning—there may be an emotional response to feedback that, at first, doesn't make sense. Feedback that is "disturbing" to the purpose aim feels bad and meaning is quick to calibrate, expending effort to clarify a purpose aim.

Feedback alerts the person to discrepancies. Although we often tend to prefer feedback that tells us how well we are doing, one way that feedback is particularly important for purpose aim function is in flagging discrepancies, alerting us we may be going "off-course" from our purpose aim. Discrepancies occur when feedback on the actual effect does not match the ideal effect represented by the purpose aim (Marken, 2002). A perceived discrepancy feeds back to the purpose aim, filtered through personal meaning to assess how important the discrepancy is. Discrepancy alerts us to scan the situation for changes that may be "disturbing" how we are enacting our purpose aim, such as doing the task incorrectly, or how the effect is being perceived by others, such as someone else in the situation misunderstanding our intent. Then compensatory intentions are generated to adjust actions to realign aim and effect (Marken, 2002). It's like a prosocial thermostat: the purpose aim sets a target temperature (anticipated effect); when the thermometer (perception) assesses the situation does not meet the criterion's threshold (one's effect is not realized, per feedback), the purpose aim turns on the furnace (intention), which "warms up" the situation (new actions).

Again, Burrow et al. (2016a) is an example: this series of studies show that purpose aims (not necessarily related to a prosocial effect) moderate "our subjective appraisals" of "how much effort" relate to climbing a mountain in a way that perceives the challenge as doable (Burrow, Hill, & Sumner, 2016): "purpose may be uniquely equipped to operate as a system that enables individuals to more accurately assess challenges and find their way through" (p. 101). Put in terms of the life momentum model, we may overestimate difficulty based solely on situational cues, but meaning *when attached to a purpose aim* interprets less discrepancy between the aim's desired effect and the effort to actualize that effect.

Similarly, Burrow and Hill (2013) had participants track their own mood (emotional feedback) while riding in subway cars as other riders of different ethnicities entered and exited at stops (disturbance). The moods of subway riders whose purpose aim was not primed were affected by the disturbance of a more ethnically diverse ridership, whereas those whose purpose aim was primed did not. In the language of the life momentum model, their purpose aim effectively counteracted the disturbance in a dynamic situation, which resulted in no effect on negative mood (Marken, 2002, 2009). The purpose aim did its job!

Feedback differs from social support. Social support is important ecologically because everyone in an ecosystem directly or indirectly depends on what others in the situation do. Social support involves receiving resources from others, whereas feedback requires the person to act first before others in the situation offer anything. We can be supported without doing anything—which is why, counterintuitively, sometimes social support may be harmful to the functioning of a purpose aim. Social supports that directly improve task performance can be antagonistic to self-regulation, a problem known as the "intentionality paradox" (Larson, 2006).

For example, a study of youth's own perceptions of purpose aims and practice found that the largest group, comprising American "socially supported" youth (37%), *consumed* the help of others to *get* credentials with little thought about what they would do with the credentials. But they felt less certain about their futures and their confidence because they were at the mercy of their supporters. On the other hand, "giver" students with altruistic purpose aims tended to report feeling not as generally well-supported. Instead, the altruism-focused students felt required to proactively seek opportunities to help others. This initiative put them in situations to garner feedback, which probably played a role in their expression of more confidence and certainty in their purpose aims (Moran, 2014).

The support is more helpful when it is specifically related to the purpose aim. Whereas the socially supported students used others' efforts to maintaining their current *status*, the altruistic students used opportunities to *develop* their purpose aim. Another study found that students with friends who cheered and helped *with the student's interests and ambitions* were 50% more likely to state an intention. Again, students with well-defined purpose aims did not wait for social supports but tended to initiate the involvement of their families, neighborhoods, and social institutions to create opportunities to pursue their specific purpose aim (Moran et al., 2013).

Too much general or performance-focused social support may weaken a youth's purpose aim because it can make the purpose aim unnecessary in a situation—the individual acts by using the support rather than following their own intention (Moran, 2014, 2016b). One study found that most youth assume a culturally well-supported, normative purpose aim, such as getting a good job in culturally valued industries (Moran, 2010). Pursuing normative purpose aims is easier because they have established support structures like a well-defined education track, internships or other early training opportunities, clear job descriptions, and the like. From a researcher perspective, well-supported normative effects make it difficult to tell if a purpose aim is functioning at all because there may be so much external support for some normative roles that a purpose aim is not needed.

The implication is that others in a situation—especially powerful individuals within the ecosystem like parents, friends, employers and teachers—need to understand clearly what they are supporting. For example, a study of teachers' perceived roles in the development of student purposes found they tended to focus on caring for the students themselves, which is a good thing to do. But some teachers, by trying to keep students comfortable in the *current* learning situation, did not support the students *stretching beyond* the here-and-now. Only about a third of teachers understood their importance in helping students, as agents of their own development, learn to think more long-term, stay encouraged toward their ambitions, and seek prosocial opportunities (Moran, 2016b).

12.6 Culture: Contributor not Context

Culture is not a context, it is an organism with its own momentum. Up to this point, I have discussed how individuals pursue their purpose aims within situations that draw from the common good's tools, understandings, and "default" behaviors of the culture. Yet I also have argued that any—and perhaps all—of the individuals in a situation may have purpose aims driving their perception to find affordances to make their own prosocial effects. These individuals also are co-producers *of* the situation. The situation is not a container, it is composed in real time by the perceptions, actions and effects of all involved. Actors with purpose aims are more self-directing in the effects they have on others. I assert that the common good also is not a container or backdrop. It plays an active role in situations and in purpose practice.

To simplify this discussion, I will focus on national culture—American, Singaporean, Chilean, Spanish, Ghanaian—because that is the level at which much cultural research has been done. However, it is important to note that some national cultures are more homogeneous (e.g., Finnish, Korean) than others that are more "melting pots" of multiple subcultures (e.g., Brazilian, American).

The life momentum model shows how culture is not a context in an ecology, it is an active "organism" in its own right. Each cultural participant is like a cell within the larger culture organism, each doing their part because no one mind can hold all of a culture's shared understandings (Moran & John-Steiner, 2003; Valsiner, 2000). Many life purpose studies done within a single culture tend not to make explicit the functions of the culture or the common good unless the study focuses on a specific subculture or ethnic group (e.g., Gloria, Castellanos, & Orozco, 2005; Kiang, 2012; Liang, White, Rhodes, Strodel, Gutowski, Mousseau, & Lund, 2017; Osai, 2016; Sharma, & De Alba, 2018; Zell, 2011) or the study is published in a multinational venue where cultural clarification is needed (e.g., Lee, Foo, Adams, Morgan, & Frewen, 2015; Nkyi, 2015). Ecologically, not explicitly addressing culture is a missed opportunity because, by conceptualizing culture as static, we fail to recognize the fluidity of culture, how its resources *flow through* individuals. Perhaps because the culture is taken for granted as available to all, there is little impetus to consider that the culture itself is making effects.

Within situations, the culture is mostly represented by the common good. One opportunity would be to explore the culture-specific dynamics of how—and how well—the common good influences the desired prosocial effects of the culture's participants. In the language of the life momentum model, this amounts to recognizing a feedback loop for the common good similar to the feedback loop already discussed for purpose aim: how does the common good regulate itself?

This cultural point-of-view is more difficult to fathom because it isn't "housed" in one person's mind. Cultural perspective is not subjective but intersubjective. Think of our individual minds linked through communication, observation, and collaboration between each other. Subjectivity focuses on what individual minds contribute (the "nodes" in a network diagram); intersubjectivity focuses on the links (the "lines" and "arrows" between nodes in a network diagram).

The culture is what we share, what moves between our minds that also becomes part of our minds. Cultures often are not homogenously distributed across and within participants, even in more ethnically homogeneous countries. As already noted, each cultural participant is "carrying"—through beliefs, perceptual lenses, emotionality, behaviors—a subset of shared cultural meanings (Valsiner, 2000). For example, not everyone understands "being American" in the same way (Malin, 2011). Although we tend to think about culture as "out there" in books, architecture, art, normative social behaviors, and the like, active culture is "in here" inside individuals as we use culturally appropriated materials in our lives (see Moran & John-Steiner, 2003).

From this view, the active role of the common good is to aggregate and disseminate the prosocial effects that individuals within the culture produce. This role is somewhat of a democratic process in that cultural participants' contributions are judged useful and worthy to perpetuate in part through those same participants' individual perceptions and decisions. But because of the specific shared meanings of participants in one culture, there may be gatekeepers, norms, laws, beliefs or other social mechanisms that may create inequality within the culture in the possibilities of different participants to make contributions that ripple beyond their own actions. Some cultures have a shared meaning that hierarchy is important (e.g., Russia), whereas other cultures endorse egalitarianism of contribution (e.g., Denmark). Some cultures endorse certainty in their shared behaviors and meanings through strict rules (e.g., Japan), whereas others are ok tolerating ambiguity (e.g., the UK). Some cultures promote a short-term orientation (e.g., Ghana), whereas others train their participants to take the long view (e.g., Germany). The most widely used cultural difference dimension is individualism-collectivism: some cultures expect their members to think about themselves in terms of a relatively independent "I" (the US is by far the most individualistic), whereas other cultures steer participants to think about the self in light of their in-group, as a "we" (e.g., China) (Hofstede & Milosevic, 2018; country examples from https://www.hofstede-insights.com/country-comparison/).

How a common good self-regulates would be influenced by these cultural dimensions as (a) internalized into subjective perspectives (how strongly the individualism or uncertainty tolerance is internalized into the self of individual cultural participants) as well as (b) externalized in social behaviors resulting from intersubjective agreed-upon understandings (such as law abidance, politeness/manners, and other normative engagements). Thus, researching purpose aims from a cultural point-of-view requires including national norms as well as individual measures to see how much study participants individually endorse these norms in their beliefs (subjectively) and "normal" behaviors (intersubjectively).

Cross-cultural studies map possibilities for purpose practice. Most culture-related research on life purpose has not taken the approach described above. Most studies have been cross-cultural comparisons of differences between two groups (e.g., Bundick & Tirri, 2014; Damon, Moran, Tirri, Araujo, & Bundick, 2009; Frost & Frost, 2000; Grouzet, Ahuvia, Kim, Ryan, Schmuck, & Kasser, 2005; Sink, Purcell, Van Keppel, & Gamper, 1997; Steger, Kashdan, Sullivan, & Lorentz, 2008). Although conceptually interesting, cross-cultural studies reinforce the idea that cultures are backdrops or containers because culture is used as a grouping variable. If we open the American jar, we get one set of ingredients for purpose; if we open the Japanese jar, we get different ingredients. In addition, cross-cultural comparisons can exacerbate in-group/out-group perspectives that can be counterproductive to prosocial effects in general (e.g., Burrow & Hill, 2013). So cross-cultural studies may not be the best research designs for understanding purpose practice.

That said, how might we reinterpret this body of research from a more dynamic perspective, considering the common good as a participant in situations? Perhaps cross-cultural findings could provide starting points for which elements of purpose practice may be more relevant in a particular ecosystem based on how shared resources and shared meanings from the common good are integrated into individual purpose aims, which could be viewed as an endorsement of culture-specific dimensions of purpose (e.g., Kawai & Moran, 2017).

First, the language used to conceptualize purpose aim provides clues to the role of purpose aims in relation to the common good and how individuals may recognize some resources versus others as affordances. This can be a big challenge for understanding purpose aim from a cultural perspective: studies often "adapt" measures created in one culture to other cultures without clearly recognizing the implicit assumptions embedded in measure design, instructions, and item contents. Prosocial motivation can be explained in part for Americans because "I receive a tax deduction," but that is not possible in most other countries. A six-country study of youth purpose required translating the concept represented by the American English word "life purpose," including its integrated dimensions of personal meaning, future intention, active engagement, and prosocial impact (Moran, 2009). To maximize the possibility that "purpose" was understood in similar ways across countries, collaborating researchers checked what terms were used in past studies and in everyday language, engaged considerable discussion with each other, and did multiple translations and back-translations. The terms chosen to use in the survey were "objective" in Spain, "ultimate achievement" in South Korea, "ideal life" in China, "life project" in Brazil, and "hopeful future" in Finland (Moran, 2018a). Each of these terms shows subtle differences in what the cultures warrant as "most important" at the collectively endorsed level. The Korean term extends the general accomplishment orientation of the culture (especially academic and workplace) to an overarching "ultimate" whole-life perspective (Shin et al., 2018). The Spanish term captures the current state of difficulty for many youth because of recent economic downturns and social upheavals, hence a focus on a goal for the youth to create their own path into the future (Folgueiras & Palou, 2018; Opazo et al., 2018 The Chinese term mirrors the culture's Confucian roots of ideal behavior and its current communist ideology of ideal societal relations (Jiang & Guo, 2018). The Brazilian term emphasizes integration of multiple aspects of life for a stable subjective perspective over the long term, which is important given Brazil's heterogeneous and volatile society and economy (Arantes et al., 2017). The Finnish term reflects the Nordic country's strong belief in individual autonomy focused on a "moral beacon" that emphasizes how individuals' futures are intertwined with the long-term prospects for all (Tirri & Kuusisto, 2016). Two special journal issues on youth purpose internationally showed further country differences in terminology for "purpose": "good prospects" in Thailand, "future life perspective" in Japan, "moving toward God" in Iran, and "inhloso kanye bizo"—Zulu for "calling"—in South Africa (see Moran, 2017, 2018a, 2018b).

Second, given a particular culture's terminology for life purpose, countries differentially value, promote and support specific contents for purpose aims. Some aims may be more likely to find affordances in the common good to help individuals pursue them. So the following should not come as a surprise: academic achievement is a primary life aim in Asian countries (Heng, Blau, Fulmer, Bi, & Pereira, 2017; Jiang & Guo, 2018; Kawai & Moran, 2017; Shin et al., 2018); economic and social justice aims are important in Spain (Folgueiras & Palou, 2018; Opazo et al., 2018); religious or spiritual aims are promoted in Iran (Hedayati et al., 2017), South Africa (Mason, 2017), and Thailand (Balthip, McSherry, Petchruschatachart, Piriyakoon-torn, & Liamputtong, 2017); national aims are paramount in China (Jiang & Guo, 2018), and family-focused aims are found nearly everywhere (Kiang & Fuligni, 2010; see special issues, Moran, 2017, 2018b). These cultural emphases suggest current normative aims that likely benefit from more extensive support from established social institutions.

Third, what the common good might "afford" individuals may depend on the subjectively perceived developmental level of the person's purpose aim and practice. The common good may set up thresholds or turning points that regulate the types of resources individuals may access based on whether their developmental level is *searching-for* versus *found-general-sense-of* versus *committed-to-specific* aim. Sense of purpose is a feeling of "having" a life direction even if the specific aim of that direction is unknown; it is associated with general confidence to move forward. Searching for purpose is actively seeking a direction, so neither aim nor direction is settled; it is associated with more uncertainty and less confidence but also more curiosity (Steger, Kawabata, Shimai, & Otake, 2008).

An interesting finding in the six-country study, which parallels other studies, has implications for the dynamics of purpose practice. In most Western countries (reviewed in Steger & Samman, 2012) as well as South Africa (Temane, Khumalo, & Wissing, 2014), searching for purpose negatively correlates with sense of purpose: someone searches for purpose because they don't yet have one. There is an implied threshold of "enough searching," in part because it is associated with unpleasantness (Steger et al., 2008). Once this threshold is passed, which seems to have a critical timing in young adulthood, the person should settle on a specific purpose aim to optimize long-term well-being (Bronk et al., 2009). "Finding" a purpose is a turning point in purpose practice moving from *developing* the purpose aim toward *using* the purpose aim to self-regulate one's life path. Once this turning point is reached, searching wastes effort that would be better spent finding situations to enact the found purpose. However, in many Asian cultures, sense and searching positively correlate (Moran, 2018a; Steger et al., 2008). Search is an ongoing part of purpose practice. One's own purpose aim is intimately entwined with others, and families or employers may be part of dialogues deciding a youth's purpose aim. How one's purpose aim is enacted in specific situations depends strongly on meaning-making through collectivist emotions like shame, transcendence, sympathy, indebtedness, and gratitude that emphasize and support belonging within the situation. One's vision of the future is never fully personal, it must consider one's in-group (Kawai & Moran, 2017). Thus, individuals who have a sense of purpose still must be sensitive to and scan for opportunities not only to enact their purpose aim but also to make sure their enactments accord with belongingness in the situation.

Fourth, the common good helps reinforce where is the boundary between *self* and *other*—who a person considers part of one's own subjectivity versus a "different" subjectivity—by defining cultural criteria for allowing or rewarding helping "others." This is an important distinction since prosocial effect comprises a benefit to others beyond oneself. This distinction also influences whether benefiting others is considered a personal choice or a moral duty and whether a person focuses on only helping others they know or also strangers (Busch & Hofer, 2011). Whether family is part of or separate from self especially is contested across countries. In most Western countries, the self comprises the individual (Markus & Kitayama, 1991), but in many Asian, African and Latinx countries, self at least partially includes one's family (Balthip et al., 2017; Busch & Hofer, 2011 Folgueiras & Palou, 2018; Heng et al., 2017; Kawai & Moran, 2017). In some cultures, wider in-groups beyond family may also be included in the self. For example, development of sense of purpose and purpose aims relate to national aims mandated through education in Iran and China (Hedayati et al., 2017; Jiang & Guo, 2018). In China, the national aim is political, in Iran it is religious. By influencing purpose aims through education—which is one of the strongest enforcers of cultural norms within the common good—these curricula both circumscribe and set clearer pathways for the individual purpose aims that contribute to the national aims. Although these two countries were part of the six-country study, such clear examples are not the only examples. For instance, the civic education movement in the United States aims to make national identity and civic purpose a bigger part of individual purpose aims (Malin et al., 2015). And as noted in news sources of record like the BBC and *The New York Times*, many countries around the world currently are turning to nationalist aims and sentiments to cohere their societies and cultures (e.g., U.K. Brexit, Turkey, Israel, Hungary, India, Brazil, U.S.).

Finally, although most of this chapter has focused on how purpose aim regulates the transformational processes of purpose practice (meaning, intention, action, perception), the common good also can regulate these processes. There likely are situations where myriad individual purpose aims and the shared common good cooperate or compete for influence. These cooperative or competitive interactions themselves may be culture specific. A study of the relationship of sense of purpose and expecting to feel positive emotions in upcoming community service showed a wide array of pathways across six countries (Moran, 2018a). Two mediated pathways were included: intrinsic motivation, which is enjoying the task, and helping identity, which is being seen by others as prosocial. In the life momentum model, expected positive emotions is part of meaning, community service is intended action and expected effect, intrinsic motivation is self-feedback one's action in self-oriented terms, and helping identity is expected feedback from others on prosocial effect. Brazilian, Spanish and American students expected to feel positively because they expected both to enjoy the action and to receive positive feedback on their efforts, with sense of purpose on its own providing no additional influence on emotions. What mattered was the here-and-now of the situation: how they would feel about the work as well as how others in the situation would feel about them. South Korean students who scored higher on sense of purpose generally tended to expect less positive emotion, unless they were recognized by others for their prosocial efforts—the visible achievement mattered, but enjoyment of the task did not. Finland's and China's pathways were opposites of each other. Students in both countries expected to feel positively about serving in the community based partly on their sense of purpose, but also partly on one but not the other mediators. Enjoying the task mattered in Finland, but being viewed as a helper person mattered in China. In Finland, students are selected for service courses in part because they already have an inner drive, whereas in China, service is part of compulsory purpose education that identifies strongly with helping behavior.

Thus, the purpose aim (at least a sense of purpose) anticipated how (a) the emotional meaning of the service situation was influenced by (b) the common good's prior normative training of students' perceptual filters that (c) resulted in the relative influence on students' perception from the feedback students gave themselves based on their actions versus from the feedback others provided on their effects. Interpreted in relation to the life momentum model, these findings suggest that the prosocial effect is visible to others and communicated through feedback to the student for sense of purpose to engage in community service situations. This held for all countries except Finland, and it may be most crucial for Japanese and Chinese students to emotionally sense others' meanings of their purpose-driven actions and effects. Brazilian, Spanish and American students may require a combination of both self-generated and other-generated feedback within the situation for their sense of purpose to distally influence the service work at all. Chinese and Finnish students, since there still was a direct effect of sense of purpose, may not need, as much as the others, the influence of enjoyment and recognition to make meaning; but if these more proximal influences occur, one would be more helpful than the other in the two countries.

What these relationship differences may mean dynamically and ecologically is that not only the focus of purpose aims but the way purpose aims are selected and the meanings by which these purpose aims might influence perception may be partially mediated by how the specific culture's common good frames and trains resources to be perceived. That is, the *linkages between* the elements of the life momentum model might differ by culture, even if the elements themselves are the same. For example, I would expect that the common good is a much stronger influencer in Asian countries because of their collectivistic orientations, but especially in China because of its government as well. In these countries, the common good and purpose aim may not be two intersecting influences on individual perception (i.e., coming from "opposite sides" of the model into the centrally located perception process). Instead, the common good may "feed" purpose aims directly, then purpose aims influence perception. This would represent a fully internalized mental representation of the culturally promoted "default" of prosocial effect.

These differences potentially could have huge effects on, for example, how education for the development of a purpose aim and practice in different countries could proceed. In some cultures, education may support only a few purpose aims because of limited options or stringent enforcement of specific effects considered "prosocial." So the cultural participants' purpose aims converge on specific aims (e.g., serve Allah, create technology) or on specific situations within which purpose practice is allowed or considered proper (e.g., religion or family or career). In other cultures, education may diverge because purpose aims might become "marketed" for consumption through programs or manuals, or no set curriculum is agreed upon, or perhaps even the concept of purpose is disputed. So the culture's participants are left to their own ingenuity to craft not only an idiosyncratic purpose aim but also an idiosyncratic purpose practice (Moran, 2019a). This second divergent approach seems to be the state of the United States currently as numerous books, programs, camps, and websites have sprung up to compete for education dollars.

Cultural-historical transformation of shared meanings into idiosyncratic meanings. Past cross-cultural studies offer hints of what matters in each culture. But it is important to go beyond reporting differences to clarify *how* cultural common goods and individual purpose aims and practices compose each other. Searching for and developing a purpose aim, and engaging that aim in everyday situations, depend on how cultural participants have developed meaning-making and perceptual filters, believe they have agency to form intentions for their own behavior, can access common good resources, can act in the presence of other cultural participants from whom they can receive feedback on their efforts. Culture influences whether purpose aim and practice are even possible at the individual level.

One direction that could be particularly helpful for directly applying the life momentum model in research is through a cultural-historical approach. Building upon the developmental work of early 20th-century Russian psychologist Lev Vygotsky and his colleagues (see Moran & John-Steiner, 2003; Valsiner, 2000), cultural-historical research has proceeded nearly independently of cross-cultural research. The cultural-historical emphasis is: how does individuals' development unfold through social interaction and cooperation using cultural tools, and how do cultural tools develop through their use by individuals? Analyses are of carefully observed processes, practices, and interactions—parent/child, expert/novice, work team—within rich environments of cultural tools, like language resources and artifacts, over a situationally important period of time (Valsiner, 2000). Thus, cultural-historical methods are well-poised for examining feedforward/feedback models like the life momentum model. In fact, this perspective's strength is the moment-by-moment interactions of the processes in purpose practice—perception, idiosyncratic meaning-making, intention, individual action, shared meanings, resources, and cultural "defaults"—that highlight culture's influence not *on* but *through* these interactions among individuals (Elhammoumi, 2001; Valsiner, 2011). Take Malin et al.'s (2014) general developmental pathway for purpose aims starting with empathy, which then becomes filtered through enactment roles, reprioritized meaningful interests, and the extension of intentions further into the future. A cultural-historical follow-up to this study would consider this generalized timeline as a "cultural default" for the U.S., but would look more closely at idiosyncratic variability in the timeline, including perhaps other sequences that are accepted in the culture but not as well supported, such as pathways that start with action instead of empathy (for example, required service-learning as an entry point to purpose aim development; Moran, 2019b; Moran & Opazo, 2019).

Although, to my knowledge, studies have not been done on life purpose practice from a cultural-historical framework, one theorist has addressed it. A life purpose aim regulates the nonlinear developmental process of each individual "always on the border of oneself and the 'world beyond'.... [I]n that process of purposive efforts, the very limits—horizons—are extended through culture....to make movement from the real (here-and-now) to the constructed (imaginary there-and-then) possible" (Valsiner, 2011, p. 215, 228). Purpose aim is the verge of present and future that is continually moving forward with the person as life goes on. It is the avant garde of one's vision of life as experienced.

Purpose aim functions in the present moment to set a trail for future moments to happen: purpose practice does not *build* momentum, it *is* momentum. In physics, momentum is the impetus gained through motion, and it equals mass times velocity, with velocity including both direction and speed. Momentum in relation to life purpose practice is the impetus of the purpose aim to make prosocial effects; prosocial effects, by supporting, maintaining, and building the culture's common good, are needed to extend time into the future. If the common good is not maintained, then there is no future for any cultural participants (as shown in the "tragedy of the commons"; Hardin, 1968). Mass is equivalent to the integration of perception, meaning, intention, opportunity, and actions; the more of these processes that are engaged in a situation, the stronger the commitment to the purpose (Moran, 2020). Individuals "loop through" numerous culturally situated experiences repeatedly over their lives, with their purpose aim "extending through culture" by finding affordances in situations through simultaneously orienting perception *toward* what is most meaningful and *away* from distractions. Velocity builds efficiency in one direction as defined by the purpose aim.

The cultural-historical approach makes explicit the feedback/feedforward interactions between individual and culture that occur in situations where individuals interact, even though these interactions may not always fully accomplish one's purpose aim (Moran & John-Steiner, 2003). Studies of life purpose in collectivistic cultures tend to make this point more than studies in the United States, the "outlier" hyper-individualistic culture (Moran, 2017). For example, the South African model of life purpose, based on a long-time African spiritual worldview, posits a driver of collective well-being through individual ethical living, although few youths currently live up to this ideal (Mason, 2017). How Japanese youth define their present actions' support of their future life perspective must consider contribution to society even though the Japanese model of contribution through lifetime employment is no longer applicable (i.e., the common good has removed a prior resource for youth to direct their lives). Still, even though youth now must compete for jobs, they are still responsible for and struggle with figuring out how their actions will contribute to the common good (Kawai & Moran, 2017).

Cultures orient their participants temporally—such as toward the past for tradition-maintaining cultures, future for innovation or change-seeking cultures, and repeating cycles for periodic or seasonal-rhythmic cultures. Based on these temporal orienta-tions, cultures set direction and rhythm for normative life trajectories (Valsiner, 2011), which provide the defaults for which purpose aims youth may choose (Moran, 2017; Moran, 2019a), how cultural participants may provide feedback on each other's contributions (Moran & Opazo, 2019), and how aims derive intentions and personal meanings (Kawai & Moran, 2017; Markus & Kitayama, 1991; Moran & John-Steiner, 2003). Since no studies have been done from a cultural-historical perspective, I speculate one possible scenario.

The United States is a large and diverse country, yet arguably its dominant temporal orientation is toward the future embracing change: tomorrow will be different than today. There is considerable pressure on youth to focus purpose aims on entrepreneurship (business or social), innovation, and social change activism. Although several traditional professions are still culturally promoted, like medicine and law, technology yet-to-be-invented is touted as one the most prosocial effects youth might pursue because "tech can save us." It could also be argued, based on reports in the news, that some tradition-maintaining purpose aims, like practicing an established religion or having children, increasingly are falling out of favor with today's youth. In the current "fast-forward" cultural mindset, feedback is rapid fire through social media and computerized testing and grades, plus students seem to require feedback more often on their efforts—every short essay must have comments, not just major papers. Shared meanings have short lives as personal idiosyncratic meanings are launched at lightning speed as memes, gifs, videos, acronyms and neologisms. Americans, especially youth, expect personal meaning and experience to dominate shared experience: what *I* think matters is what matters the most. Even children are seen as parental self-fulfillment (if enjoyed) or nuisances (if not) rather than a continuance of family or society. Because of the perceived rapid pace of cultural developments, there is little time to intend before needing to act, or the opportunity may be lost. Hence, we see slogans like "Just do it!" and "Move fast and break things." There is little stability—it is 24-hour motion. I have suggested elsewhere that this whirlwind cultural environment, in which youth feel like social institutions are unreliable, may be why life purpose as a developmental milestone has arisen now (Moran, 2019a). If everything is constantly in motion, then the world increasingly can seem absurd; meaning-making cannot keep up. If the culture's common good no longer can provide pathways, youth must become trailblazers. Perhaps this chaotic moment in American—and perhaps world—history is why so many young people are stepping up to fight for equality and respect, address gun control and climate change, and start their own organizations.

12.7   Plurality: Blending Cultures

I have discussed how purposes and common goods both have feedforward links to each other as well as feedback loops through the other to regulate their own influence on prosocial effect. The life momentum model diagram focuses on one person's purpose aim interacting with one culture's common good. This diagram can be linked to the same diagram representing other situational participants and cultural participants interacting through perception, action, effect and the common good. But many people living today experience a globalized world. Globalization means that one person may experience—perhaps simultaneously—the influences of more than one culture. Indeed, individuals may experience more than one culture inside themselves because they or their parents immigrated. Increasingly more everyday situations may be examples of plurality—multiple cultures interacting or perhaps even blending.

Interactions among multiple cultures. A metaphor of life purpose aims and practices I have used in the past is a cultural tapestry: the warp is the shared culture through which individuals weave their specific purpose aims to compose the weft (Moran, 2017). To extend this metaphor, what if the threads represent individuals from *different* cultures? The tapestry is not cultural but multicultural and perhaps intercultural.

This depiction reinforces that culture is not external to us but inside us: we carry culture with us, and our psychology is expansive enough to be able to carry more than one. What's more, in theory, "mobile culture"—ideas, theories, beliefs, understandings—that we carry wherever we go can be shared with others from different cultures, potentially without risk to our original culture if participants in situations, instead of maintaining in-group biases, practice curiosity, open-mindedness, humility, and gratitude. But based on social and political unrest in 2020, we're not there yet. It may be that our current historical moment is a realignment or reorganization of meaning-making and social relations, both which directly influence what "prosocial effect" entails.

During modern history, national culture provides a default worldview to help cultural participants cohere experiences into a life narrative of "what it means to be" American or Korean or Chilean (e.g., Malin, 2011) and to help the country cohere a history and a blueprint for "how the world works" through the common good (Moran, 2019a). Globalization, multinational capitalism, migration, trade, and technology are breaking down traditional national meanings. This institutional breakdown may feel like an individual breakdown: anxiety, depression and suicide have risen since the 1990s (Twenge, 2011). Navigating multiple cultures creates new stresses—uncertainty, inequality, speed of change, loss of shared meaning (Moran, 2019a)—that may challenge someone's capacity to adapt (De Vogli, 2004). Individuals may experience social turbulence (Conning, 2019; Moran, 2017) and lower personal well-being (Fitzsimmons, Liao, & Thomas, 2017) while they negotiate these challenges (Moran, 2019a).

Yet, these challenges also are when a purpose aim can be particularly helpful by providing psychological coherence, focus, and control amidst the cultural and social turbulence (De Vogli, 2004; Moran, 2019a). Intercultural experiences can make purpose practice more perceivable by individuals because the intersection of two or more cultures highlights one's own "default" meanings that other cultures' meanings may challenge. Cultural interaction expands the possible meanings that could define or strengthen the importance of one's own aim (Moran, 2019a; Moran et al., 2013). Dialogue, tolerance, curiosity, and appreciation of differences can sensitize perception to new types of affordances, which expands opportunities to enact one's purpose aim (Cooper, Jackson, Azmitia, & Lopez, 1998; Kashdan & Steger, 2007; Kiang & Fuligni, 2010; Sumner, Turner, & Burrow, 2018).

Intercultural blending. Cultural blending can occur when individuals interact with others from different cultures (Valsiner, 2000) and absorb new ideas and insights within themselves (Bronk & Finch, 2010; Cooper et al., 1998; Fitzsimmons et al., 2017; Martinez & Dukes, 1997). Going beyond examining how cultures differentiate individuals (cross-cultural) or how cultures and individuals compose each other (cultural-historical), the intercultural approach focuses on how cultures influence other cultures through increased interaction between individuals from diverse backgrounds. Humans are learning organisms. Once individuals from different cultures start interacting, the cultures are likely to become blended, both in individuals' minds as they integrate ideas from multiple sources, and in artifacts such as fusion foods, arts and science collaborations.

One culture does not directly affect another culture in an abstract way. Rather, cultures must be learned by, and operate simultaneously within, a specific individual (bicultural). Or cultures must be enacted through interactions between individuals from different cultures (multicultural). Even encountering artifacts from another culture is still an interaction between two individuals: the author, artist, scientist, architect who made the artifact, and the individual who used the artifact.

In the life momentum model, if each diagram represents one individual, then interculturality equates with one individual's purpose aim being linked to more than one common good. The arrows through perception and effect to the common goods of different cultures represent bridges, also called "straddles" (Carter, 2006) or "weak ties" (Granovetter, 1983). As more individuals create these bridges, the connections between cultures strengthen. Connections between and within cultures of relatively equal strength may represent the integration of separate culture's common goods into a large multicultural or global common good. What, if any, integration occurs depends on specific dynamic features of the situation. More field research is needed.

Considerable research has started to examine multiple cultures at once, including in relation to sense of purpose and purpose aims and practice (see Moran, 2017, 2018b, special issues). A few intercultural papers address ethnic diversity related to sense of purpose and purpose practice at least to the extent that people from different backgrounds were put into the same situation (e.g., Burrow & Hill, 2013; Burrow et al., 2014). Both sense of purpose and writing about one's specific purpose aim seemed to overcome in-group bias so that individuals of one ethnicity did not experience negative mood when surrounded by individuals of another ethnicity. Another study surveyed youth in 4-H on how willing they were to increase the ethnic diversity of the program, which on average was strongly positively endorsed, especially among youth who were curious (Sumner et al., 2018). This finding suggests that younger people who have not overlearned in-group bias may be more open to bridging cultural differences and to leading as bridgers to show others how to integrate multiple cultural perspectives as affordances for one's own purpose practice.

Surprisingly, intercultural blending has tended to show more spreading of individuation than communitarianism (see special issues, Moran, 2017, 2018b). Youth in many countries are experiencing turbulence between traditional and modern practices, as the internet and media bring the worldwide influences into their communities. For example, although Thailand promotes Twelve Core Values that strongly relate to meaning, intention and prosociality, its culture is modernizing, becoming more urban, literate, educated, and tech-savvy. Generation gaps have arisen in religious observation, academic achievement, and family integrity, such that leaders are looking to individual youths' development of purpose aims to counteract these negative trends (Balthip et al., 2017). In Mongolia, education, career, and political opportunities for young women have greatly expanded through the country's growing market economy and Internet connections, although these cultural transformations have been slow to impact individual women's life purpose aims so far (Bespalov, Prudnikova, Nyamdorj, & Vlasov, 2017). In Iran, despite centralized religious and educational institutions to follow Islamic moral tenets to prioritize collective well-being, more than half of youth report purpose aims oriented toward hedonistic and personal economic well-being rather than or in addition to serving Allah, in part in response to economic crises of the last decade (Hedayati et al., 2017).

Individual life purpose aims may be replacing shared worldviews as a guiding force for prosocial behavior (Moran, 2019a). This global "ripple effect" from collectivistic toward individuated mechanisms of social structuring is one of the reasons that the life momentum model requires individuals to have a purpose aim focused on prosocial effect and contribution. If a purpose aim is defined solely around self-benefit, then cultures can become individualistic in the extreme, and individuals forget that the resources they all draw from are shared and can be lost (Moran, 2019a). If individuation is not countered with concern for others and the common good, then the rise of individual purpose aims may reduce, not expand, opportunities for contributions because social interaction occurs less (Moran, 2019a).

12.8 Manifesto: All of Us Moving Forward, Intertwined by Purpose Aims

Here are a few takeaways from this exploration of the life momentum model of purpose aim and purpose practice.

First, we need to rethink purpose as something we *do* not something we *have* or we *are*, and recognize that purpose practice is not easy. There is not a recipe to "get purpose"—we have to cook it up ourselves through lived experience. Despite the abundance of correlations between sense of purpose and well-being measures, purpose practice may not always be "fun" or have a "happy" ending. Why not? One reason is because purpose aims don't have an ending. They perpetually reorient us to use our energies toward prosocial effects. Another reason is because often a purpose aim entails passion (Vallerand, 2008)—not in the colloquial meaning of intense excitement, but in the traditional meaning of suffering for a beloved. Purpose practice focuses us on an aim of utmost importance to us, which we are willing to struggl to realize, even when it's difficult (Zhang, Shi, Liu, & Miao, 2013). We stay the course. Exemplary, passionate purpose aims include: from a career perspective, the "starving artist" or "dedicated scientist" who forgoes having children to "birth" creative pursuits; from a family perspective, the traditional view of parents as "sacrificing" so their children's lives may be better; and from a social change perspective, many activists like Martin Luther King, Cesar Chavez, Mahatma Gandhi, Margaret Sanger—continuing today with Greta Thunberg—who endure threats, trolling, and other adversity for their purpose aim. Strangely, these exemplars do not necessarily describe their efforts as suffering (Colby & Damon, 1992). Sometimes they enjoy it, or at least don't feel the pain as setbacks, because the aim is so important to them that it overrides the suffering.

Second, we need to help youth understand how amazing purpose practice can be. Purpose practice is powerful in (a) its ability to influence perception that generates a cascade of processes to increase the likelihood of producing a prosocial effect, *and* (b) its ability to sustain itself by simultaneously orienting us toward fruitful situations, steering us away from irrelevant ones, and counteracting disturbances that try to throw us off-kilter. But purpose practice is also fragile. If not cultivated and repeatedly made salient in everyday life, it can be overwhelmed by extrinsic incentives in our lives, mimicry of others' aims rather than pursuing our own, overlearned habits, and the general background noise of modern societies. Teachers want to help their students develop a purpose aim and practice, but they need more guidance on how a purpose aim actually functions, not just how its defined, categorized, or divided into components or dimensions (Moran, 2016b).

Third, for understanding purpose, perspective matters. From our own perspective on our own purpose aims, purpose is not a cause of our own behavior. But from other people's perspectives, the prosocial effects of our purpose aims can be causes of their behavior. McKnight and Kashdan (2009) state purpose is a "causal agent." Dynamically, it is not. A cause is a stimulus or event *outside* us that gives rise to a response in or by us. But my purpose aim is *inside* me, part of my own psychology providing *self*-direction (Marken, 2009). Why should we care about this distinction? Because much psychology research today uses study designs that may erroneously give the environment "credit" for our behavior, when actually we are not pawns of the environment. We are drivers, producers, sentient planners. Neuroscience supports this claim: our brains anticipate how to move us forward. Cause and purpose aim are confused because if others in a situation see me act after a specific stimulus in a way that would be considered normative as a reaction to the stimulus, then my action is attributed to—"caused by"—the external stimulus (Marken, 2009). But if I have a purpose aim functioning in the situation, then this finding would be an error. If my purpose is aligned with the normative reaction to the stimulus, it's unclear whether the attribution should go to the external stimulus or to me. If my purpose is not aligned with the normative reaction, then there may be no correlation. Not taking into account that purpose aims may be functioning, not only in research studies but in everyday situations, means we are not understanding human psychology very well.

Finally, researchers need to develop both new measures and new analytical techniques that can capture and examine purpose aim more dynamically within purpose practice. The life momentum model requires researchers to make explicit that individuals in a situation may have a purpose aim functioning, helping them construe a situation idiosyncratically based on the prosocial effect they want to make. Furthermore, knowing only a purpose aim is being practiced may be insufficient because it is *what* the actual mental representation of a specific prosocial effect is that generates intentions. Not only does the specific purpose aim help interpret what happens within the specific situation, but also it could help project how individuals are likely to move forward into new situations (Valsiner, 2011).

As a last thought, I wonder if our focus on life purpose in the early 21st century is cultural development in an "in-between" stage. In many places in the world, many people have become less constrained by collective rules, norms, institutions, and traditions that have guided us. Now we have personal choice among options: we select what guides us. In some cultures, our options may have become overwhelming to the point of confusion. Many of the former "pre-set" categorical developmental milestones or identity markers have become continuous options, partially by our choice—sex, gender, sexual orientation, marriage, parenthood, education, job/career, timing and method of death. A life purpose can help us organize these and other choices by making our considerations more meaningful and intentional in relation to how we matter to each other's well-being and our collective well-being. We need to play a stronger role in encouraging and promoting each other's purpose aims toward prosocial effects. We are all connected, even if our connections are not salient in every moment. We are producers of the ecosystems we live in, and purpose can make us better contributors. We create culture as culture creates us.

References

Arantes, V., Araujo, U., Pinheiro, V., Marimon, M. M., & Sastre, G. (2017). Youth purpose through the lens of the theory of organizing models of thinking. *Journal of Moral Education, 46*(3), 245–257. https://doi.org/10.1080/03057240.2017.1345725.

Balthip, K., McSherry, W., Petchruschatachart, U., Piriyakoontorn, S., & Liamputtong, P. (2017). Enhancing life purpose among Thai adolescents. *Journal of Moral Education, 46*(3), 295–307. https://doi.org/10.1080/03057240.2017.1347089.

Bespalov, A., Prudnikova, M., Nyamdorj, B., & Vlasov, M. (2017). Life aspirations, values and moral foundations in Mongolian Youth. *Journal of Moral Education, 46*(3), 258–271. https://doi.org/10.1080/03057240.2017.1347087.

Bronfenbrenner, U. (1979). *The ecology of human development: Experiments by nature and design.* Cambridge, MA: Harvard University Press.

Bronk, K. C. (2012). A grounded theory of noble youth purpose. *Journal of Adolescent Research, 27*(1), 78–109. https://doi.org/10.1177/0743558411412958.

Bronk, K. C. (2014). *Purpose in life.* Dordrecht, The Netherlands: Springer.

Bronk, K. C., & Finch, W. H. (2010). Adolescent characteristics by type of long-term aim in life. *Applied Developmental Science, 14*(1), 35–44. https://doi.org/10.1080/10888690903510331.

Bronk, K. C., Hill, P. L., Lapsley, D. K., Talib, T. L., & Finch, H. (2009). Purpose, hope, and life satisfaction in three age groups. *The Journal of Positive Psychology, 4*(6), 500–510. https://doi.org/10.1080/17439760903271439.

Bundick, M., & Tirri, K. (2014). Student perceptions of teacher support and competencies for fostering youth purpose and positive youth development: Perspectives from two countries. *Applied Developmental Science, 18*(3), 148–162. https://doi.org/10.1080/10888691.2014.924357.

Burrow, A. L., & Hill, P. L. (2013). Derailed by diversity? Purpose buffers the relationship between ethnic composition on trains and passenger negative mood. *Personality and Social Psychology Bulletin, 39*(12), 1610–1619. https://doi.org/10.1177/0146167213499377.

Burrow, A. L., Hill, P. L., Ratner, K., & Fuller-Rowell, T. E. (2018a). Derailment: Conceptualization, measurement, and adjustment correlates of perceived change in self and direction. *Journal of Personality and Social Psychology, 118*(3), 584–601. https://doi.org/10.1037/pspp0000209.

Burrow, A. L., Hill, P. L., Ratner, K., & Sumner, R. (2018b). A better tomorrow: Toward a stronger science of youth purpose. *Research in Human Development, 15*(2), 167–180. https://doi.org/10.1080/15427609.2018.1445926.

Burrow, A. L., & Spreng, R. N. (2016). Waiting with purpose: A reliable but small association between purpose in life and impulsivity. *Personality and Individual Differences, 90,* 187–189. https://doi.org/10.1016/j.paid.2015.11.010.

Burrow, A. L., Hill, P. L., & Sumner, R. (2016). Leveling mountains: Purpose attenuates links between perceptions of effort and steepness. *Personality and Social Psychology Bulletin, 42*(1), 94–103. https://doi.org/10.1177/0146167215615404.

Burrow, A. L., Stanley, M., Sumner, R., & Hill, P. (2014). Purpose in life as a resource for increasing comfort with ethnic diversity. *Personality and Social Psychology Bulletin, 40*(11), 15-7-1516. https://doi.org/10.1177/0146167214549540.

Busch, H., & Hofer, J. (2011). Identity, prosocial behavior, and generative concern in German and Cameroonian Nso adolescents. *Journal of Adolescence, 34,* 629–638. https://doi.org/10.1016/j.adolescence.2010.09.009.

Carter, P. L. (2006). Straddling boundaries: Identity, culture, and school. *Sociology of Education, 79,* 304–328. https://doi.org/10.1177/003804070607900402.

Colby, A., & Damon, W. (1992). *Some do care: Contemporary lives of moral commitment.* New York: The Free Press.

Coles, R. (1993). *The call of service.* Boston, MA: Houghton Mifflin.

Conning, A. S. (2019, November). *How people learn to think globally.* Paper presented at the Association for Moral Education annual conference, Seattle, WA.

Cooper, C. R., Jackson, J. F., Azmitia, M., & Lopez, E. M. (1998). Multiple selves, multiple worlds: Three useful strategies for research with ethnic minority youth on identity, relationships, and opportunity structures. In V. C. McLoyd & L. Steinberg (Eds.), *Studying minority adolescents: Conceptual, methodological, and theoretical issues* (pp. 111–125). Mahwah, NJ: Erlbaum.

Costin, V., & Vignoles, V. L. (2019). Meaning is about mattering: Evaluating coherence, purpose, and existential mattering as precursors of meaning in life judgments. *Journal of Personality and Social Psychology, 118*(4), 864–884. https://doi.org/10.1037/pspp0000225.

Damon, W. (2008). *The path to purpose: Helping our children find their calling in life.* New York: Free Press.

Damon, W., Moran, S., Tirri, K., Araujo, U. F., & Bundick, M. J. (2009). *Finding purpose in three societies: Cultural and developmental analyses.* Philadelphia, PA: Paper presented at the International Positive Psychology First World Congress.

De Vogli, R. (2004). *Change, psychosocial stress and health in an era of globalization.* Paper prepared for the project 'Health and Social Upheaval', UCLA. Retrieved from http://discovery.ucl.ac.uk/2051/1/Change_Stress_Health.pdf.

Elhammoumi, M. (2001). Lost—or merely domesticated? The boom in socio-historicocultural theory emphasizes some concepts and overlooks others. In S. Chaiklin (Ed.), *The theory and practice of cultural-historical psychology* (pp. 200–217). Aarhus, Denmark: Aarhus University Press.

Fitzsimmons, S. R., Liao, Y., & Thomas, D. C. (2017). From crossing cultures to straddling them: An empirical examination of outcomes for multicultural employees. *Journal of International Business Studies, 48,* 63–89. https://doi.org/10.1057/s41267-016-0053-9.

Folgueiras, P., & Palou, B. (2018). An exploratory study of aspirations for change and their effect on purpose among Catalan university students. *Journal of Moral Education, 47*(2), 186–200. https://doi.org/10.1080/03057240.2018.1433643.

Frankl, V. E. (1959). *Man's search for meaning.* New York: Washington Square Press.

Frost, K. M., & Frost, C. J. (2000). Romanian and American life aspirations in relations to psychological well-being. *Journal of Cross-Cultural Psychology, 31*(6), 726–751. https://doi.org/10.1177/0022022100031006004.

George, L. S., & Park, C. L. (2016). Meaning in life as comprehension, purpose, and mattering: Integration and new research questions. *Review of General Psychology, 20*(3), 205–230. https://doi.org/10.1037/gpr0000077.

Gibson, E. J., & Pick, A. D. (2000). *Perceptual learning and development: An ecological approach to perceptual learning and development.* Oxford, UK: Oxford University Press.

Gloria, A. M., Castellanos, J., & Orozco, V. (2005). Perceived educational barriers, cultural fit, coping responses, and psychological well-being of Latina undergraduates. *Hispanic Journal of Behavioral Sciences, 27*(2), 161–183. https://doi.org/10.1177/0739986305275097.

Granovetter, M. (1983). The strength of weak ties: A network theory revisited. *Sociological Theory, 1,* 203–233. https://doi.org/10.2307/202051.

Grouzet, F. M. E., Ahuvia, A., Kim, Y., Ryan, R. M., Schmuck, P., Kasser, T., et al. (2005). The structure of goal contents across 15 cultures. *Journal of Personality and Social Psychology, 89*(5), 800–816. https://doi.org/10.1037/0022-3514.89.5.800.

Hardin, G. (1968). The tragedy of the commons. *Science, 162,* 1243–1248. https://doi.org/10.1126/science.162.3859.1243.

Hedayati, N., Kuusisto, E., Gholami, K., & Tirri, K. (2017). Life purposes of Iranian secondary school students. *Journal of Moral Education, 46*(3), 283–294. https://doi.org/10.1080/03057240.2017.1350148.

Heft, H. (2013). An ecological approach to psychology. *Review of General Psychology, 17*(2), 162–167. https://doi.org/10.1037/a0032928.

Heng, M. A., Blau, I., Fulmer, G., Bi, X., & Pereira, A. (2017). Adolescents finding purpose: Comparing purpose and life satisfaction in the context of Singaporean and Israeli moral education. *Journal of Moral Education, 46*(3), 308–322. https://doi.org/10.1080/03057240.2017.1345724.

Hill, P. L., Burrow, A. L., & Sumner, R. A. (2013). Addressing important questions in the field of adolescent purpose. *Child Development Perspectives, 7,* 232–236. https://doi.org/10.1111/cdep.12048.

Hill, P. L., Burrow, A. L., Brandenberger, J. W., Lapsley, D. K., & Quaranto, J. C. (2010). Collegiate purpose orientations and well-being in adulthood. *Journal of Applied Developmental Psychology, 31,* 173–179. https://doi.org/10.1016/j.appdev.2009.12.001.

Hofstede, G., & Milosevic, D. (2018). Dimensionalizing cultures: The Hofstede model in context. *Online readings in psychology and culture, 2*(1), 8.

Jiang, F., & Guo, D. (2018). Are Chinese student teachers' life purposes associated with their perceptions of how much their university supports community service work? *Journal of Moral Education, 47*(2), 201–216. https://doi.org/10.1080/03057240.2018.1430023.

Johnson, S. K., Tirrell, J. M., Callina, K. S., & Weiner, M. B. (2018). Configurations of young people's important life goals and their associations with thriving. *Research in Human Development, 15*(2), 139–166. https://doi.org/10.1080/15427609.2018.1441576.

Kashdan, T. B., & Steger, M. F. (2007). Curiosity and pathways to well-being and meaning in life: Traits, states, and everyday behaviors. *Motivations and Emotion, 31,* 159–173. https://doi.org/10.1007/s11031-007-9068-7.

Kawai, T., & Moran, S. (2017). How do future life perspective and present action work in Japanese youth development? *Journal of Moral Education, 46*(3), 323–336. https://doi.org/10.1080/03057240.2017.1350150.

Keyes, C. L. M. (2011). Authentic purpose: The spiritual infrastructure of life. *Journal of Management, Spirituality & Religion, 8*(4), 281–297. https://doi.org/10.1080/14766086.2011.630133.

Kiang, L. (2012). Deriving daily purpose through daily events and role fulfillment among Asian American youth. *Journal of Research on Adolescence, 22*(1), 185–198. https://doi.org/10.1111/j.1532-7795.2011.00767.x.

Kiang, L., & Fuligni, A. J. (2010). Meaning in life as a mediator of ethnic identity and adjustment among adolescents from Latin, Asian, and European American backgrounds. *Journal of Youth and Adolescence, 39*(11), 1253–1265. https://doi.org/10.1007/s10964-009-9475-z.

King, L. A., & Hicks, J. A. (2009). Meaning in life as a subjective judgment and a lived experience. *Social and Personality Psychology Compass, 3*(4), 638–653. https://doi.org/10.1111/j.1751-9004.2009.00193.x.

Larson, R. (2006). Positive youth development, willful adolescents, and mentoring. *Journal of Community Psychology, 34,* 677–689. https://doi.org/10.1002/jcop.20123.

Lee, J. N. T., Foo, K., Adams, A., Morgan, R., & Frewen, A. (2015). Strengths of character, orientations to happiness, life satisfaction and purpose in Singapore. *Journal of Tropical Psychology, 5,* 1–21. https://doi.org/10.1017/jtp.2015.2.

Lewin, K. (1951). *Field theory in social science: Selected theoretical papers.* New York: Harper & Brothers. (Reprinted 1997 by the American Psychological Association).

Liang, B., White, A., Rhodes, H., Strodel, R., Gutowski, E., Mousseau, A. M. D., et al. (2017). Pathways to purpose among impoverished youth from the Guatemala city dump community. *Community Psychology in Global Perspective, 3*(2), 1–21.

Lichtwarck-Aschoff, A., Van Geert, P., Bosma, H., & Kunnen, S. (2008). Time and identity: A framework for research and theory formation. *Developmental Review, 28,* 370–400. https://doi.org/10.1016/j.dr.2008.04.001.

Loeb, P. R. (2010). *Soul of a citizen: Living with conviction in challenge times.* New York: St. Martin's Griffin.

Malin, H. (2011). America as a philosophy, Implications for the development of American identity among today's youth. *Applied Developmental Science, 15*(2), 54–60. https://doi.org/10.1080/10888691.2011.560805.

Malin, H. (2015). Arts participation as a context for youth purpose. *Studies in Arts Education, 56*(3), 268–280. https://doi.org/10.1080/00393541.2015.11518968.

Malin, H., Ballard, P. J., & Damon, W. (2015). Civic purpose: An integrated construct for understanding civic development in adolescence. *Human Development, 58,* 103–130. https://doi.org/10.1159/000381655.

Malin, H., Reilly, T. S., Quinn, B., & Moran, S. (2014). Adolescent purpose development: Exploring empathy, discovering roles, shifting priorities, and creating pathways. *Journal of Research on Adolescence, 24*(1), 186–199. https://doi.org/10.1111/jora.12051.

Marken, R. S. (2002). *More mind readings: Methods and models in the study of purpose.* St. Louis, MO: newview.

Marken, R. S. (2009). You say you had a revolution: Methodological foundations of closed-loop psychology. *Journal of General Psychology, 13*(2), 137–145. https://doi.org/10.1037/a0015106.

Markus, H. R., & Kitayama, S. (1991). Culture and the self: Implications for cognition, emotion, and motivation. *Psychological Review, 98,* 224–253. https://doi.org/10.1037/0033-295X.98.2.224.

Martela, F., & Steger, M. F. (2016). The three meanings of meaning in life: Distinguishing coherence, purpose, and significance. *The Journal of Positive Psychology, 11*(5), 531–545. https://doi.org/10.1080/17439760.2015.1137623.

Martinez, R. O., & Dukes, R. O. (1997). The effects of ethnic identity, ethnicity, and gender on adolescent well-being. *Journal of Youth and Adolescence, 26,* 503–516. https://doi.org/10.1023/A:1024525821078.

Mason, H. (2017). *Inhloso kanye bizo*: Exploring South African university students' conceptions and enactment of purpose. *Journal of Moral Education, 46*(3), 272–282. https://doi.org/10.1080/03057240.2017.1345723.

McKnight, P. E., & Kashdan, T. B. (2009). Purpose in life as a system that creates and sustains health and well-being: An integrative, testable theory. *Review of General Psychology, 13*, 242–251. https://doi.org/10.1037/a0017152.

Molasso, W. R. (2006). Measuring a student's sense of purpose in life. *Michigan Journal of College Student Development, 12*(1), 15–24.

Moran, S. (2009). Purpose: Giftedness in intrapersonal intelligence. *High Ability Studies, 20*(2), 143–159. https://doi.org/10.1080/13598130903358501.

Moran, S. (2010). Changing the world: Tolerance and creativity aspirations among American youth. *High Ability Studies, 21*(2), 117–132. https://doi.org/10.1080/13598139.2010.525342.

Moran, S. (2014). Youth's own understandings of purpose: Are there distinct "cultures of purpose"? *Applied Developmental Science, 18*(3), 1–13. https://doi.org/10.1080/10888691.2014.924359.

Moran, S. (2016a). *Ethical ripples of creativity and innovation.* Basingstoke, UK: Palgrave Macmillan.

Moran, S. (2016b). What do teachers think about youth purpose? *The Journal of Education for Teaching, 42*(5), 582–601. https://doi.org/10.1080/02607476.2016.1226556.

Moran, S. (2017). Youth purpose worldwide: A tapestry of possibilities. *Journal of Moral Education, 46*(3), 231–244. https://doi.org/10.1080/03057240.2017.1355297.

Moran, S. (2018a). *Educating for life purpose and prosocial action: A six-nation perspective.* Cambridge, MA: Civic & Moral Education Initiative, Harvard Graduate School of Education.

Moran, S. (2018b). Purpose-in-action education. *Journal of Moral Education, 47*(2), 145–158. https://doi.org/10.1080/03057240.2018.1444001.

Moran, S. (2019a). Is personal life purpose replacing shared worldview as youths increasingly individuate? Implications for educators. *International Journal of Learning, Teaching and Educational Research, 18*(5), 8–23. https://doi.org/10.26803/ijler.18.5.2.

Moran, S. (2019b). Youth life purpose: Evaluating service-learning via development of lifelong 'radar' for community contribution. In P. Aramburuzabala, L. McIlrath, & H. Opazo (Eds.), *Embedding service-learning in European higher education* (pp. 51–66). London, UK: Routledge.

Moran, S. (2020). Life purpose in youth: Turning potential into a lifelong pursuit of prosocial contribution. *Journal for the Education of the Gifted, 43*(1), 38–60. https://doi.org/10.1177/016 2353219897844.

Moran, S., Bundick, M. J., Malin, H., & Reilly, T. S. (2013). How supportive of their *specific* purposes do youth believe their family and friends are? *Journal of Adolescent Research, 28*(3), 348–377. https://doi.org/10.1177/0743558412457816.

Moran, S., & Garcia, R. L. (2019). How does US college students' sense of life purpose relate to their emotional expectations of being a volunteer in the community as part of a service-learning course? *Bordón, Journal of Education, 71*(3), 45–62.

Moran, S., & Gardner, H. (2018). Hill, skill and will: A multiple intelligences perspective. In L. Meltzer (Ed.), *Understanding executive function: Implications and opportunities for the classroom* (2nd ed., pp. 19–40). New York: Guilford Press.

Moran, S., & John-Steiner, V. (2003). Creativity in the making: Vygotsky's contribution to the dialectic of creativity and development. In K. Sawyer, V. John-Steiner, S. Moran, R. J. Sternberg, D. H. Feldman, J. Nakamura, & M. Csikszentmihalyi (co-authors), *Creativity and development* (pp. 61–90). New York: Oxford University Press.

Moran, S., & Opazo, H. (2019). How service-learning mentors teachers' life purpose toward long-term community impact. *The Chronicle of Mentoring & Coaching, 2*(1), 762–767.

Nkyi, A. K. (2015). Purpose in life among senior high school students in Ghana. *Journal of Global Research in Education and Social Science, 3*(4), 187–197.

Oliner, S. P., & Oliner, P. M. (1988). *The altruistic personality: Rescuers of Jews in Nazi Europe.* New York: Free Press.

Opazo, H., Aramburuzabala, P., & Ramirez, Ch. (2018). Emotions related to Spanish student-teachers' changes in life purposes following service-learning participation. *Journal of Moral Education, 47*(2), 217–230. https://doi.org/10.1080/03057240.2018.1438992.

Osai, E. R. (2016). *On purpose: Motivational and contextual predictors of purpose and positive engagement among urban-residing, African American youth.* Dissertation, University of Michigan, Ann Arbor, MI.

Quinn, B. (2014). Other-oriented purpose: The potential roles of beliefs about the world and other people. *Youth & Society, 46*(6), 779–800. https://doi.org/10.1177/0044118X12452435.

Ryff, C. D. (1989). Happiness is everything, or is it? Explorations on the meaning of psychological well-being. *Journal of Personality and Social Psychology, 57,* 1069–1081. https://doi.org/10.1037/0022-3514.57.6.1069.

Sharma, G., & De Alba, E. (2018). Sense of purpose among female students belonging to minority ethnic and Buddhist backgrounds. *Journal of College and Character, 19*(2), 137–151. https://doi.org/10.1080/2194587X.2018.1445644.

Shin, H., Kim, M.-Y., Hwang, H., & Lee, B.-T. (2018). Effects of intrinsic motivation and informative feedback in service-learning on the development of college students' life purpose. *Journal of Moral Education, 47*(2), 159–174. https://doi.org/10.1080/03057240.2017.1419943.

Shippen, T., & Moran, S. (2014). *Stability and turbulence of purpose during decision-making.* Washington, DC: Paper at the annual meeting of the American Psychological Association.

Sink, C. A., Purcell, M. A., Van Keppel, J. R., Jr., & Gamper, H. (1997). *Meaning and purpose in Russian, Swiss, and American adolescents.* York, UK: Paper presented at the British Educational Research Association annual conference.

Steger, M. F., Frazier, P., Oishi, S., & Kaler, M. (2006). The Meaning in Life Questionnaire: Assessing the presence of and search for meaning in life. *Journal of Counseling Psychology, 53,* 80–93. https://doi.org/10.1037/0022-0167.53.1.80.

Steger, M. F., Kashdan, T. B., Sullivan, B. A., & Lorentz, D. (2008a). Understanding the search for meaning in life: Personality, cognitive style, and the dynamic between seeking and experiencing meaning. *Journal of Personality, 76*(2), 199–228. https://doi.org/10.1111/j.1467-6494.2007.00484.x.

Steger, M. F., Kawabata, Y., Shimai, S., & Otake, K. (2008b). The meaningful life in Japan and the United States: Levels and correlates of meaning in life. *Journal of Research in Personality, 42,* 660–678. https://doi.org/10.1016/j.jrp.2007.09.003.

Steger, M. F., & Samman, E. (2012). Assessing meaning in life on an international scale. *International Journal of Wellbeing, 2*(3), 182–195. https://doi.org/10.5502/ijw.v2.i3.2.

Stoddard, S. A., & Pierce, J. (2015). Promoting positive future expectations during adolescence: The role of assets. *American Journal of Community Psychology, 56,* 332–341. https://doi.org/10.1007/s10464-015-9754-7.

Stoddard, S. A., Zimmerman, M. A., & Bauermeister, J. A. (2012). Thinking about the future as a way to succeed in the present: A longitudinal study of future orientation and violent behaviors among African American youth. *American Journal of Community Psychology, 48*(3–4), 238–246. https://doi.org/10.1007/s10464-010-9383-0.

Sumner, R., Turner, A., & Burrow, A. L. (2018). Diversity and inclusion as essential elements of 4-H youth development programs. *Journal of Youth Development, 13*(4), 68–80. https://doi.org/10.5195/jyd.2018.586.

Temane, L., Khumalo, I. P., & Wissing, M. P. (2014). Validation of the meaning in life questionnaire in a South African context. *Journal of Psychology in Africa, 24*(1), 51–60. https://doi.org/10.1080/14330237.2014.904088.

Tirri, K., & Kuusisto, E. (2016). Finnish student teachers' perceptions on the role of purpose in teaching. *Journal of Education for Teaching, 42*(5), 532–540. https://doi.org/10.1080/02607476.2016.1226552.

Twenge, J. M. (2011). Generational differences in mental health: Are children and adolescents suffering more, or less? *American Journal of Orthopsychiatry, 81*(4), 469–472. https://doi.org/10.1111/j.1939-0025.2011.01115.x.

Vallerand, R. J. (2008). On the psychology of passion: In search of what makes people's lives most worth living. *Canadian Psychology, 49*(1), 1–13. https://doi.org/10.1037/0708-5591.49.1.1.

Valsiner, J. (2000). *Culture and human development.* Thousand Oaks, CA: Sage.

Valsiner, J. (2011). The development of individual purposes: Creating actuality through novelty. In L. A. Jensen (Ed.), *Bridging cultural and developmental approaches to psychology* (pp. 212–232). New York: Oxford University Press.

Van Geert, P. (1998). We almost had a great future behind us: The contribution of non-linear dynamics to developmental-science-in-the-making. *Developmental Science, 1,* 143–159. https://doi.org/10.1111/1467-7687.00020.

Waddington, D. I. (2010). Building on treacherous ground: Sense-of-purpose research and demarcating problematic purposes. *The Alberta Journal of Educational Research, 56*(1), 82–94.

Yeager, D. S., & Bundick, M. J. (2009). The role of purposeful work goals in promoting meaning in life and in schoolwork during adolescence. *Journal of Adolescent Research, 24*(4), 423–452. https://doi.org/10.1177/0743558409336749.

Yeager, D. S., Henderson, M., Paunesku, D., Walton, G., Spitzer, B., D'Mello, S., et al. (2014). Boring but important: A self-transcendent purpose for learning fosters academic self-regulation. *Journal of Personality and Social Psychology, 107,* 559–580. https://doi.org/10.1037/a0037637.

Zell, M. C. (2011). Achieving a college education: The psychological experiences of Latino/a community college students. *Journal of Hispanic Higher Education, 9*(2), 167–186. https://doi.org/10.1177/1538192709343102.

Zhang, S., Shi, R., Liu, X., & Miao, D. (2013). Passion for a leisure activity, presence of meaning, and search for meaning: The mediating role of emotion. *Social Indicators Research, 115,* 1123–1135. https://doi.org/10.1007/s11205-013-0260-8.

Chapter 13
Youth Purpose: A Translational Research Agenda

Kendall Cotton Bronk and Caleb Mitchell

Abstract Psychological research on purpose conducted in the past 15–20 years has considerably advanced our understanding of the construct. However, there are at least two questions that have not been as adequately explored: *How can we foster purpose in the lives of young people,* and *what does purpose look like among diverse groups of youth?* This chapter reviews a series of studies that have sought to explore these questions. For instance, we include a discussion of two empirically-tested interventions that help young people search for and identify their purpose in life. Design logic and lessons gleaned from these studies are addressed. In addition, the chapter outlines studies of purpose with young people from low-socioeconomic areas in the United States, with street children living in Liberia, and with European college students living amidst a serious economic downturn. Findings and implications from this line of research are also discussed. The chapter concludes with a discussion of topics future researchers of youth purpose should explore.

Keywords Purpose in life · Positive youth development · Positive psychological interventions · Adolescents

Since roughly 2000, when psychological research on purpose got underway in earnest, research has significantly advanced our understanding of this important construct. Research has explored varied conceptions of purpose, positive correlates of a life lived with purpose, and even the developmental trajectory of the construct (see Bronk, 2013 for a review of research on these topics and others). However, research has yet to address at least two important dimensions of purpose. *How can we foster purpose in the lives of young people,* and *what does purpose look like among diverse groups of youth?* This chapter reviews a series of studies, conducted at the Claremont Graduate University's Adolescent Moral Development lab at Claremont Graduate University (CGU; http://www.amdcgu.com), that explore these questions.

K. C. Bronk (✉) · C. Mitchell
Claremont Graduate University, Claremont, CA, USA
e-mail: Kendall.Bronk@cgu.edu
URL: https://www.kendallcottonbronk.com

Before diving into the particulars of this research, however, it is helpful to introduce our conception of purpose.

13.1 Purpose Defined

The working definition that has guided our work and other's work suggests purpose refers to a long-term, forward-looking intention to accomplish aims that are both meaningful to the self and of consequence to the world beyond the self (Damon, Menon, & Bronk, 2003). This definition features three primary dimensions. First, a purpose in life is an intention. It is a far-horizon goal of sorts that provides direction to future plans. In this way, purpose is forward-looking. Second, a purpose in life is personally meaningful. Individuals' most significant values and beliefs generally serve as the foundation of their purpose in life. Consequently, individuals eagerly invest time, energy, and other resources toward its pursuit. In other words, individuals do not merely dream about their purposes; they act on them. Third, in addition to being important to the individual, purpose is also of consequence to the world beyond the individual. It is directed toward the broader world. This part of the definition distinguishes our conception of purpose from some other conceptions of the construct. Whereas most conceptions of purpose incorporate the first two criteria (a far-horizon, goal-directed aim that is personally meaningful), not all include the third criteria (*inspired by a desire to make a difference in the broader world*). The beyond-the-self dimension, however, is a critical part of the construct. Research finds it is responsible for many of the positive experiences and outcomes associated with the construct (Damon, 2008). For instance, compared to others, individuals who demonstrate this beyond-the-self dimension are more likely to possess well-integrated personality dispositions (Mariano & Valliant, 2012) and more likely to report that their lives are satisfying (Bronk & Finch, 2010).

Based on this conception of purpose, the construct is relevant to individuals from adolescence onward. Not until roughly the second decade of life do most young people, at least in Western cultures, develop the cognitive abilities that enable the hypothetical-deductive reasoning and abstract thought required to support the search for purpose (Damon, 2008; Piaget, 1964). Consequently, although children are likely to engage in meaningful activities, they are unlikely to develop an enduring purpose in life (Bronk, 2012).

Not only are adolescents cognitively equipped to lead lives of purpose, but they are also often eager to do so. Early purpose formation coincides with identity development, which is the key developmental milestone of the adolescent and young adult years (Damon, 2008; Erikson, 1968, 1980), and research finds that purpose formation and identity development—at least for some young people—are intertwined and mutually-reinforcing processes, whereby growth in one encourages growth in the other (Bronk, 2011; Burrow & Hill, 2011; Hill & Burrow, 2012). Perhaps because of adolescents' developmental preparedness for purpose, at least some studies find (e.g. Bronk et al., 2009) they report that identifying their purpose is a satisfying experience. Given that committing to a purpose in life is consistently associated with reports of satisfaction, it makes sense to begin cultivating purpose as early in the lifespan as possible. In short, although individuals can—and do– discover and lead lives of purpose into adulthood, adolescence marks a stage ripe for purpose formation. For this reason, much of our work has focused on purpose among youth.

Our work on youth purpose has a strong applied focus. Rather than merely describing and understanding how purposes form, we also seek to encourage their development. Accordingly, in addition to sharing our findings in academic books and peer-reviewed journals, we also share our findings in blogs, television news programs, and newspaper articles. Translating our scientific understanding into practical information people can use to help youth discover and lead lives of purpose is core to what we do.

13.2 Cultivating Purpose

The applied nature of our work is evident in the two questions that have guided our work over the past few years. The first is, *how can we intentionally cultivate purpose among youth?* A large and growing body of research points to the many benefits of leading a life of purpose. For instance, studies find that purpose is associated with a wide range of physical health benefits, including better sleep, less chronic pain, and even longevity (Hill & Turiano, 2014; Kass et al., 1991; Krause, 2009; Ryff, Singer, & Love, 2004; Turner, Smith, & Ong, 2017). Research similarly finds that purpose is associated with a variety of psychological indicators of health, including hope, happiness, and life satisfaction (Bronk et al., 2009; French & Joseph, 1999; Gillham et al., 2011). Although much of this work is correlational in nature, emerging research suggests the relationship may be causal, whereby leading a life of purpose contributes to better physical health. More specifically, recent empirical studies have concluded that leading a life of purpose changes individuals' genomic make-up in a health-sustaining way (Fredrickson et al., 2015). The different ways we experience life influences our genetic expression, and leading a life of purpose elicits a favorable profile of gene expression in immune cells (Kitayama, Akutsu, Uchida, & Cole, 2016). In other words, beyond merely coexisting with healthy outcomes, recent research suggests the presence of purpose helps support them.

Despite the benefits associated with leading a life of purpose, the experience is relatively rare. Although more research is this area is warranted, existing research suggests only about 1 in 10 early adolescents, 1 in 5 late adolescents, and 1 in 3 college-aged youth report having a clear purpose in their lives (Damon, 2008). Because purpose appears to develop alongside identity and because identity development begins in adolescence (Bronk, 2011; Damon, 2008; Erikson, 1968, 1980; Sumner, Burrow, & Hill, 2015), it may be the case that rates of purpose increase further into adulthood as by then, more people have developed a stable sense of identity. In addition, these relatively low rates of purpose may be a function of the way we conceptualize purposes. As noted above, our conception of purpose is more stringent than some others (e.g. Ryff & Singer, 1998).

Purpose toolkit. Taking these two findings together—that leading a life of purpose contributes to beneficial outcomes and that it is a relatively rare experience for youth—led us to investigate ways of intentionally cultivating purpose. Our approach to this effort was shaped, in large part, by happenstance. Early longitudinal research into purpose, of which the first author was a part, explored the nature and prevalence of purpose among North American youth. As part of this work, researchers gathered Time 1 surveys from youth across the United States and Canada (Bundick, 2011). Months later, a subset of these individuals was randomly selected to participate in interviews about the nature of their purpose in life. Interviewers were surprised by youths' eagerness to talk about issues related to purpose. Several of the interviewees asked to have the recordings sent to them; others requested the transcripts. Members of the research team began to wonder if the one-time, 45-minute interview probing purpose might have served as an informal intervention of sorts. With that in mind, following the Time 2 survey collection effort, which took place months after the interview, interviewees' scores were compared with the non-interviewees' scores, and youth who had been interviewed exhibited significantly higher purpose scores!

Although it was promising to learn that the interview was an effective, albeit unintentional, purpose-fostering tool, there were clearly problems with using this approach to help large numbers of youth discover meaningful purposes for their lives. Interviewing youth is a time-consuming and unwieldy effort. It requires trained interviewers, parental permission, and face-to-face encounters. Consequently, although conducting interviews may be a useful approach to helping small numbers of youth discover their purpose, it would not be a feasible approach to cultivating purpose among larger numbers of young people.

To expand our impact, we decided to explore online purpose-fostering options (Bronk et al., 2019). Our aim was to translate the interview protocol into a set of online activities young people could complete to relatively quickly and easily explore and ultimately discover their purpose in life. We created two online toolkits, which we tested against a third Control Toolkit. Each of the three toolkits invited youth to log-on to a website once a day for three days over the course of a week to complete between 15 and 20 min of online activities each time. Before, immediately after, and a week after completing the online activities, youth completed surveys designed to assess the extent to which they were actively searching for a purpose and the extent to which they had identified a purpose for their lives. Change-sensitive measures, including the Search for Purpose Inventory (Dubon, Riches, Benavides, & Bronk, in preparation) and the Claremont Purpose Scale (Bronk, Riches, & Mangan, 2018), were created to assess changes in the search for purpose and identified purpose levels, respectively. In addition, youth in each of the three conditions completed measures of gratitude, hope, and prosocial intentions.

The Purpose Toolkit featured activities that sought to cultivate each component of the construct. Accordingly, activities were designed to help youth (1) reflect on the long-term aims that mattered most to them, (2) contemplate their personally significant values and beliefs, (3) and consider how they could use their talents to contribute to the world beyond themselves. Following the logic of the interview, participants logged into the website and completed a set of online activities that encouraged them to consider the broader world and their role in it (Reilly & Damon, 2013). In one such activity, they were presented with a quotation about the beyond-the-self dimension of purpose and asked to reflect on and write about what they would change about the world, if they could change anything they wanted. In another activity, youth completed a Q-sort, in which they identified the values (e.g., caring for my family, contributing to my community, living my life in accordance with my religious beliefs, creating something new, preserving the environment) that were most important to them. Following this, they wrote about why each of their top 3 values was so important to them and how each shaped their future plans. Yet another activity presented youth with a brief clip of comedian Jimmy Fallon talking about his purpose in life. Afterward, they were asked to write about the way they hoped to leave their mark on the world. Youth who had trouble identifying ways of contributing were encouraged to send emails to 5 adults who knew them well, including to family friends, employers, coaches, mentors, teachers, etc. Emails asked the adults to answer 3 questions about the youth: *What do you think I really enjoy doing? What do you think I'm particularly good at? How do you think I'll leave my mark?* Responses helped youth identify possible purposes.

Gratitude toolkit. Rather than fostering purpose directly, the second toolkit, the Gratitude Toolkit, sought to cultivate purpose indirectly, via gratitude. Theoretical research suggests youth focused on the blessings in their lives are inclined to consider ways of giving back (Damon, 2008). Other scholars have similarly argued that the recognition that other people have helped them triggers an urge to repay either the benefactor or others, to alleviate the uncomfortable sense of indebtedness (Trivers, 1971). The prosocial behavior that results from a grateful state is referred to as upstream reciprocity, which includes direct upstream reciprocity (where individuals pay back the person who helped them) and indirect upstream reciprocity (where individuals pay the favor forward to another individual or group; Nowak & Roch, 2007). Whether helping those who helped them or helping others, grateful individuals are more likely than their peers to contribute to the world beyond themselves (McCullough, Emmons, & Tsang, 2002), and the relationship between gratitude and contribution appears to be a causal one where gratitude leads to prosocial action (Bartlett & DeSteno, 2006; Froh, Bono, & Emmons, 2010; Tsang, 2007). We were curious to see if the self-transcendent action inspired by grateful thinking might manifest as purpose.

To empirically test this possibility, activities in the Gratitude Toolkit were designed to cultivate a grateful mindset. In one activity, youth completed an abridged version of the Three Good Things exercise (Seligman, Steen, Park, & Peterson, 2005), during which they were asked to list 3 things they were grateful for each day. In another activity, youth were introduced to the concept of benefit appraisals, which encouraged them to recognize that with each act of gratitude: (1) the recipient receives some benefit, (2) the helper incurs some cost (e.g., time, energy, other personal resources), and (3) the intention behind the act is geared toward assisting the recipient. Empirical research finds that reminding individuals of this appraisal process enhances feelings of gratitude (Froh et al., 2014). Another activity asked youth to take a "Gratitude Walk," during which they were instructed to reflect on the blessings in their lives for at least 5 min. Yet another activity featured a brief video clip that introduced the benefits of practicing (Seligman et al., 2005) and expressing gratitude (Toepfer & Walker, 2009). After this, participants were asked to write a letter of gratitude to someone who had helped them.

In addition to designing the Purpose and Gratitude Toolkits, we also created a Control Toolkit, which consisted of activities designed to enhance memory strategies. One activity presented a brief video clip that taught youth how to make up stories that would help them remember lists of items. Another activity encouraged youth to practice "location memory" and another instructed youth in how to use the MAPS (Music, Association, Picturing, Stories) strategy for remembering discrete pieces of information.

Participants included 224 youth who were randomly assigned to complete one of the three toolkits during a one-week period ($n = 79$ Purpose Toolkit; $n = 73$ Gratitude Toolkit; $n = 71$ Control Toolkit). Results suggest that from pre-test to post-test, participants who completed the Purpose and Gratitude Toolkits, but not the Control Toolkit, demonstrated significant increases in their search for purpose and in the extent to which they reported having identified a purpose for their lives. For individuals in both experimental conditions, levels of identified purpose did not change from the post- to lagged-post-test, which suggests the effects of the week-long intervention endured for at least another week. Interestingly, in addition to showing increases in both the search for purpose and identified purpose, youth in the Gratitude Toolkit condition also demonstrated significant increases in gratitude, hope, and prosocial intentions (Baumsteiger, Mangan, Bronk, & Bono, 2019). Youth in the Purpose Toolkit and Control conditions did not show these same increases, suggesting there may be some advantages to cultivating purpose indirectly via gratitude.

Interestingly, other researchers have similarly found that cultivating purpose indirectly can be effective. For instance, experiences of awe incline individuals to connect with the world beyond the self, and this can take the form of discovering a purpose for their lives (Shiota, Keltner, & Mossman, 2007). These indirect approaches to cultivating purpose may be effective because being asked directly to reflect on one's purpose can be intimidating, especially for individuals who do not yet know exactly what it is. Approaching the topic indirectly—either through reminding individuals of the blessings in their lives or by having them experience a sense of vastness—may be less threatening ways of encouraging young people to consider how they want to contribute to the broader world.

13.3 Purpose Among Diverse Groups of Youth

The research on interventions that foster purpose paints a promising picture. To help more youth discover meaningful purposes in life, we needed to understand how purpose develops among individuals from different cultures and contexts. Toward that end, the second question our work has recently explored is, *what does purpose look like among diverse groups of young people?* Although scientific research on purpose has increased dramatically over the past 15 years (Bronk, 2013), most studies have focused on purpose among middle-class, primarily European-American youth growing up in the United States. The bidirectional interactions between person and context conceptualized by the relational developmental systems model (Lerner, 2004; Lerner et al., 2019) suggest the process of purpose development is likely to vary among youth from different socioeconomic, ethnic, and cultural backgrounds. To gain a fuller sense of what purpose entails among diverse groups of young people, our lab conducted three additional studies.

Purpose amidst the Great Recession. Although the relational developmental systems theory predicts that both proximal and distal contexts are likely to influence purpose development (Lerner, 2004), research has most commonly focused on the role of proximal contexts (e.g., families, schools). We were eager to build on this research by examining how broader political and economic forces influenced purpose formation.

In particular, we sought to understand what effect the Great Recession had on young people's views of the future and their purposes in life (Bronk, Leontopoulou, & McConchie, 2018). Other purpose researchers have similarly been interested in understanding the effects of this dramatic economic downturn on individuals' purposes in life. A recent study concluded that although health and well-being scores were somewhat lower for a sample of US individuals post-recession than for a sample of US individuals pre-recession, rates of purpose among the two samples did not differ (Kirsch, Love, Radler, & Ryff, 2019). In other words, although the downturn appears to have been associated with lower levels of some dimensions of well-being, it was not associated with lower levels of purpose.

The Great Recession ended in the United States in 2009, but it lasted through 2016 in Greece. Young people, especially those in the second and third decades of life, are particularly likely to be negatively influenced by economic downturns, such as the Great Recession (Sherrod, 2017). Ready to enter fulltime employment, they often struggle to find work, and all too often, they end up trapped in a cycle of unemployment or underemployment.

To gain a fuller sense of how youth with purpose navigated the worldwide economic downturn known as the Great Recession, members of our lab (Bronk, Leontopolou, & McConchie, 2018) conducted a mixed methods study with late adolescents ($M_{age} = 21.5$, $SD = 1.8$). The study sought to address two related questions: (1) *compared to their peers, were youth with a well-developed sense of purpose better equipped to thrive in the midst of an economic downturn,* and (2) *if they were, how did having a purpose help them thrive?* Surveys were administered to identify youth with a strong sense of purpose and to examine how purpose was related to indicators of well-being, including optimism, resilience, and positive future expectations. Following quantitative data collection, a subset of respondents was invited to participate in interviews. Specifically, youth who scored at least one standard deviation above and one standard deviation below the mean purpose score were invited to participate in interviews. This extreme groups design enabled us to compare the effects of the recession on youth with and without purpose.

Quantitative findings provided evidence that youth with a clear sense of purpose were thriving despite the economic downturn. Purpose was associated with higher rates of optimism, resilience, and positive future expectations. Mediational analyses indicated resilience meditated the relationship between purpose and positive future expectations, suggesting that those with a stronger purpose maintained positive future expectations by way of their resilience in the face of adversity. Optimism was also found to partially mediate the relationship between purpose and future expectations, suggesting that a sense of optimism helped, to a degree, those with a stronger sense of purpose maintain more positive future expectations. Taken together, survey results suggested youth with purpose were weathering the economic downturn better than individuals without purpose.

Interviews shed light on why this might be the case. More specifically, qualitative findings revealed that youth with above-average purpose scores felt efficacious about their ability to navigate a successful future, despite the economic downturn. Consequently, they focused on finding jobs that enabled them to grow and served as a source of joy and meaning. Youth with below-average purpose scores, on the other hand, felt the future was futile, and consequently, they sought jobs primarily as a means of survival. Related to these different professional-orientations, high-purpose youth were reluctant to leave Greece to find work, whereas low-purpose youth reported being eager to do so. High-purpose youth managed to remain hopeful by focusing on how they could help, support, and contribute to their friends, family, communities, and country, and at times, by tuning out the negative economic news. Taken together, results suggest that a purpose in life can serve a powerfully protective role. From a practical perspective, findings suggest one way of helping youth weather economic down- turns may be to cultivate purpose. Doing so is likely to benefit not only the young people, but also the families, communities, and even countries to which these young people choose to contribute.

Purpose among Low-income Youth. In addition to wanting to learn more about the role economic forces play in purpose formation, we were also eager to understand how socioeconomic status influenced purpose. Research and theory both suggest socioeconomic status is likely to influence purpose development (Manstead, 2018; Sumner, Burrow, & Hill, 2018)—the question is how?

Positive youth development scholars argue that indicators of thriving, including purpose, should be available to all young people, including those from low-income backgrounds (Benson, 2006; Damon, 2004; Lerner, 2004). In addition, Austrian neurologist and psychiatrist Viktor Frankl (1959) provided a particularly compelling example of someone who discovered purpose in an extremely under-resourced setting. As a concentration camp inmate, he thought deeply about his purpose and the importance of leading lives of purpose more generally. At the same time, Maslow's (1943) classic theory of the hierarchy of needs suggests something as self-actualizing as a purpose in life should not develop until after individuals have been able to meet their basic needs. Empirical research on purpose, and the closely related meaning construct, lends support to both of these diverging theoretical perspectives (e.g., Moran, Bundick, Malin, & Reilly, 2013; Oishi & Diener, 2014).

To gain a better sense of exactly how socioeconomic status interacts with purpose development, we conducted a mixed methods study guided by three questions (Bronk, Mitchell, Hite, Mehoke, & Cheung, in press 2020): *How prevalent is purpose among youth from low-income backgrounds? What indicators of well-being is purpose associated with among youth from low-income backgrounds? How do youth from low-income backgrounds discover meaningful purposes in life?* As a point of comparison, data collected for this study came from youth from two different high schools in southern California. One high school served primarily youth from low-income backgrounds and the other served youth from primarily middle-income backgrounds. We included a middle-income sample to enable us to determine the relative prevalence of purpose among youth in this population; we did not intend to suggest middle-income youth are a standard against which others should be compared.

Based on quantitative findings, no difference in the rate of purpose between the two samples emerged. In other words, youth from the low-income community were as likely as youth from the middle-income community to report leading lives of purpose. In addition, results suggest purpose among youth from low- and middle-income backgrounds is associated with largely the same indicators of well-being. Across both samples, purpose was positively associated with hope, life satisfaction, prosocial intentions, peer support, positive affect, self-rated health, and feelings of safety, and it was negatively related to depression and stress. No relationship was observed between purpose and sleep quality or between purpose and engagement in exercise. Taken together, these results suggest purpose acts as a protective factor across these domains, regardless of youths' socioeconomic backgrounds.

Although the quantitative results pointed to similarities in the experience of purpose, themes that emerged from the qualitative data highlighted some interesting differences. Across slightly more than half the youth in the low-income sample, a fairly consistent purpose-discovery process emerged. Perhaps not surprisingly, most youth from the low-income community talked about encountering personal hardships (e.g., financial hardships, racial and gender bias, health issues) that might have derailed their pursuit of purpose. However, in some cases, rather than thwarting purpose, these hardships instead served as catalysts for its development. This occurred when youth were able to connect their hardships in the past to opportunities for meaningful action in the future. Not all personal hardships inspired purpose. It was only when youth who experienced personal hardships *also* had access to developmental assets, most commonly familial support, like-minded peers, and religious belief systems, that purpose developed. In other words, when youth from the low-income community had access to developmental assets, they were able to connect personal hardships in the past to opportunities for meaningful action in the future, and, in so doing, they discovered purpose. We looked for evidence of this same purpose-discovery process among youth in the middle-income sample, and we only found one instance of it.

From an applied perspective, these findings provide some of the first empirical evidence for the way youth from low-income backgrounds discover purposes in life.

These findings, coupled with knowledge that purpose can serve as an important source of resiliency for youth living in poverty (Machell, Disaboto, & Kashdan, 2016), provide direction to extracurricular, in-school, and other programs that seek to foster purpose among young people. More specifically, findings suggest that rather than trying to ignore or avoid potential obstacles to purpose formation, effective purpose-fostering programs should help youth identify personally significant ways of addressing the hardships in their lives. This emergent process is supported by recent research that identifies other significant pathways, including social support, passion identification, and faith, in the development of purpose among young people living in poverty (Gutowski, White, Liang, Diamonti, & Berado, 2017; Liang et al., 2017; Moran, Bundick, Malin, & Reilly, 2013). In addition, learning that purpose is most likely to blossom in the presence not only of hardships but also of contextual nutrients further highlights the need to build developmental assets in under-served communities.

Purpose and PYD among Liberian street-children. The previous study shed light on what purpose development among youth growing up in low-resourced communities in the United States entails. We wondered if poverty would have the same effects on purpose development among youth from other countries. Recently, there has been a push for internationalizing investigations of positive youth development by studying youth from the majority world—or the roughly 80% of the world's population that lives on less than $10 a day (Lerner et al., 2019; Sherrod, 2017). Research on youth in these nations is relatively sparse, yet such nations are where the majority of the world's youth live and where global populations of young people are increasing the fastest. Majority world youth face challenges not posed to youth from industrialized nations, suggesting results from studies in industrialized nations are not clearly, or even generally, applicable to youth in majority world contexts (Lerner et al., 2019).

To learn more about what purpose and other indicators of positive youth development look like among youth in the majority world, members of our lab (Bronk, Blom, & McConchie, 2019) conducted a mixed-methods study of early adolescents ($M_{age} = 10.93$, $SD = 1.35$), most of whom were living on the streets in Liberia (Blom, Bronk, Sullivan, McConchie, Ballesteros, & Farello, in press, 2020). Over the past roughly forty years, the country has suffered two catastrophic civil wars and a regional Ebola outbreak. These events decimated Liberia's critical institutions and infrastructure (Economist, 2017; UN Human Development Report, 2006; World Bank Group, 2011). Recognizing the extreme challenges confronting Liberian youth and the general breakdown of institutions that historically supported the healthy development of Liberia's young citizens (e.g., families, schools, churches), a sport for development program called L.A.C.E.S. (Life and Change Experienced Through Sport; www.laces.org) was established in the country in 2007. Sport for development programs, like L.A.C.E.S., utilize sport or physical activity to promote positive change, encourage social inclusion, and build peace among youth (Blom et al., 2015; Coalter, 2007; Lyras & Peachey, 2011). The United Nations (2014) recognizes sport for development programs as potentially effective grassroots approaches to fostering positive youth development around the globe.

All study participants were enrolled in L.A.C.E.S. Youth remain in the sport for development program for several years, and each year programming runs 3 days a week, 40 weeks a year. As such, youth have prolonged contact with the program, and the program has the opportunity to have a lasting effect on its young participants. The program has religious roots, and in addition to cultivating Christian beliefs, it focuses on cultivating purpose and other indicators of positive development.

The study was designed to answer three questions: (1) *Does participation in L.A.C.E.S. increase purpose and other indicators of positive development (e.g. social responsibility, close personal relationships, and peace) among Liberian youth living on the streets?* (2) *If so, how does L.A.C.E.S. cultivate purpose and these other important indicators of positive youth development? And,* (3) *what experiences, relationships, and conditions cultivate and stymy the growth of purpose and healthy development more generally among Liberian youth?* These questions were answered through surveys, interviews, and a photojournalistic methodology.

To answer the first question, regarding whether L.A.C.E.S. cultivated purpose and other indicators of positive youth development, participants completed surveys at the beginning and end of the program year. Results suggested that participation in the L.A.C.E.S. program did contribute to increases in purpose and other indicators of positive development (e.g. increased social responsibility, closeness to program coaches, and attenuated attitudes toward violence). To answer the second question, regarding how the program was effective, youth participated in interviews in which they reported that the program helped them discover their purpose and flourish in part by providing character building lessons. L.A.C.E.S. programming featured lessons designed to build socioemotional skills (e.g., respecting others, being honest), and, for a number of youths, this was their primary source of education in such matters. Providing positive role models—especially in the form of coaches—offering instrumental support (e.g., access to food), helping the youth get along better with their peers, and providing a foundation of a religious belief system were other ways youth reported the program helped support their healthy development.

To address the third research question, regarding the supports for the growth of purpose and positive development more generally among Liberian early adolescents, youth also participated in a photojournalistic study, in which they took pictures of the people, places, and experiences that supported and thwarted their purpose and other indicators of healthy development. Youth spent an afternoon with their L.A.C.E.S. coach taking pictures in their community. Afterward, they shared the pictures with researchers and explained how each of the subjects supported or detracted from their pursuit of purpose and healthy development. Many of the same things that supported their healthy development when present, detracted from it when they were absent. For instance, some of the most common objects in pictures were basic resources (e.g., clean drinking water, adequate food, safe places to sleep). Youth who had access to these things noted that they helped support flourishing, and youth who lacked access noted their absence detracted from flourishing. In addition, youth astutely identified access to education and supportive adults as key supports to purpose formation and healthy development.

Although this was a pilot study, we learned a good deal from the investigation. For instance, we learned that grassroots, sports programs can effectively foster purpose and other indicators of positive development in majority world contexts. We also learned that some of the same things that help youth in middle-class communities discover purpose and thrive (e.g., supportive adults) are important to the positive youth development of Liberian youth. At the same time, we learned that important differences existed, as well. For instance, although youth in middle class contexts generally take access to basic needs for granted, youth in Liberia do not. They recognize that these things, including clean drinking water, sufficient food, and a safe place to sleep, are essential to leading lives of purpose and to their healthy development more generally. This study also served to underscore the need to gain a fuller understanding of what the purposes and positive development of majority world youth entail.

13.4   Conclusion

Our research—and others'—has shed important light on how we can help cultivate purpose in youth and on what purposes look like among diverse groups of young people. However, there is much still to learn.

In the coming years, additional research on several important aspects of purpose is warranted. For instance, to date research has focused on individual purposes; what might a collective sense of purpose look like? Political groups share a purpose, as do groups supporting particular forms of social change, sports teams, and religious congregations. We have launched a study of family purpose, and some of the questions we are examining include: what do collective family purposes look like, how do they form, and how do they endure across generations? We also want to explore how individuals in these families pursue their individual purposes along with their familial ones. Our study represents only one aim in this direction, however. More research on family and other forms of collective purpose is needed.

In addition to examining collective purposes, we also need to examine individual purposes among youth living in diverse locales. In particular, more purpose research featuring young people from majority world countries is needed. The world's youth population is increasingly located in majority world countries (UNFPA, 2014), which means to fully understand what youth purpose looks like and how it shapes young people's lives, this is increasingly where we need to look.

Adolescent and young adult cancer survivors represent another group of young people worthy of research on purpose. Studies find that when individuals perceive a shortened future time horizon, they are more likely to reflect on the things that give their lives meaning (Carstensen, Isaacowitz, & Charles, 1999; Feifel, 1969). Most of the time, this happens naturally, as when individuals age (e.g., Carstensen et al., 1999; Nissim et al., 2012), but when young people receive a cancer diagnosis, they too are likely to perceive a shorter future time horizon (Little & Sayers, 2004). Existing research suggests that young people with purpose are more likely to smoothly navigate a cancer diagnosis (Scheier & Carver, 2001); might it also be the case that being diagnosed with cancer inclines young people to develop a purpose in life? Given that adolescent youth are increasingly likely to survive a cancer diagnosis, exploring this possibility is warranted.

Finally, our research and others' (e.g. Bundick, 2012) have established that it is possible to intentionally cultivate purpose. However, we still know little about how to effectively integrate purpose-fostering programs into schools in large-scale ways. How can we create cultures of purpose in secondary schools? What kinds of activities most effectively and practically, given the scheduling constraints of public education, help larger numbers of young people across this country and beyond discover and lead productive lives of purpose? Empirical investigations into novel approaches to cultivating purpose and rigorous evaluations of existing purpose-fostering programs are needed.

References

Bartlett, M. Y., & DeSteno, D. (2006). Gratitude and prosocial behavior: Helping when it costs you. *Psychological Science, 17*, 319–325.

Baumsteiger, R., Mangan, S., Bronk, K. C., & Bono, G. (2019). An integrative intervention for cultivating gratitude among adolescents and young adults. *The Journal of Positive Psychology.* https://doi.org/10.1080/17439760.2019.1579356.

Baumsteiger, R., Riches, B., Mangan, S., McConchie, J., & Bronk, K. C. (revise & resubmit, 2019). What matters?: A methodological investigation of values and purpose among adolescents and emerging adults. *The Journal of Positive Psychology.*

Benson, P. L. (2006). *All kids are our kids: What communities can do to raise caring and responsible children and adolescents* (2nd ed.). San Francisco: Jossey Bass.

Blom, L. C., Judge, L., Whitley, M. A., Gerstein, L., Huffman, A., & Hillyer, S. (2015). Sport for development and peace: Experiences conducting domesticand international programs. *Journal of Sport Psychology in Action, 6*(1), 1–16.

Blom, L., Bronk, K. C., Sullivan, M., McConchie, J., Ballesteros, J., & Farello, A. (under review). Peace indicators in Liberian youth: Effectiveness of sport for development programming.

Bronk, K. C. (2011). Portraits of purpose: The role of purpose in identity formation. *New Directions for Youth Development, 132*, 31–44.

Bronk, K. C. (2012). A grounded theory of youth purpose. *Journal of Adolescent Research, 27*, 78–109. https://doi.org/10.1177/0743558411412958.

Bronk, K. C. (2013). *Purpose in life: A key component of optimal youth development.* New York, NY: Springer.

Bronk, K. C., Baumsteiger, R., Mangan, S. Riches, B., Dubon, V., Benavides, C., & Bono, G. (in press, 2019). Fostering purpose among adolescents: Effective online interventions. *Journal of Character Education.*

Bronk, K. C., Blom, L. C., & McConchie, J. (2019, March). *Fostering peace, purpose, and positive development among youth in Liberia.* Paper presentation for the Biennial Meeting of the Society for Child Development, Baltimore, MD.

Bronk, K. C., & Finch, H. (2010). Adolescent characteristics by type of long-term aim in life. *Applied Developmental Science, 14*(1), 1–10.

Bronk, K. C., Hill, P. L., Lapsley, D., Talib, T., & Finch, W. H. (2009). Purpose, hope, and life satisfaction in three age groups. *The Journal of Positive Psychology, 4*, 500–510.

Bronk, K. C., Leontopolou, S., & McConchie, J. (2018a). Youth purpose during the Great Recession: A mixed-methods study. *The Journal of Positive Psychology, 14,* 405–416.

Bronk, K. C., Mitchell, C., Hite, B., Mehoke, S., & Cheung, R. (2020). Purpose among youth from middle- and low-income backgrounds. *Child Development, in press.*

Bronk, K. C., Riches, B., & Mangan, S. (2018b). Claremont purpose scale: A measure that assesses three dimensions of purpose. *Research in Human Development, 15,* 101–117. https://doi.org/10.1080/15427609.2018.1441577.

Bundick, M. J. (2011). The benefits of reflecting on and discussing purpose in life in emerging adulthood. *New Directions in Youth Development, 132,* 89–104. https://doi.org/10.1002/yd.430.

Burrow, A., & Hill, P. L. (2011). Purpose as a form of identity capital for positive youth adjustment. *Developmental Psychology, 47,* 1196–1206.

Carstensen, L. L., Isaacowitz, D. M., & Charles, S. T. (1999). Taking time seriously: A theory of socioemotional selectivity. *American Psychologist, 54,* 165–181. https://doi.org/10.1037/0003-066X.54.3.165.

Coalter, F. (2007). *A wider social role for sport: Who's keeping score?.* London: Routledge.

Damon, W. (2004). What is positive youth development? *ANNALS of the American Academy of Political and Social Science.* https://doi.org/10.1177/0002716203260092.

Damon, W. (2008). *The path to purpose: Helping our children find their calling in life.* New York, NY: Free Press.

Damon, W., Menon, J., & Bronk, K. C. (2003). The development of purpose during adolescence. *Applied Developmental Science, 7,* 119–128. https://doi.org/10.1207/s1532480xads0703_2.

Dubon, V. X., Riches, B., Benavides, C., & Bronk, K. C. (in preparation). Validating a searching for purpose scale.

Economist (2017). *The legacy of Ma Ellen: Praise for the women who put Liberia back on its feet.* https://www.economist.com/leaders/2017/10/05/praise-for-the-woman-who-put-liberia-back-on-its-feet.

Erikson, E. H. (1968). *Identity: Youth and crisis* (pp. 91–141). New York, NY: W.W. Norton & Company.

Erikson, E. H. (1980). *Identity and the life cycle.* New York, NY: W.W. Norton & Company.

Feifel, H. (1969). Perception of Death. *Annals of The New York Academy Of Sciences, 164*(3 Care of Patie), 669–674. http://dx.doi.org/10.1111/j.1749-6632.1969.tb14082.x.

Frankl, V. (1959). *Man's search for meaning.* Boston, MA: Beacon Press.

Fredrickson, B. L., Grewen, K. M., Algoe, S. B., Firestine, A. M., Arevalo, J. M., Ma, J., et al. (2015). Psychological well-being and the human conserved transcriptional response to adversity. *PLoS ONE, 10,* e0121839. https://doi.org/10.1371/journal.pone.0121839.

French, S., & Joseph, S. (1999). Religiosity and its association with happiness, purpose in life, and self-actualization. *Mental Health, Religion, and Culture, 2,* 117–120.

Froh, J. J., Bono, G., & Emmons, R. (2010). Being grateful is beyond good manners: Gratitude and motivation to contribute to society among early adolescents. *Motivation and Emotion, 34,* 144–157. https://doi.org/10.1007/s11031-010-9163-z.

Froh, J. J., Bono, G., Fan, J., Emmons, R. A., Henderson, K., Harris, C., et al. (2014). Nice thinking! An educational intervention that teaches children how to think gratefully. *School Psychology Review, 43,* 132–152.

Gillham, J., Adams-Deutsch, Z., Werner, J., Reivich, K., Coulter-Heindl, V., Linkins, M. ... Seligman, M. E. P. (2011). Character strengths predict subjective well-being during adolescence. *The Journal of Positive Psychology, 6,* 31–44. https://doi.org/10.1080/17439760.2010.536773.

Gutowski, E., White, A., Liang, B., Diamonti, A. J., & Berado, D. (2017). How stress influences purpose development: The importance of social support. *Journal of Adolescent Research, 33*(2), 571–597. https://doi.org/10.1177/0743558417737754.

Hill, P. L., & Burrow, A. L. (2012). Viewing purpose through an Eriksonian lens. *Identity: An International Journal of Theory and Research, 12,* 74–91.

Hill, P. L., & Turiano, N. A. (2014). Purpose in life as a predictor of mortality across adulthood. *Psychological Science, 25,* 1482–1486. https://doi.org/10.1177/0956797614531799.

Kass, J. D., Friedman, R., Leserman, J., Caudill, M., Zuttermeister, P. C., & Benson, H. (1991). An inventory of positive psychological attitudes with potential relevance to health outcomes: Validation and preliminary testing. *Behavioral Medicine, 17,* 121–129.

Kirsch, J. A., Love, G. D., Radler, B. T., & Ryff, C. D. (2019). Scientific imperatives vis-à-vis growing inequalities in America. *American Psychologist, 74*(7), 764–777.

Kitayama, S., Akutsu, S., Uchida, Y., & Cole, S. W. (2016). Work, meaning, and gene regulation: Findings from a Japanese information technology firm. *Psychoneuroendocrinology, 72,* 175–181. https://doi.org/10.1016/j.psyneuen.2016.07.004.

Krause, N. (2009). Meaning in life and mortality. *The Journals of Gerontology, Series B: Psychological Sciences and Social Sciences, 64,* 517–527. https://doi.org/10.1093/geronb/gbp047.

Lerner, R. (2004). Diversity in individual—context relations as the basis for positive development across the lifespan: A developmental systems perspective for theory, research, and application. The 2004 Society for the Study of Human Development Presidential Address. *Research in Human Development, 1,* 327–346.

Lerner, R. M., Tirrell, J. M., Dowling, E. M., Geldhof, G. J., Gestsdóttir, S., Lerner, J. V. … Sim, A. T. R. (2019). The end of the beginning: Evidence and absences studying positive youth development in a global context. *Adolescent Research Review, 4,* 1–19.

Liang, B., White, A., Rhodes, H., Strodel, R., Gutowski, E., DeSilva Mousseau, A. M., et al. (2017). Pathways to purpose among impoverished youth from the Guatemala City Dump Community. *Community Psychology in Global Perspective, 3,* 1–21.

Little, M., & Sayers, E. (2004). While there's life …. Hope and the experience of cancer. *Social Science and Medicine, 59*(6), 1329–1337. http://dx.doi.org/10.1016/j.socscimed.2004.01.014.

Lyras, A., & Peachey, J. W. (2011). Integrating sport-for-development theory and praxis. *Sport Management Review, 14*(4), 311–326.

Machell, K. A., Disabato, D. J., & Kashdan, T. B. (2016). Buffering the negative impact of poverty on youth: The power of purpose in life. *Social Indicators Research, 126,* 845–861.

Mangan, S., Baumsteger, R., & Bronk, K. C. (2020). Recommendations for positive psychology interventions in school settings. *The Journal of Positive Psychology, in press.*

Manstead, A. S. R. (2018). The psychology of social class: How socioeconomic status impacts thoughts, feelings, and behavior. *British Journal of Social Psychology, 57,* 267–291.

Mariano, J. M., & Valliant, G. E. (2012). Youth purpose among the 'greatest generation'. *Journal of Positive Psychology, 7*(4), 281–293.

Maslow, A. H. (1943). A theory of human motivation. *Psychological Review, 50*(4), 370–396. https://doi.org/10.1037/h0054346.

McCullough, M. E., Emmons, R. A., & Tsang, J. (2002). The grateful disposition: A conceptual and empirical topography. *Journal of Personality and Social Psychology, 82,* 112–127. https://doi.org/10.1037//0022-3514.82.1.112.

Moran, S., Bundick, M. J., Malin, H., & Reilly, T. S. (2013). How supportive of their *specific* purposes do youth believe their friends and family are? *Journal of Adolescent Research, 28,* 348–377.

Nissim, R., Rennie, D., Fleming, S., Hales, S., Gagliese, L., & Rodin, G. (2012). Goals set in the land of the living/dying: A longitudinal study of patients living with advanced cancer. *Death Studies, 36,* 360–390. https://doi.org/10.1080/07481187.2011.553324.

Nowak, M., & Roch, S. (2007). Upstream reciprocity and the evolution of gratitude. *Proceedings of the Royal Society of London, Series B: Biological Sciences, 274,* 605–609. https://doi.org/10.1098/rspb.2006.0125.

Oishi, S., & Diener, E. (2014). Residents of poor nations have a greater sense of meaning in life than residents of wealthy nations. *Psychological Science, 25*(2), 422–430. https://doi.org/10.1177/0956797613507286.

Papanastasiou, S., Ntafouli, M., & Kourtidou, D. (2016). The state of the children in Greece report 2016. *Hellenic National Committee for UNICEF 2016.* Available from https://www.unicef.gr/uploads/filemanager/PDF/2016/children-in-greece-2016-eng.pdf.

Piaget, J. (1964). Cognitive development in children: Development and learning. *Journal of Research in Science Teaching, 2,* 176–186. https://doi.org/10.1002/tea.3660020306.

Reilly, T., & Damon, W. (2013). Understanding purpose through interviews. In J. Froh & A. C. Parks (Eds.), *Activities for teaching positive psychology: A guide for instructors* (pp. 45–52). Washington DC: American Psychological Association.

Ryff, C. D., Singer, B., & Love, G. D. (2004). Positive health: Connecting well-being with biology. *Philosophical Transactions: Biological Sciences, 359,* 1383–1394.

Ryff, C. D., & Singer, B. (1998). The contours of positive human health. *Psychological Inquiry, 9*(1), 1–28. https://doi.org/10.1207/s15327965pli0901_1.

Scheier, M. F., & Carver, C. S. (2001). Adapting to cancer: The importance of hope and purpose. In A. Baum & B. L. Andersen (Eds.), *Psychosocial interventions for cancer* (pp. 15–36). American Psychological Association. https://doi.org/10.1037/10402-002.

Seligman, M. E. P., Steen, T. A., Park, N., & Peterson, C. (2005). Positive psychology progress: Empirical validation of interventions. *American Psychologist, 60,* 410–421. https://doi.org/10.1037/0003-066x.60.5.410.

Sherrod, L. (2017). Foreword. In A. C. Peterson, S. H. Koller, F. Motti-Stefanidi, & S. Verma (Eds.), *Positive youth development in global contexts of social and economic change* (pp. 15–17). New York, NY: Routledge.

Shiota, M., Keltner, D., & Mossman, A. (2007). The nature of awe: Elicitors, appraisals, and effects on self-concept. *Cognition and Emotion, 21*(5), 944–963. https://doi.org/10.1080/02699930600923668.

Sumner, R., Burrow, A. L., & Hill, P. L. (2015). Identity and purpose as predictors of subjective well-being in emerging adulthood. *Emerging Adulthood, 3*(1), 46–54.

Sumner, R., Burrow, A. L., & Hill, P. L. (2018). The development of purpose in life among adolescents who experience marginalization: Potential opportunities and obstacles. *American Psychologist, 73,* 740–752.

Toepfer, S. M., & Walker, K. (2009). Letters of gratitude: Improving well-being through expressive writing. *Journal of Writing Research, 1,* 181–198. https://doi.org/10.17239/jowr-2009.01.03.1.

Trivers, R. L. (1971). The evolution of reciprocal altruism. *The Quarterly Review of Biology, 46,* 35–57.

Tsang, J. (2007). Gratitude for small and large favors: A behavioral test. *The Journal of Positive Psychology, 2,* 157–167. https://doi.org/10.1080/17439760701229019.

Turner, A. D., Smith, C. E., & Ong, J. (2017). Is purpose in life associated with lower sleep disturbance in older adults? *Sleep Science and Practice, 1,* 14. https://doi.org/10.1186/s41606-017-0015-6.

UN Human Development Report. (2006). *Liberia.* http://www.undp.org/content/dam/liberia/docs/docs/NHDR_LIBERIA_2006.pdf.

UNFPA (2014). *The power of 1.8 billion: Adolescents, youth, and the transformation of the future.* State of world population: Harvard University. Accessed online at https://www.unfpa.org/sites/default/files/pub-pdf/EN-SWOP14-Report_FINAL-web.pdf.

United Nations Office of Sport and Development of Peace. (2014). Annual Report. Accessed online 1 July 2020https://www.un.org/sport/sites/www.un.org.sport/files/ckfiles/files/UNOSDP%20Annual%20Report%202014%20web(1).pdf.

World Bank Group (2011). *Options for the development of Liberia's energy sector.* http://siteresources.worldbank.org/EXTRAFRRegTOPENERGY/Resources/717305-1266139.

Discussion: The Burdens and Promises of Purpose Inquiry

Anthony L. Burrow and Patrick L. Hill

Abstract We close this volume by inviting readers to reflect on some of the foundational principles threaded throughout the previous chapters. Conceptual and empirical challenges that remain ahead for purpose researchers are discussed, but with an effort to construe them as opportunities to gain further insight and truly advance of the field. We leverage relevant examples from the previous chapters to serve as useful starting points for future research opportunities. We then present four enduring questions about purpose that we anticipate will require collective and sustained investment into the scientific study of this salubrious sense in people's lives.

> I leave Sisyphus at the foot of the mountain! One always finds one's burden again.
>
> … One must imagine Sisyphus happy.
>
> –Albert Camus (1965)

We hope that through the previous chapters readers have discerned some foundational principles common across scholarship on purposeful living. We highlight three such principles in our final remarks that approximate the themed meetings we have hosted over the years, which brought together the collection of authors contributing to this volume. First, curiosity about the nature of purpose is as ancient as it is nascent. Centuries of discourse on the value of imbuing one's life with purpose provide important footing for testing it as a rich and meaningful resource for a range of outcomes desired in contemporary life. A second principle is that the study of purpose concerns issues ranging from the personal and self-focused to the collective and social. As such, the degree to which people cultivate and feel purpose in their lives stands to reveal as much about their own identities, vocational interests, and well-being as it does about the place they grew up, their relationships with others, and their willingness to contribute to society. A third and final principle—perhaps

A. L. Burrow (✉)
Department of Human Development, Cornell University, Ithaca, NY, USA

P. L. Hill
Department of Psychological and Brain Sciences, Washington University in St. Louis, St. Louis, MO, USA

© Springer Nature Switzerland AG 2020
A. L. Burrow and P. Hill (eds.), *The Ecology of Purposeful Living Across the Lifespan*,
https://doi.org/10.1007/978-3-030-52078-6

one that should be most evident to readers—is that a fuller view of purposeful living emerges when it accounts for both people and the ecologies that surround them. The diverse research questions asked, methods used, and inferences drawn by those who have contributed chapters demonstrate how considering both individuals and environments together yields greater insight about the value of purpose than either considered alone. Thus, grappling in a serious way with the old and the new, the personal and the collective, and the essential connections between people and their contexts are compulsory tasks of any researcher striving to reveal transcendent truths about purpose.

Consistently attending to these core principles might appear burdensome, mundane, or redundant for those dedicated to the study of purpose. Doing so may appear especially daunting when viewed against the backdrop of common critiques about the science of purpose itself, including its elusive definition and measurement, abstruse routes by which individuals acquire or discover it, or the paucity of agreed-upon mechanisms by which its known benefits arise. Even *we* have often questioned how collective generations of inspired thinkers and careful researchers have not yet fully resolved seemingly basic and foundational questions about purpose! Still, we have found happiness in collaborating to inquire purpose and its role in people's lives—a happiness that does not depend entirely on providing definitive answers. This happiness instead stems from simply knowing we are contributing to a grander process. The work of those who have contributed to this volume iterates on the ideas of pioneering philosophers, which together informs the questions empirical scientists who will follow might ask. This hopeful vision is perhaps best articulated by the philosopher Seneca, who wrote (Seneca & Hine, 2010):

> The time will come when diligent research over long periods will bring to light things which now lie hidden. A single lifetime, even though entirely devoted to the sky, would not be enough for the investigation of so vast a subject... And so this knowledge will be unfolded only through long successive ages. There will come a time when our descendants will be amazed that we did not know things that are so plain to them... Many discoveries are reserved for ages still to come, when memory of us will have been effaced.

Suffice it to say, we trust in the scientific process and the contributions we make to it. We accept our role and will not tire in our efforts to learn more about what it means to live purposefully, because to us, the effort *is* the joy. Just as Albert Camus persuasively recasts how observers should imagine the endless attempts of the mythological Sisyphus to push his boulder forever upwards—from an obligatory labor into a happy engagement—we believe engaging in the study of purpose, in and of itself, represents a worthwhile and happy endeavor. Therefore we, too, continue to embrace our burdens in this work by imagining them as opportunities to learn more about what underlies the salubrious sense of purpose.

To close then, we would like to say a bit more about the work that lies ahead. Our aim is help in illuminate some of the persistent challenges and opportunities in this field. Specifically, we want to highlight four enduring questions to inspire new theorizing and careful analysis of purpose across the lifespan. We believe that working through these questions, in large-part by building from the foundations afforded by clear examples within the preceding chapters, will ultimately strengthen the science of purpose.

The first challenge requires contending with the possibility that a purposeful life is not necessarily an easy life. Amidst accumulating evidence situating purpose as a valuable resource for positive outcomes, one should not lose sight of what is and is not true about this resource. Several chapters included in this volume confer support for the idea that purposeful living is not free from strain or stress. Rogers, for example, provides cases of young people leveraging a sense of purpose to better navigate experiences of oppression or marginalization, but not removing the occurrence of these experiences altogether. Likewise, MacTavish describes leaving the mobile-home park to find a goal-directed life can represent a formidable and ongoing challenge. These insights resemble an emerging set of findings from daily process studies that show that purposeful people do, in fact, report everyday stressors—and in some cases even more than less purposeful peers (Hill, Sin, Turiano, Burrow, & Almeida, 2018). That their days are not entirely stress-free is an important discernment because it enables seeing that it may be in how purposeful individuals cope with stressors when they occur that matters, not the absence of stress itself. What might it mean for a broader understanding of this construct, if a purposeful life is not inherently comfortable to those living it? Future work might explore how purposeful individuals perceive and understand the challenges they face.

A second enduring question of purpose involves its acquisition. If we believe a sense of purpose is worth having, how should people obtain it? Much is made of the uniquely human capacity to 'find' or discover one's purpose. Indeed, Frankl's foundational writings about our ability (and need) to find purpose in the most heinous of conditions has inspired a great many to rigorously search for it no matter their situation. But some scholars have questioned whether this linguistic framing potentially oversells the amount of agency individuals have (or perceive themselves having) in acquiring it (e.g., Colby, 2020; O'Keefe, Dweck, & Walton, 2018). In his chapter, Larson's discussion of purpose development among youth suggests purpose may not be found purely by volition, but rather through carefully curated and intentional interactions with people and program features designed to develop this sense over time. The importance of this person-context relationship is further instantiated by Yu and Deutsch's detailing of how meaningful relationships with adults afford a rich experiential scaffolding that may direct youths' engagement in roles that become identified as purposeful. While we do not intend to undermine its role in purpose development, researchers should exercise caution in suggesting that agency is the only route to purpose. Likewise, they should make clear that agency alone will not always lead to purpose in certain contexts (Sumner, Burrow, & Hill, 2018). Even as many individuals do look for and explore what gives their life purpose, Sumner reminds us that there may also be important conditions (social, demographic, or otherwise) that constrain what purposes they consider viable for themselves. Of course, carefully designed interventions have been shown to bolster a *sense* of purpose, at least temporarily (e.g., Bronk, et al., 2019; Yeager, et al., 2014). However, these manipulations do not claim to have moved individuals from a state of not having purpose to possessing one. More research must contend with the discrepancy between our recognition of the value of purpose for our most cherished outcomes and the paucity of clear strategies for ensuring those who seek it ultimately obtain it (Burrow, Hill, Ratner, & Sumner, 2018). Continuing to list the benefits of purpose without offering greater insight into how people can obtain it risks scrubbing clean a glass wall that allows those on one side to better see—but not grasp—the reward on the other.

Of course, in order to confirm that a person has acquired purpose, or has developed it in substantial quantity, a sound method for reliably assessing it is needed. Relatedly, a third enduring question asks how should purpose be measured? Authors contributing to this book have reported on a diverse a range of purpose measures; indeed, many are available within the field. While the variety of options may create flexibility in measuring purpose with a wide range of populations and across different kinds of contexts, it also risks the potential for slippage in the ways in which researchers are operationalizing the same construct. Kiang, Malin, and Sandoz clearly articulated this in their discussion of the importance of aligning theory with proper measurement in order to aid consistent interpretation of empirical findings. This concern is clearly not unique to the study of purpose. But, given the renewed appreciation purpose is enjoying within the psychological literature, it is worth asking whether a singular and definitive purpose measure could be of use to researchers working across different developmental periods. The benefits to researchers of having a common measure of purpose could be enormous, if it generated greater confidence that the correlates and consequences of purpose found under study are not attributable to differences in the devices used to detect them. Yet, it also raises important questions about whether purpose should be expected to manifest the same at different developmental periods. Without clarity on how to measure purpose, we risk a disorganized field that may miss important insights gleaned by those assessing things differently. By centering measurement, the field stands to enhance coherence and gain substantial organization.

A fourth enduring question concerns how research regarding purpose as a felt sense can be integrated with research on the aspirational content of one's purpose. Renowned psychologist Edward Thorndike wrote, "Psychology helps to measure the probability that an aim is attainable." Applied to an individual's sense of purpose in life, psychological measures stand to tell us how likely they are to accomplish what they set out to. But of course, a bit more is needed for researchers to fully capitalize on this potential, namely, knowing what the content of their purpose actually is. Put plainly, we must move beyond isolated investigations into either the extent to which individuals sense purpose in their lives or exploring what their purpose actually entails, and instead attend to both simultaneously. As made abundantly clear throughout this book, purpose is a resource for greater psychosocial adjustment, health, and well-being. Yet, whether these benefits persist across differences in the content of one's aspirations reflects a critical blind spot within the purpose literature. Furthermore, we must think about how well what a person intends to accomplish resonates with what is supported by their environment. Ecological systems perspectives (Bronfenbrenner, 1979, 1989; Bronfenbrenner & Morris, 2006) could provide useful for considering contextualization. Greater alignment between a one's purpose content and their ecological niche may orchestrate greater support for purpose-related efforts (McKnight & Kashdan, 2009), thus amplifying the likelihood of positive outcomes.

These questions, and the constellation of others they likely inspire, await unhurried answers. We anticipate pursuing these answers will be as enjoyable as their discovery. As the discovered benefits of purpose continue to accumulate through increasingly rigorous study, ensuring that all people wanting to experience it can do so seems like a worthy aim. Yet, we believe that the study of purpose is more beneficial when people and their environments are tethered. Doing so removes unproductive guesswork in having to imagine how well findings translate to the real lives of people. To be certain, mapping the ecology of purpose across the lifespan will not be easily accomplished, as most things worth achieving rarely are. And sometimes, as we have found, those who pick up an idea will be burdened with having to restart the charge from the beginning. But if Camus' revisioning of Sisyphus is to be useful, then we can presume there is opportunity even at the bottom of the mountain, and happiness in store for those who endeavor to ascend it.

References

Bronfenbrenner, U. (1979). *The ecology of human development: Experiments by nature and design.* Cambridge, Mass.: Harvard University Press.

Bronfenbrenner, U. (1989). Ecological systems theory. *Annals of Child Development., 6,* 187–249.

Bronfenbrenner, U., & Morris, P. A. (2006). The bioecological model of human development. In R. M. Lerner, W. Damon, R. M. Lerner, & W. Damon (Eds.), *Handbook of child psychology: Theoretical models of human development* (pp. 793–828). Hoboken, NJ, US: John Wiley & Sons Inc.

Bronk, K. C., Baumsteiger, R., Mangan, S., Riches, B., Dubon, V., Benavides, C., et al. (2019). Fostering purpose among young adults: Effective online interventions. *Journal of Character Education, 15*(2), 21–38.

Burrow, A. L., Hill, P. L., Ratner, K., & Sumner, R. (2018). A better tomorrow: Toward a stronger science of youth purpose. *Research in Human Development, 15*(2), 167–180.

Camus, A. (1965). *The myth of Sisyphus, and other essays.* London: H. Hamilton.

Colby, A. (2020). Purpose as a unifying goal for higher education. *Journal of College and Character, 21*(1), 21–29.

Hill, P. L., Sin, N. L., Turiano, N. A., Burrow, A. L., & Almeida, D. M. (2018). Sense of purpose moderates the associations between daily stressors and daily well-being. *Annals of Behavioral Medicine, 52*(8), 724–729.

McKnight, P. E., & Kashdan, T. B. (2009). Purpose in life as a system that creates and sustains health and well-being: An integrative, testable theory. *Review of General Psychology, 13*(3), 242–251. https://doi.org/10.1037/a0017152.

O'Keefe, P. A., Dweck, C. S., & Walton, G. M. (2018). Implicit theories of interest: Finding your passion or developing it? *Psychological Science, 29*(10), 1653–1664.

Seneca, L. A., & Hine, H. M. (2010). *Natural questions.* Chicago: The University of Chicago Press.

Sumner, R., Burrow, A. L., & Hill, P. L. (2018). The development of purpose in life among adolescents who experience marginalization: Potential opportunities and obstacles. *American Psychologist, 73*(6), 740–752.

Yeager, D. S., Henderson, M. D., Paunesku, D., Walton, G. M., D'Mello, S., Spitzer, B. J., et al. (2014). Boring but important: A self-transcendent purpose for learning fosters academic self-regulation. *Journal of Personality and Social Psychology, 107*(4), 559–580.

© Springer Nature Switzerland AG 2020   255
A. L. Burrow and P. Hill (eds.), *The Ecology of Purposeful Living Across the Lifespan,*
https://doi.org/10.1007/978-3-030-52078-6

CPSIA information can be obtained
at www.ICGtesting.com
Printed in the USA
LVHW050709251021
701442LV00002B/150